# EQUINE DENTISTRY

# EQUINE DENTISTRY

EDITED BY

## GORDON J BAKER
## JACK EASLEY

W. B. SAUNDERS COMPANY LTD

Edinburgh • London • New York • Oxford • Philadelphia • St Louis • Sydney • Toronto 1999

WB SAUNDERS
An imprint of Elsevier Science Limited

First published 1999
Reprinted 2000, 2002, 2003 (twice)

ISBN 0 7020 23922

**British Library Cataloguing in Publication Data**
A catalogue record for this book is available from the British Library

**Library of Congress Cataloging in Publication Data**
A catalog record for this book is available from the Library of Congress

**Note**
Medical knowledge is constantly changing. As new information becomes
available, changes in treatment, procedures, equipment and the use of drugs
become necessary. The editors, authors, contributors and the publishers have,
as far as it is possible, taken care to ensure that the information given in this
text is accurate and up to date. However, readers are strongly advised to
confirm that the information, especially with regard to drug usage, complies
with the latest legislation and standards of practice.

your source for books,
journals and multimedia
in the health sciences
**www.elsevierhealth.com**

The
publisher's
policy is to use
paper manufactured
from sustainable forests

Typeset by EXPO Holdings, Malaysia
Printed in China
C/05

# CONTENTS

Contributors     vii

Preface and Acknowledgements     ix

## SECTION 1
## MORPHOLOGY

1. **Dental Anatomy**     3
   *P M Dixon*

2. **Dental Physiology**     29
   *G J Baker*

3. **Ageing**     35
   *S Muylle*

## SECTION 2
## DENTAL DISEASE AND PATHOLOGY

4. **Abnormalities of Development and Eruption**     49
   *G J Baker*

5. **Oral and Dental Trauma**     60
   *T R C Greet*

6. **Abnormalities of Wear and Periodontal Disease**     70
   *G J Baker*

7. **Endodontic Disease**     79
   *G J Baker*

8. **Oral and Dental Tumours**     85
   *D C Knottenbelt*

## SECTION 3
## DIAGNOSIS OF DENTAL DISORDERS

9. **Dental and Oral Examination**     107
   *Jack Easley*

10. **Systemic Effects of Dental Disease**     127
    *D C Knottenbelt*

11. **Dental Imaging**     139
    *C Gibbs*

## SECTION 4
## TREATMENT OF DENTAL DISORDERS

12. **Equine Dental Instrumentation**     173
    *W L Scrutchfield*

13. **Dental Prophylaxis**     185
    *W L Scrutchfield*

14. **Basic Equine Orthodontics**     206
    *Jack Easley*

15. **Equine Tooth Removal (Exodontia)**     220
    *Jack Easley*

16. **Endodontic Therapy**     250
    *G J Baker*

17. **Mandibular and Maxillary Fracture Osteosynthesis**     259
    *H R Crabill and C Honnas*

Index     271

# CONTRIBUTORS

**G J Baker**
BVSc, PhD, MRCVS, Diplomate ACVS
227 LAC
University of Illinois
Urbana
IL, 61802
USA

**Mark Crabill**
DVM
Las Colinas Veterinary Clinic
Equine Medical & Surgical Centre
6112 N. O'Connor Boulevard
Irving
TX 75039
USA

**PM Dixon**
MVB, PhD, MRCVS
Department of Veterinary Clinical Studies
University of Edinburgh
Easter Bush Vet Centre
Easter Bush, Roslin
Midlothian EH25 9RG
UK

**Jack Easley**
DVM, MS, Diplomate ABVP (Equine)
328 Comanche Road
Shelbyville
KY, 40065
USA

**Christine Gibbs**
BVSc, DVR, PhD, MRCVS
Stoneleigh
Ropers Lane
Wrington
Bristol, BS40 5NF
UK

**Tim R C Greet**
BVMS, MVM, CertEO, DESTS, FRCVS
Beaufort Cottage Stables
High Street
Newmarket
Suffolk, CB8 8JS
UK

**C Honnas**
DVM, MS, Diplomate ACVS
Texas A&M University
College of Veterinary Medicine
College Station
TX, 77843-4461
USA

**Derek C Knottenbelt**
BVM&S, DVM&S, MRCVS
Division of Equine Studies
University of Liverpool
Leahurst, Neston
Wirral
Merseyside L64 7TE
UK

**S Muylle**
DVM
Department of Morphology
Faculty of Veterinary Medicine
Salisburylaan 133
B-Mereleke
Belgium

**WL Scrutchfield**
DVM, MS, Diplomate ACVIM
2111 Arrington Road
College Station
TX, 77845
USA

# PREFACE AND ACKNOWLEDGEMENTS

This textbook could not have been produced without the encouragement and help of many people. We thank our families for their patience and support throughout the writing, editing, and production. We were fortunate to have so many quality colleagues to contribute many chapters in this work. We hope that covering the many topics by worldwide authors has given us a chance to present a thorough documentation of the art and science of Equine Veterinary Dentistry.

We are indebted to the excellence and patience of the editing and production staff of Harcourt Brace (W. B. Saunders, London) and, in particular, to Catriona Byres, Deborah Russell, and to Emily Pillars for their skill in keeping us on–what we hope will prove to be–the right track. We are grateful for the enthusiastic support and work of the staff of the Word Processing and Biomedical Communications Centers of the University of Illinois College of Veterinary Medicine.

Our own interest and enthusiasm for this subject is based on a total of some fifty years of observing, working, "wrestling," and studying the processes of dental structure, function, malfunction, pathology, and the treatment of tooth disorders in the horse. For these experiences, we thank the many colleagues, outside our co-authors, who have been willing to share their ideas with us and to those who have referred cases to us to investigate and treat. We remember with thanks, our equine patients – the creatures who have made it possible to learn, acquire knowledge, demonstrate, and enjoy this exciting profession. It has also been a great pleasure to work with owners and trainers who continually remind us that, just when you think you've seen "it" and understand "it," something else comes along to, in some cases, shed a new or different understanding on a problem or, in other cases, to present a new problem that still awaits a complete investigation.

It also became clear to us, as we worked through the text, that a number of "principles and processes" that have been covered in previous articles and textbook chapters do not hold true under severe scrutiny, i.e., we certainly do not know or understand many things–at best, we only think we know.

> The things we know
> The things we think we know
> The things we don't think we know
> The things we wish we knew
> The things we hope to know
> The things we WILL know
>
> *Dr Steve Kneller, University of Illinois,*
> *College of Veterinary Medicine, 1996*

Consequently, we would like to present this text to our audience, of veterinarians in practice, in research, to veterinary students in training, and to others with an interest in the biology of the lives of horses not as a complete text but, as in all scientific efforts, as a work in progress. It is our sincere hope the information presented in this text will not only benefit the veterinary profession and interest of equine dentistry but more importantly provide the care and consideration our equine friends so rightly deserve. We would encourage readers to commit their views to paper or to cyber space and send us their thoughts, ideas, and suggestions.

A number of the illustrations have been viewed in other media, and we thank the authors, editors, and publishers for permission to use them in this work. This text has four sections: Morphology, Dental Disease and Pathology, Diagnosis of Dental Disorders and Treatment of Dental Disorders, and a total of seventeen chapters. Relevant references follow each chapter and they may be used as a source for further reading and study.

We believe that the use of the modified Triadan numbering system for tooth identification has advantages over traditional nomenclature. It is easier to say or to write 101 than upper right I (incisor) 1. We have used the Triadan system where applicable throughout the text. In some discussions and comments, however, as the reader will see, there is a place for other descriptive terms–the incisors (i.e., all twelve of them in the adult horse), premolars, molars, canine teeth and cheek teeth.

Gordon J Baker,
*University of Illinois,*
*Urbana, Illinois*

Jack Easley,
*Shelbyville, Kentucky*

February 1999

# MORPHOLOGY

# DENTAL ANATOMY

PM Dixon, MVB, PhD, MRCVS, Department of Veterinary Clinical Studies, Easter Bush Veterinary Centre, Easter Bush, Midlothian, Scotland.

## INTRODUCTION

### EQUINE DENTAL NOMENCLATURE

Adult mammals have four types of teeth, termed incisors, canines, premolars (PM) and molars (M), in a rostrocaudal order.[1] Teeth embedded in the incisive (premaxilla) bone are by definition termed incisors (I). The most rostral tooth in the maxillary bone is the canine (C). All teeth caudal to this tooth (site) are molars. If replaced they are deciduous molars, if not they are permanent molars.[1] Each type of tooth has certain morphological characteristics and specific functions. Incisor teeth are specialized for the prehension and cutting of food. The canine teeth are for defence and offence (for capture of prey in carnivores). Equine premolars (PM) 2–4 and the three molars (M) (collectively termed cheek teeth) function as grinders for mastication. The occlusal or masticatory surface is the area of tooth in contact with the opposing tooth; the term coronal refers to the crown. The anatomical crown is that part of the tooth covered by enamel and in brachydont (short crowned) teeth is usually the same as the clinical crown, i.e. the erupted aspect of the tooth. However, in equine teeth (hypsodont – long crowned) especially young teeth, most of the crown is termed unerupted or reserve crown, with a smaller length (about 10–15 per cent in young adult horses) of clinical crown. The term coronal is used when referring to direction toward the occlusal surface.

Apical refers to the area of tooth furthest away from the occlusal surface, i.e. the area where the roots develop and is the opposite of coronal. Lingual refers to the medial aspect (area closest to the tongue) of all the lower teeth while palatal refers to the same aspect of the upper cheek teeth. Buccal (aspect closest to cheeks) refers to the lateral aspect of both upper and lower (cheek) teeth, while labial refers to the rostral and rostrolateral aspect of teeth (incisors only in horses) close to the lips. The terms proximal, approximal or interproximal all refer to the area of teeth that face the adjoining teeth (in the same arcade or arch). Less commonly used terms in equine dentistry are the terms mesial and distal which refer respectively to the surfaces of teeth that face toward and away from an imaginary line between the central incisors.

### EVOLUTION OF EQUINE TEETH

The precursor of the modern horse *Equus caballus* was a small animal named Hyracotherium (also known as dawn horse or Eohippus) that lived in South America in the Eocene era some 50–70 million years ago.[2] This animal lived on succulent plants that caused little dental wear and it could satisfactorily prehend and masticate this type of food with its short-crowned (brachydont) teeth that were similar to most omnivore or carnivore (e.g. human or canine) teeth. However, subsequent major climatic changes, with secondary changes in vegetation, resulted in much of South America becoming covered with coarse grassland such as the Steppes and Tundra. Some descendants of Hyracotherium evolved to survive on this coarse grass diet. These evolutionary changes included the very significant development of cecal digestion that, along with the development of a rumen in other ungulate species, allowed mammals to utilize microbes within their gastrointestinal tract to help digest cellulose. This major foodstuff became abundant over much of the earth, but intrinsic mammalian gastrointestinal enzymes could not degrade it for digestion.

Subsequent to the development of cecal digestion to utilize cellulose containing foodstuffs, the ingestion of large quantities of coarse foodstuffs that contained abrasive silicates (which is harder than enamel) both as small particles of biogenic silica in leaves[2] and as larger particles in soil attached to roots and lower stems, for prolonged periods (up to 16.5 hours/day) placed additional demands on the teeth of these equine precursors. Hyracotherium plucked its food with its lips rather than with its shovel shaped incisors.[2] In contrast, its successors developed specialized incisor teeth for efficient low grazing of grasses, but the prehension of this type of foodstuff caused increased incisor wear. It is interesting that other herbivores such as cattle developed a dental pad, with loss of the upper incisors, thus preventing them grazing the shortest, most nutritious forage. Following ingestion, the necessary grinding down of this coarse foodstuff to a small particle size (the average length of fibers in equine feces is just 3.7 mm)[3] to allow more efficient endogenous and microbial digestion, causes even higher degrees of wear on the cheek teeth. However, unlike ruminants that can regurgitate their food for further chewing, horses have only one opportunity to grind their foodstuffs effectively.

A compensatory evolutionary change was the development of hypsodonty, with the long reserve crown of the cheek teeth embedded in the alveoli of the maxillae and mandibles, that deepened to accommodate this development. Brachydont teeth (permanent dentition) erupt fully prior to maturity and are normally long and hard enough to survive for the life of the individual because they are not subjected to prolonged and high levels of dietary abrasive forces. In contrast, hypsodont teeth erupt over most of the horse's life at a rate of 2–3 mm/year[4,5] which is similar to the rate of attrition (wear) on the occlusal surface of the tooth, provided that the horse is on a grass (or some alternative fibrous diet, e.g. hay or silage) rather than being fed high levels of concentrate food.

The latter type of diet will reduce occlusal wear and also restrict the range of lateral chewing actions,[6] however, the teeth will continue to erupt at the normal rate and thus dental overgrowths can occur. Both brachydont and hypsodont teeth have a limited growth period and thus are termed anelodont teeth. A further progression of this evolutionary development for coping with highly abrasive diets (e.g. in some rodents and rabbits) is the presence of teeth that continually grow throughout all of the animal's life, termed elodont teeth. Horses also enhanced the efficiency of their chewing by evolving complex premolars that resemble molars, i.e. molarization of PM 2–4. Hyracotherium had four premolars and three molars in each jaw, but PM 1 later became much smaller and nonfunctional ('wolf tooth') or absent.

Brachydont teeth have a distinct neck between the crown and root, a feature that could not be present in permanent hypsodont teeth that have a prolonged eruption period. At eruption, hypsodont teeth have no true roots and in this text the term root specifically refers to the apical area which is enamel free.[7,8] The terms apical or periapical are much more appropriate to describe this area of equine teeth that, for example, commonly develop infections in the mandibular second and third cheek teeth, even prior to the development of any roots. Research shows that 25 per cent of equine mandibular cheek teeth have no root development even at 12 months following eruption.[9]

Because of the marked wear on the surface of hypsodont teeth, exposure on the occlusal surface of enamel, and also of dentin and cement (cementum) is inevitable and leads to the presence of alternate layers of these three calcified dental tissues on the occlusal surface. This is in contrast to the sole presence of enamel on the occlusal surface of brachydont teeth. The presence of infolding of the peripheral enamel, and also of enamel cups (infundibula) in the upper cheek teeth and in all incisors also increases the amount and irregularity of exposed enamel ridges on the occlusal surface. This feature confers additional advantages to the hypsodont host and therefore a permanently irregular occlusal surface that is advantageous in the grinding of coarse fibrous foodstuffs is created by a self-sharpening mechanism.

Further evolutionary adaptations to grazing by the horse's ancestors were the development of limited rostrocaudal movement and restricted opening of the temporomandibular joint, and the development of powerful mandibular muscles, in particular the masseters and medial pterygoideus, to enable the necessary prolonged and powerful side-to-side grinding jaw movements that are characteristic of equidae. These primitive horses, that also developed a larger body size and a single toe allowing increased speed, later migrated up to North America and hence by the Greenland Bridge (which then connected Alaska and Asia) to Asia and Europe, where they evolved into the modern horse (*Equus caballus*).

# EMBRYOLOGY OF TEETH

Dental development (dentogenesis) involves several processes including epithelial–mesenchymal interaction, growth, remodeling and calcification of tissues until a tooth is fully developed.[10,11,12] During dental development, the tooth germ undergoes a series of distinct, consecutive events termed the initiating, morphogenetic and cytodifferentiative phases. These phases occur in all types of mammalian dentition,[13] however, their timing and termination vary, i.e. compared to brachydont teeth hypsodont teeth have a delayed termination of the morphogenetic and cytodifferentiative stages, while in elodont teeth, these stages proceed at the apical region throughout all of the animal's life.

Tooth formation begins by the development of a horseshoe-shaped epithelial thickening along the lateral margin of the fetal oral cavity. This epithelial thickening, termed the primary

epithelial band, invaginates into the underlying mesenchymal tissue to form two distinct ridges, the vestibular lamina and caudal to it, the dental lamina. The dental lamina produces a series of epithelial swellings called tooth buds along its buccal margin. This stage is known as the bud stage of tooth development (Fig. 1.1). At this stage, a mesenchymal cell proliferation develops beneath the hollow ectodermal tooth bud and invaginates into the tooth bud which now develops into an inverted cap-shaped structure called the enamel organ. This is called the cap stage of dental development (Fig. 1.1).

All deciduous teeth and the permanent molars develop from the enamel organ of the dental laminae. However, permanent incisors, canines and premolars are formed from separate enamel organs that are derived from lingual (medial) extensions of the dental laminae of the deciduous teeth (Fig. 1.1). Consequently, the deciduous incisors will be displaced labially (toward lips) by the erupting permanent incisors.

With formation of the enamel organ, the mesenchymal cells continue to proliferate within the concave aspect of the enamel organ and are now termed the dental papilla that is later responsible for dentin and pulp formation. These cells now also extend peripherally, as a structure termed the dental sac (follicle) which surrounds and protects the enamel organ and dental papilla until tooth eruption (Fig. 1.2).[14,1] The enamel organ, dental papilla and dental sac are together termed the tooth germ, with each germ responsible for an individual tooth.

The enamel organ proliferates further and, in brachydont dentition, assumes a bell shape, which is termed the bell stage of dental development. At this stage, the concavity of the enamel organ increases while the mesenchymal cells of the dental papilla invaginate further into its hollow aspect (Fig. 1.1). In equine teeth, invaginations of enamel epithelium, that will later become infundibula, develop from the convex aspect of the 'bell' into the papilla (one per incisor and two per upper cheek tooth). Equine cheek teeth have multiple cusps (raised occlusal areas) that arise from protrusions on the convex aspect of the bell. The brachydont enamel organ is circular on

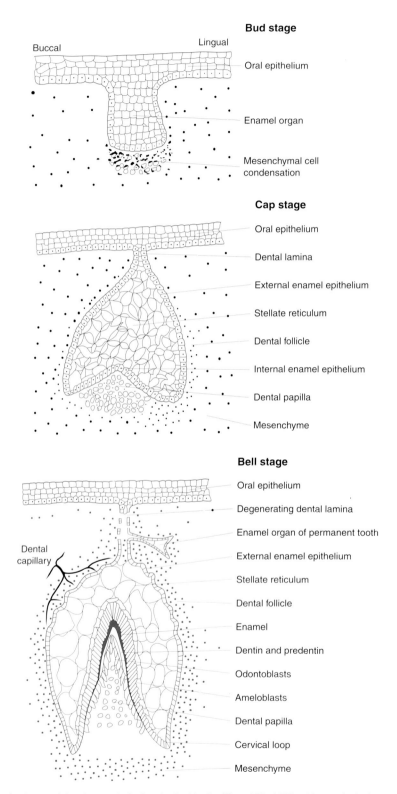

**Figure 1.1.** Three early stages of development of a brachydont tooth. (From Kilic 1995, with permission).

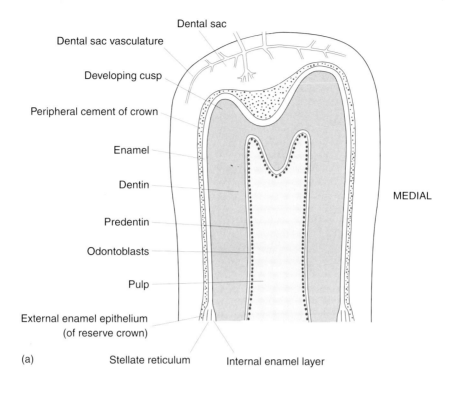

Dental sac

Dental sac vasculature

Developing cusp

Peripheral cement of crown

Enamel

Dentin

MEDIAL

Predentin

Odontoblasts

Pulp

External enamel epithelium
(of reserve crown)

(a)

Stellate reticulum  Internal enamel layer

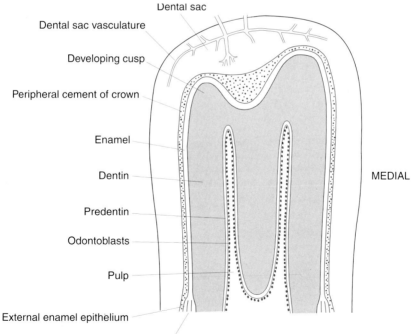

Dental sac

Dental sac vasculature

Developing cusp

Peripheral cement of crown

Enamel

Dentin

MEDIAL

Predentin

Odontoblasts

Pulp

External enamel epithelium

(b)  Internal enamel epithelium

**Figure 1.2.** Two stages of the development of a multicusped hypsodont tooth without an infundibulum (i.e. a lower cheek tooth) showing the presence of coronal cement and enamel that are covered by the dental sac. The large common pulp chamber (a) later develops two horns (b) due to deposition of dentin by the odontoblasts within the pulp chamber.

transverse section, however the enamel organ of equine cheek teeth develop infoldings[15] that later produce the infoldings of peripheral enamel.

Most cytodifferentiative events in the tooth germs occur during the transitional period between the cap and bell stages. The cells lining the concave aspect of the enamel organ become the internal enamel epithelium and the cells lining the convex aspect of the enamel organ form the external enamel epithelium.[11] Between them lies a third layer of star-shaped cells with large intracellular spaces, the stellate reticulum (Fig. 1.1) that has nutritive and mechanical functions in enamel development. The cells of the internal dental epithelium develop into tall columnar cells with large, proximally located nuclei. This induces alterations at the molecular level in the underlying dental papilla whose uppermost cells now rapidly enlarge, becoming odontoblasts. The first dentin layer is now laid down along the basal membrane which then disintegrates. These changes reciprocally induce the overlying internal enamel epithelial cells to differentiate into ameloblasts which now begin to produce enamel.[16]

After they initially deposit a structureless enamel layer, the ameloblasts migrate away from the dentinal surface and form a projection termed Tomes' process at their distal surface. Secretions from the proximal aspect of Tomes' process form interprismatic enamel and secretions from the surface of Tomes' process form the enamel prisms. The development of enamel and dentin (and later also cement) occurs in two consecutive phases, the secretion of extracellular matrix of mucopolysaccharides and organic fibers that is followed by its mineralization.[17,18]

Odontoblasts, like ameloblasts and cementoblasts (that produce cement) are end cells, meaning that they cannot further differentiate into other cell types. During dentin deposition, the basal aspects of odontoblasts gradually become thinner and form long fine cytoplasmic extensions termed odontoblast processes that remain in the dental tubule while the odontoblast cell body remains at the surface of the developing dentin in the pulp cavity.[12]

In multicusped teeth (such as equine cheek teeth) mineralization starts independently at each cusp tip (Figs 1.2, 1.3 and 1.4) and then

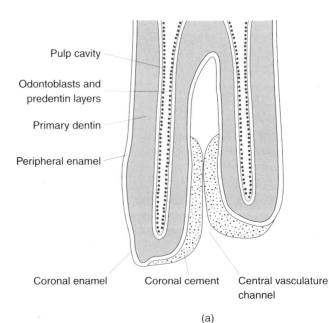

Pulp cavity

Odontoblasts and predentin layers

Primary dentin

Peripheral enamel

Coronal enamel          Coronal cement          Central vasculature channel

(a)

**Figure 1.3.** The crown and occlusal surface of a multicusped hypsodont tooth with an infundibulum (i.e. an upper cheek tooth) (a) immediately prior to eruption, (b) immediately following eruption showing loss of the dental sac over the occlusal surface and (c) following wear of the primary occlusal surface to expose the secondary occlusal surface that is the permanent occlusal surface in hypsodont teeth.

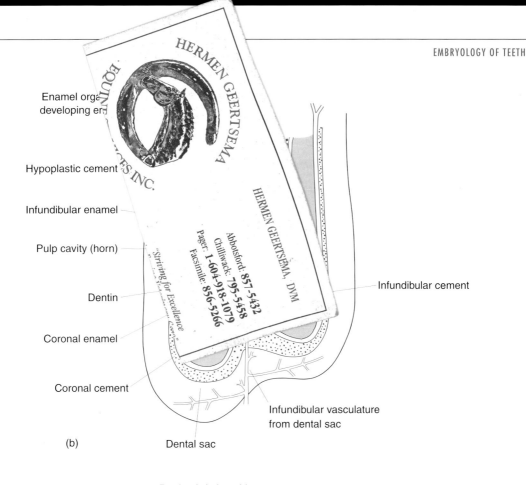

Enamel organ and
developing en...

Hypoplastic cement...

Infundibular enamel

Pulp cavity (horn)

Dentin

Coronal enamel

Coronal cement

Infundibular cement

Infundibular vasculature
from dental sac

(b)                    Dental sac

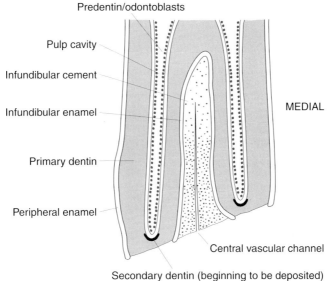

Predentin/odontoblasts

Pulp cavity

Infundibular cement

Infundibular enamel

Primary dentin

Peripheral enamel

MEDIAL

Central vascular channel

(c)          Secondary dentin (beginning to be deposited)

**Figure 1.3.** *continued.*

merges as calcification progresses down toward the amelodentinal junction.[1] As dentin and enamel deposition continues, odontoblasts and ameloblasts move in opposite directions and thus avoid becoming entrapped in their own secretions. Radiography has shown the calcification of equine deciduous cheek teeth buds (three in each quadrant) to have begun by

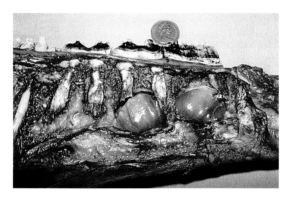

**Figure 1.4.** Dissected hemimandible of a yearling thoroughbred showing the tooth germs of the first and second mandibular cheek teeth developing beneath, and causing resorption of, their temporary counterparts. Through the soft tissue of the surrounding dental sac it can be seen that the more developed second cheek tooth germ has calcification of the coronal aspects of the developing enamel cusps.

the 120th day of fetal life and to be completed by 240 days.[19] The deciduous PM 2 germs are largest, indicating that they develop first. Calcification of the first permanent tooth begins about 6 months later.[19]

In brachydont teeth, vascularization begins at the periphery of the tooth germs at the early cap stage and blood vessels continue to ramify into the dental sac and extend into the dental papilla.[12] Until this stage, the enamel epithelium is supplied by small mesenchymal capillaries. Once dentinal and enamel mineralization begins, the connection between the enamel epithelium and the dental papilla is completely lost. The developing enamel now obtains its blood supply from the vasculature of the surrounding dental sac (Fig. 1.3).

After crown formation is completed in brachydont teeth, the external and internal enamel epithelial cells at the cervical region proliferate down over the dental papilla as a double layer of cells (Fig. 1.2) that at this site are termed Hertwig's epithelial root sheath. This epithelium induces the underlying mesenchymal cells to differentiate into odontoblasts which produce dentin.[12] With the progressive distal disintegration of Hertwig's epithelial root sheath, the dental sac cells come into direct contact with dentin. Interaction between these two tissues

now induces cells of the dental sac to convert into cemental-forming cells, i.e. cementoblasts and then to lay down cement.[10,14] In equine teeth this cement deposition occurs over all of the crown, latterly over the future occlusal surface, just prior to eruption (Fig. 1.3).[15] When the crown has reached its full length, the epithelial root sheath disintegrates and no further enamel can be formed.

In the infundibula of the upper cheek teeth and all incisors, cement deposition proceeds by cementoblasts solely nourished by vasculature of the dental sac (Fig. 1.3) because, as previously noted, the underlying infundibular enamel totally isolates it from the pulp cavity vasculature. Immediately after eruption, the soft tissue of the dental sac is quickly destroyed. Infundibular cement no longer has any blood supply (Fig. 1.3) and can now be regarded as an inert or 'dead' tissue. Consequently, the term 'infundibular necrosis' or 'infundibular cement necrosis' that has been used to describe caries (dissolution of the inorganic dental tissues) of infundibular cement is inappropriate as necrosis implies death of living cells.[4]

## DENTAL STRUCTURES
### ENAMEL

Enamel is the hardest and most dense substance in the body. Due to its high mineral content (96–98 per cent) it is almost translucent, but gains its color from the underlying dentin. Much of the small organic component of enamel is composed of the keratin family of proteins, in contrast to the proteins of dentin and cement that are largely collagenous. In the equine tooth, coronal enamel (except on the occlusal surface) is usually covered by peripheral cement, except at the rostral aspect of the incisors where the cement is usually worn away, thus exposing the shiny underlying enamel. Enamel, with its high mineral content and absence of cellular inclusions (unlike dentin or cement) can also be regarded as almost an inert or 'dead' tissue. Therefore, as the ameloblasts die off once the tooth is fully formed, it has no ability to repair itself. Enamel is almost fully composed of impure hydroxyapatite crystals (Fig. 1.5) which are larger than the equivalent crystals of dentin, cement or bone. These crystals are arranged both into structured prisms which may be contained in a prism sheath and also into less structured interprismatic enamel. Different species and even different areas of teeth in an individual can have different shaped prisms or different arrangements of prismatic and interprismatic enamel which can form the basis for enamel classification.

Equine enamel is composed of two main types termed Equine Types 1 and 2 enamel, with small amounts of Equine Type 3 enamel.[20] Equine Type 1 enamel is present on the medial aspect of the enamel folds (at the amelodentinal [enamel–dentin] junction). It is composed of prisms that are rounded or oval in cross-section and lie in parallel rows between flat plates of dense interprismatic enamel (Figs 1.5 and 1.6). Equine Type 2 enamel is present on the periphery of the enamel layer (at the amelocemental [enamel–cement] junction) and is composed solely of enamel prisms ranging from 'horse-shoe' to 'keyhole' shape (Fig. 1.7) with no interprismatic enamel. Equine Type 3 enamel is composed of prisms completely surrounded by large quantities of interprismatic enamel in a honeycomb-like structure and is inconsistently

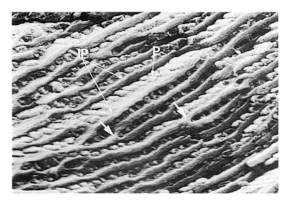

**Figure 1.6.** Scanning electron micrograph of Equine Type 1 enamel showing interprismatic plates (IP) alternating with rows of prisms (P). Note the convergence and branching (↓) of some of the interprismatic enamel plates. ×1450. (From Kilic 1995,[26] with permission).

present as a thin layer at both the amelodentinal and amelocemental junctions (Fig. 1.7).

The distributions of Equine Type 1 and 2 enamels vary throughout the teeth, with Equine Type 2 enamel increasing in thickness in the peripheral enamel folds (ridges) and decreasing where the folds invaginate toward the center of the tooth (Figs 1.8 and 1.9). Almost all enamel folds contain both Types 1 and 2 enamel. However, increased amounts of Equine Type 1

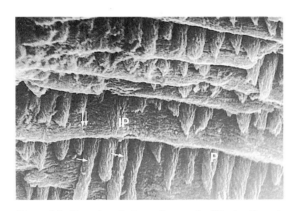

**Figure 1.5.** Scanning electron micrograph of Equine Type 1 enamel. This shows parallel rows of rounded enamel prisms lying on flat plates of interprismatic enamel. The enamel crystals within the enamel prisms (↓) are oriented parallel to the long axes of the prisms, while the enamel prisms of the interprismatic enamel plates are oriented at right angles to the prisms (↓↓). ×2720. (From Kilic et al. 1997,[25] with permission of the editor of the *Equine Veterinary Journal*).

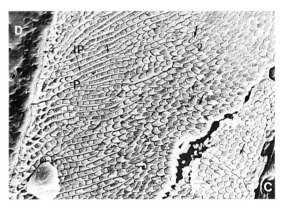

**Figure 1.7.** Scanning electron micrograph of a section of an equine tooth showing dentin (D) enamel and cement (C). A thin layer of Equine Type 3 enamel is visible on the left (3) at the junction with dentin. Adjacent to this area is a wider layer of Equine Type 1 enamel (1) showing interprismatic enamel (IP) (that is contiguous with Type 3 enamel and enamel prisms (P). To the right is a wider layer of Equine Type 2 enamel (2) that in this area has horseshoe-shaped prisms (↓). ×482. (From Kilic et al. 1997,[25] with permission of the editor of the *Equine Veterinary Journal*).

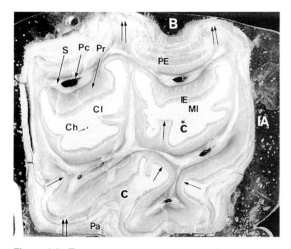

**Figure 1.8.** Transverse section, just beneath the occlusal surface of a methyl methacrylate embedded upper MI of an 18-year-old horse. The mesial (rostral) infundibulum (MI) and the caudal (distal) infundibulum (CI) are surrounded by infundibular enamel (IE) and the infundibular cement has a central channel (Ch). Five pulp cavities (Pc) are present and are surrounded by areas of secondary dentin (S) that in turn are surrounded by primary dentin (Pr). Both the peripheral enamel (PE) and infundibular enamel (IE) are thicker at the palatal (Pa) and buccal (B) aspects than at the interdental aspects (IA). Additionally, the enamel is thicker in ridges (↓↓) than in invaginations (↓). ×4. (From Kilic 1995,[26] with permission).

enamel are present in the upper cheek teeth, almost equal amounts of Equine Type 1 and 2 occur in the lower cheek teeth, whereas incisor enamel is composed almost solely of Equine Type 2 enamel. Equine Type 1 prisms are oriented at angles of approximately 45 degrees to both the amelodentinal junction and the occlusal surface, but Equine Type 2 enamel prisms are oriented at a wide variety of oblique angles.[20]

Although enamel is the hardest substance in the mammalian body it is brittle. The closely packed prisms of Equine Type 1 enamel form a composite structure with dense interprismatic plates that confer very strong wear resistance. However these often parallel rows of enamel prisms and interprismatic enamel are subject to cracking along the prismatic and interprismatic lines. One adaptive process to prevent such cracks that is particularly noticeable in Equine Type 2 enamel is the presence of enamel decussation (which means interweaving changes of direction of groups of enamel prisms) (Fig. 1.10). In contrast Equine Type 1 enamel contains no decussation. Equine incisors are smaller and flatter than cheek teeth, have less support from adjacent teeth and yet undergo great mechanical stresses during

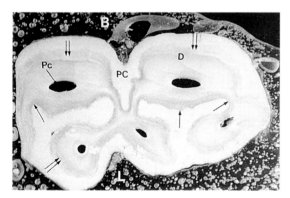

**Figure 1.9.** Transverse section, 2 cm beneath the occlusal surface of a methyl methacrylate embedded lower fourth cheek tooth of an 8-year-old horse. The enamel (peripheral only) is thickest (↓↓) in regions that are parallel to the long axis of the mandible, and thinnest (↓) in invaginations of enamel. One peripheral infolding is apparent on the buccal (B) aspect, while two deeper infoldings are present on the lingual (L) aspect. ×4. (From Kilic 1995,[26] with permission). PC, peripheral cement; D, dentin.

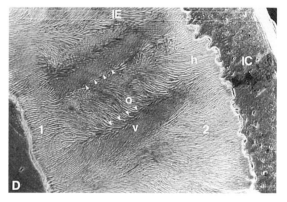

**Figure 1.10.** Scanning electron micrograph of a section of an equine incisor tooth, showing dentin (D), infundibular enamel (IE) and infundibular cement (IC). A thin layer of Equine Type 1 enamel is present on the left (1). The bulk of the enamel is Equine Type 2 (2) and this is oriented at a wide variety of angles including horizontally (h), obliquely (o) and vertically (v) relative to the occlusal surface. The bands of enamel oriented obliquely and vertically form alternating bands that are oriented perpendicular to the amelodentinal and amelocemental junctions with their junctions demarcated by grooves (▲▲▲▲). ×131. (From Kilic et al. 1997b,[25] with permission of the editor of the Equine Veterinary Journal).

prehension that could readily cause enamel cracks. Therefore it is not surprising that they are largely composed of Equine Type 2 enamel prisms. Cheek teeth primarily have the grinding function and so the presence of enamel that confers high wear resistance is more essential, and this in turn is fulfilled by the higher amounts of Equine Type 1 enamel in cheek teeth.[20]

In equine cheek teeth both peripheral and infundibular enamel are about three times thicker in areas where they are parallel to the long axis of the maxilla or mandible than where perpendicular to this axis.[20] However, enamel thickness remains constant throughout the length of the teeth, therefore, as the animal ages the enamel thickness remains constant at the different sites in the transverse plane. Enamel may have evolved to become thinner in certain regions of the tooth in response to localized reduced masticatory forces.

## DENTIN

The bulk of the tooth is composed of dentin, a cream-colored calcified tissue composed of approximately 70 per cent minerals (mainly hydroxyapatite crystals) and 30 per cent organic components (including collagen fibers and mucopolysaccharides) and water. The latter content is obvious in dried equine teeth specimens because the dentin (and also cement) will develop cracks. The mechanical properties, including tensile strength and compressibility of dentin are highly influenced by the arrangements and relationships of its matrix collagen fibers (Fig. 1.11), other organic components and calcified components with the heterogeneity of its structure contributing to its overall strength.[21] High-powered examination of equine dentin shows that it contains both calcified fibers and calcospherites. In equine teeth, the presence of dentin (and also cement) interspersed between the hard but brittle enamel layers forms a laminated structure (like safety glass) and allows the two, softer calcified tissues to act as 'crack stoppers' for the enamel[21] as well as creating an irregular occlusal surface.

Dentin can be divided into two main types, primary and secondary dentin, and the latter

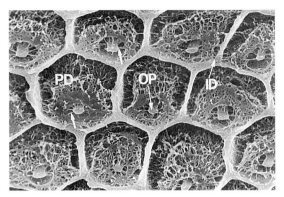

**Figure 1.11.** Scanning electron micrograph of partially decalcified dentin. The hexagonal shaped intertubular dentin (ID) has a compact appearance. A network of collagenous fibers is apparent in the fully decalcified peritubular dentin (PD) and these fibrils are attached to the odontoblast processes (OP). ×2020. (From Kilic 1995,[26] with permission).

can be further subdivided into regular (physiological) and irregular (pathological, reparative or tertiary) dentin.[22,23] Even when morphologically in the resting phase, odontoblasts remain capable of synthesizing dentin throughout their lives if appropriately stimulated[12,24] and in the equine tooth odontoblasts synthesize regular secondary dentin throughout life that gradually occludes the pulp cavity (Fig. 1.12). This process has great practical significance because the occlusal surface of equine teeth would otherwise develop pulpar exposure due to normal attrition on the occlusal aspect. With insults, such as traumatic injury, infection or excessive attrition, primary dentin can respond by developing sclerosis of the primary dentinal tubules to prevent micro-organisms or their molecular products gaining access to the pulp, a defensive feature that is additional to the deposition of reparative (irregular) secondary dentin.

As noted, the cream color of dentin largely contributes to the color of brachydont teeth. Because equine primary dentin contains very high levels of heavily mineralized peritubular dentin, it too has an almost translucent appearance similar to enamel. In contrast, the less mineralized regular secondary dentin (produced at the site of the former pulp cavity) has a dull opaque appearance. It also absorbs pigment from food which gives it a dark brown color that is obvious in the so called 'dental star' of

MORPHOLOGY

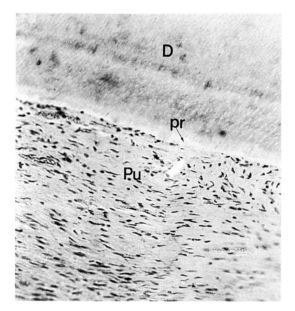

**Figure 1.12.** Light micrograph of a decalcified equine cheek tooth showing mineralized dentin (D), a thin layer of predentin (pr) and the pulp (Pu) which contains cells – odontoblasts on the surface of the predentin and fibroblast-like cells within the remaining pulp. ×64. (From Kilic 1995,[26] with permission).

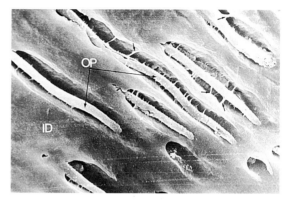

**Figure 1.13.** Scanning electron micrograph of an untreated dentinal section showing a longitudinal profile of dentinal tubules containing odontoblast processes (OP) that are attached to the intertubular dentin (ID) by calcified fibrils (↓). ×1010. (From Kilic *et al.* 1997,[28] with permission of the editor of the *Equine Veterinary Journal*).

incisors or in the brown linear areas of secondary dentin that occur on the occlusal surface of cheek teeth that are in wear.

Dentin is composed of several distinct structures including dentinal tubules (which are the outstanding histological feature of dentin), peritubular dentin (which forms the tubule walls), intertubular dentin (that lies between the tubules) and odontoblast processes. Dentinal tubules extend from the pulp cavity across the width of the tooth to the amelodentinal junction. The odontoblasts reside in the pulp cavity but their odontoblast processes extend through the dental tubules (Figs 1.11 and 1.13) as far as the enamel, sometimes subdividing into two or three tubules and displaying a sharp curvature just before reaching the amelodentinal junction. There is a debate on whether the odontoblast processes reach as far as the amelodentinal junction in other species, but in the horse it appears that they do so.[25] Because it contains odontoblast processes in its tubules, dentin is considered as a living tissue. There is an intimate association between the pulp and dentin, which act as a single functional unit, and thus the term

pulpo-dentinal complex is appropriately used for these two tissues.

In brachydont species, odontoblast processes or their surrounding fluid can convey pain signals from insulted (e.g. excessive heat or cold, trauma, infection) dentin to the pulp by incompletely understood mechanisms. In horses, where exposed dentin constitutes a major part of the occlusal surface, it is unclear if such pain-producing mechanisms exist. It is interesting that on the occlusal surface of equine teeth, apparently intact odontoblast-like processes are visible protruding from the dentinal tubules of primary and regular secondary dentin (Fig. 1.14), even though this area is constantly exposed to oral microbial and biochemical insults.[25] The most likely explanation for their apparently undamaged morphology is that they have become calcified. However, even if micro-organisms could enter patent dentinal tubules on the occlusal surface, they could not reach the pulp cavity because at the coronal aspect of the pulp cavity, all dentinal tubules are fully sealed by a layer of irregular secondary dentin.[26] When irregular (reparative) secondary dentin is present on the occlusal surface, it contains no odontoblast processes as the dentinal tubules of this less organized dentin are fully obliterated.

Peritubular dentin (Fig. 1.11) has a higher mineral content than intertubular dentin and

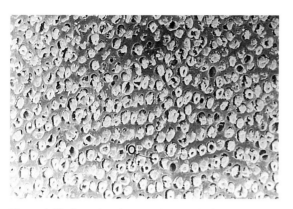

**Figure 1.14.** Scanning electron micrograph of the occlusal surface of an equine cheek tooth showing regular secondary dentin. Almost all of the dentinal tubules contain protruding odontoblast processes (OP) which are believed to be calcified, and many which are hollow. ×1010. (From Kilic 1995,[26] with permission).

therefore has a greater resistance to wear. A transitional region exists between equine primary and secondary dentin where peritubular dentin is absent. Regular secondary dentin which contains no peritubular dentin is therefore more susceptible to attrition than primary dentin. Similarly dentin near the amelodentinal junction contains the lowest amounts of peritubular dentin and would theoretically be expected to wear faster, however it is protected from excessive wear by the adjacent enamel.

## PULP

The histology of equine teeth pulp has not yet been fully evaluated and most information is derived from the literature on brachydont teeth. Pulp is a soft tissue within the dental pulp cavities that contains connective tissue, including fibroblasts, thick collagen and a network of fine reticulin fibers. It is contiguous with the periodontal connective tissue at the apical foramen. Peripherally, a thin layer of predentin (that becomes thinner in older brachydont teeth) lies between the dentin and pulp (Fig. 1.12). The bodies of the odontoblasts lie on the predentin, with their cytoplasmic processes extending into the dentinal tubules.

At eruption, equine permanent teeth possess a large common pulp that is contiguous with the surrounding primordial pulp that surrounds the developing apices. This pulp is surrounded only by a thin layer of enamel. With deposition of apical dentin and cement, root formation is complete in all equine cheek teeth by 2 years, but the two separate pulp canals (with two to three long pulp horns in each) may not develop until 5 to 6 years following mandibular cheek tooth eruption.[9] The above features have significant implications for endodontic therapy.

Unlike brachydont teeth, hypsodont teeth need to continue to lay down much secondary dentin over a prolonged period (most of their life) in order to prevent occlusal pulp exposure. Consequently, in order to supply the metabolically active odontoblasts, the apical foramina through which the tooth vasculature passes into the pulp must remain dilated ('open') for a prolonged period, although progressive reduction in foramen size does occur with age.[27] Kirkland *et al.* found constricted ('closed') apical foramina in equine mandibular cheek at 5 to 8 years after eruption, with development of two apical foramina in the rostral (mesial) root.[9] This is in contrast to the apical foramina of brachydont teeth which become more rapidly and extensively constricted ('closed') by deposition of secondary dentin within the pulp canal[1] and externally by cement deposition.

A practical result of these features is that pulp exposure in mature brachydont teeth will usually cause pulpitis that will compress and constrict the limited pulpar vasculature usually leading to pulp necrosis and death of the tooth. However, in hypsodont teeth, especially when young, the dilated apices and good blood supply may allow the pulp to withstand such inflammation. Local macrophages within the pulp, along with extravasated white blood cells and their molecules can control such pulpar infection. Additionally, the odontoblasts laying down secondary dentin can also lay down reparative dentin in response to infection of the overlying dentin or following traumatic pulp exposure. In the absence of sufficient local odontoblasts, adjacent undifferentiated connective tissue cells or fibroblasts in the pulp can transform into odontoblasts and lay down reparative dentin.

15

As well as the coronal aspect of the equine pulp cavity being progressively (fully) occluded with secondary dentin, the continued but slower similar deposition over all of the pulp cavity walls causes the overall pulp size to reduce with age. A practical consequence of this is that in younger (e.g. less than 7 to 8-year-old) horses the cheek teeth are somewhat shell-like, and may fracture if cut with shears, whereas in older horses, the large amount of secondary dentin that has been laid down makes the teeth more solid and less likely to shatter when cut. With age, the pulp of brachydont teeth loses much of its vasculature, fibroblasts and odontoblasts while its collagen content increases.

## CEMENT

Cement (cementum) is a white or cream colored calcified dental tissue with mechanical characteristics and a histological appearance similar to bone. It contains about 65 per cent inorganic (again mainly impure hydroxyapatite crystals) and 35 per cent organic and water components. Similar to dentin, its high organic content, including widespread collagen fibers gives it flexibility. The organic component of cement is comprised mainly of collagen fibers that include small intrinsic fibrils (produced by cementoblasts) and larger extrinsic fibers (produced by fibroblasts of the periodontal membrane) some of which form tight bundles termed Sharpey's fibers (median 2.5 microns in diameter in horses) that cross the periodontal space to become anchored in the alveolar bone (Figs 1.15, 1.16 and 1.17).[28]

Like dentin, cement (of subgingival area only, i.e. of reserve crown and roots) is a living tissue with its cells (cementoblasts) nourished by vasculature of the periodontal ligament. Cement and its periodontal membrane can be considered as a single functional unit.[29] However after eruption onto the clinical crown, cementoblasts now lose their blood supply from the periodontium and therefore cement on the clinical (erupted) crown can be regarded as an inert tissue. Cement is the most adaptable of the calcified dental tissues and can be quickly deposited (within the alveolus only) in response

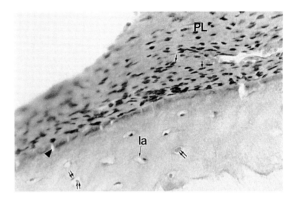

**Figure 1.15.** Light microscopy of the periphery of an upper cheek tooth showing the periodontal ligament (PL) containing fibroblast-like cells (↓). The adjacent peripheral cement contains lacunae (la) of the cementoblasts (↓↓). Projections of the periodontal ligament into the cementum (▲) probably represent Sharpey's fibers. ×1000. (From Kilic *et al.* 1997d,[30] with permission of the editor of the *Equine Veterinary Journal*).

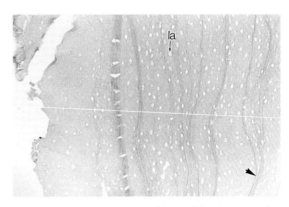

**Figure 1.16.** Light micrograph of the peripheral cement of the deep reserve crown (adjacent to the apex) of a recently erupted cheek tooth. This contains wavy incremental lines (↓) between successive depositions of cement that have occurred even at this early stage of tooth growth. Cementoblast lacunae (la) are present at all levels of the cement. ×44. (From Kilic 1995,[26] with permission).

to insults such as infection or trauma.[29] In hypsodont teeth cement covers all of the crown (including the occlusal surface transiently after eruption) and fills the infundibula.

Cement deposition continues throughout the life of the tooth, both around the roots (root cement) and also around the reserve crown (coronal cement) of hypsodont teeth, to allow new Sharpey's fibers (Figs 1.15 and 1.17) to

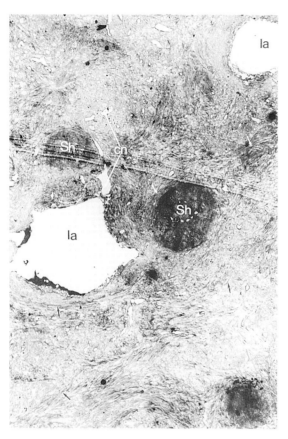

**Figure 1.17.** Transmission electron micrograph of peripheral cement of a cheek tooth. This shows irregularly shaped lacunae (la) and their canaliculae (cn) but the cementoblasts have been lost during sample preparation. The dense Sharpey's fibers (Sh) have been transversely sectioned. The intrinsic fibrils of the cement (↓) are also apparent. ×2150. (From Kilic *et al.* 1997,[30] with permission of the editor of the *Equine Veterinary Journal*).

nants exposed at the occlusal surface may eventually be composed only of roots (dentin and cement) with surrounding heavy cemental deposits. As this remnant contains no enamel it becomes smooth on its occlusal surface 'smooth mouth' and wears away quickly.

There is little peripheral cement in incisors and canines, but much greater amounts in cheek teeth, where its thickness varies greatly, largely depending on the degree of infolding of peripheral enamel. It is thickest in deeply infolded areas, especially in the two folds on the medial aspect of the lower cheek teeth (Fig. 1.9). At these sites, especially toward the tooth apex, this thick peripheral cement can be fully enclosed by these deep enamel folds and resemble infundibula.

The infundibula (in all incisors and the upper cheek teeth) are usually incompletely filled by (infundibular) cement (Fig. 1.18). Kilic *et al.* found that in addition to the 24 per cent of (upper) cheek teeth that had gross caries (mineralized dental tissue dissolution) of their infundibular cement, a further 65 per cent of horses had one or more small central vascular channels in this cement.[28,30] These extended from the occlusal surface to a variable depth

be laid down, a process necessary to allow the prolonged eruption of hypsodont teeth. However no further cement can be deposited in infundibular cement that has no blood supply following tooth eruption, nor likewise on the cement of the clinical crown. The main functions of peripheral cement are to provide anchorage for fibers of the periodontal ligament that support (with some flexibility) the tooth in the alveolus, protect the underlying dentin at the dental apex and, particularly in older hypsodont teeth, contribute to the size and strength of the remaining tooth to compensate for crown wear.[26,27] In some aged horses, the dental rem-

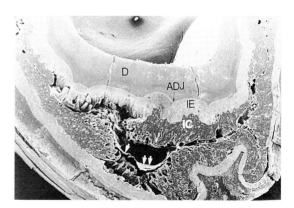

**Figure 1.18.** Scanning electron micrograph of the deep infundibular area of an upper cheek tooth of a 14 year-old horse. This section contains dentin (D), an amelodentinal junction (ADJ), infundibular enamel (IE) and infundibular cement (IC). The infundibular cement shows extensive hypoplasia, with the large central defect partially lined by shrunken organic tissue (↓) and also exposure of the infundibular enamel in several areas. ×10.6. (From Kilic *et al.* 1997,[30] with permission of the editor of the *Equine Veterinary Journal*).

and contained smaller lateral channels extending as far as the infundibular enamel. This type of cement hypoplasia was termed 'central infundibular cemental hypoplasia' (Fig. 1.18). In addition, some infundibula had linear areas of cement hypoplasia at the enamel junction termed 'junctional cemental hypoplasia'.[28] As this latter cemental hypoplasia was commonly recorded in incisors, that in general show little evidence of caries, this histological feature is consequently not believed to be clinically significant.[28]

## THE OCCLUSAL SURFACE

At eruption the crowns of equine teeth including the occlusal surface are fully covered by coronal cement, which in turn covers a thin layer of coronal enamel. With normal occlusal wear, the coronal cement and coronal enamel are very soon worn away thus exposing the secondary occlusal surface of these teeth, which in fact is the permanent occlusal surface of hypsodont teeth (Fig. 1.3). The wear process on the occlusal surface is a complex phenomenon depending on many factors including the type of diet, e.g. in the winter outdoor horses may be forced to graze lower and thus ingest more soil-covered roots and leaves, or even eat the roots of plants such as nettles (M. Booth, personal communication, 1996) thus greatly increasing the amount of silicates that are ingested. When grazing is scarce they may also eat bushes such as gorse. The duration of eating also varies according to the season from up to 13 hours/day in summer to 16.5 hours/day in winter in outdoor horses (M. Booth, personal communication, 1996). While eating hay, horses and ponies had 58–66 chews/minute, with 4200 chews/kg dry matter[31] while at grass they have 100–105 chewing movements per minute.[32] Dental attrition also depends on the force and the direction of the chewing action, the sizes, shapes and angles of the opposing occlusal surfaces and the relationship of opposing cusps and crest patterns to the occlusal motion. Consequently, painful oral disorders can cause changes in the direction and forces of chewing and thus will affect the wear patterns of cheek teeth. Focal areas of reduced wear will lead to overgrowths.

The occlusal surfaces of equine enamel contain differing wear patterns including polished areas, small local fractures, pit striations and depressions. Most large striations are perpendicular to the long axis of the dental arcades (the buccolingual plane) and appear to be caused by the normal side-to-side chewing motion of the cheek teeth grinding down small ingested phytoliths. In these deep grooves, scanning electron microscopy shows that prismatic enamel is more deeply worn than interprismatic enamel, confirming that the former is softer. Additionally, some shorter striations are present on the occlusal surface of equine teeth which are parallel to the buccolingual plane (at right angles to the normal chewing direction) and it is suggested that these striations occur due to ingested phytoliths during the crushing phase of chewing.[30]

The softer dentin on the occlusal surface wears quicker than the surrounding enamel and therefore the dentinal surface becomes depressed. The depth of these depressions is directly related to the area of the dentin, with larger exposed areas more deeply recessed. In contrast, smaller exposed areas, being better protected by the surrounding enamel have less wear. Therefore, the orientation and invaginations of the enamel folds play an important role in dividing the occlusal surface of dentin into smaller areas and thus protecting it from excessive attrition. In this respect, the lower cheek teeth have three very deep infoldings of enamel, two on the medial (lingual) aspect and one on the buccal aspect. The upper cheek teeth have less peripheral enamel infolding, however they contain two enamel infundibula which further subdivide and compartmentalize their occlusal dentin thus protecting it.[30]

## GROSS ANATOMY OF EQUINE TEETH
### INCISORS

The deciduous central, middle (intermediate) and corner incisors erupt at birth or within a few days, 4 to 6 weeks and 6 to 9 months respectively.[33] Deciduous incisors are whiter and contain wider and shallower infundibula than their permanent successors, which erupt on their lingual aspect. As noted, the eruption of both deciduous and permanent teeth can be used to estimate the age of horses up to 5 years old with a reasonable degree of accuracy (See Chapter 3).[34,35]

### The dental formulae of deciduous and permanent teeth in horses are

Deciduous teeth: 2 (Incisors 3/3, Canine 0/0, Molars 3/3) = 24 teeth

Permanent teeth: 2 (Incisors 3/3, Canine 1/1 or 0/0, Premolar 3/3 or 4/4, Molar 3/3) = 36 to 44 teeth, depending on the presence and number of canine teeth or premolar 1 (wolf teeth).[36]

The Triadan system of dental nomenclature utilizes three digits to identify each tooth, the first digit refers to the quadrant, with 1 for upper right, 2 for upper left, 3 for lower left and 4 for lower right (Fig. 1.19).[38]

Adult horses also have twelve incisors in total, six in each arcade. The upper incisor teeth are embedded in the incisive bone and the lower incisors in the rostral mandible. Incisor teeth are curved convexly on their labial aspect (concavely on their lingual aspect) and taper in uniformly from the occlusal surface toward the apex (unlike equine deciduous and all brachydont incisors that have a distinct neck). Therefore with age, spaces will eventually develop between equine permanent incisors. The fully developed incisor arcade in a young

adult horse has an almost semicircular appearance, which gradually becomes shallower with age, due to alteration of teeth shape caused by progressive wear.[4,38] The occlusal angle of incisors also changes from almost vertical apposition in the young horse to an increasing angle of incidence with age.

Equine incisor teeth also develop certain wear-related macroscopic features which have also been traditionally utilized for estimating age[35] that are discussed in detail in Chapter 3. The infundibulum present in all incisors is termed the incisal cup. This funnel-like structure is oval in shape and about 10 mm deep when the tooth first erupts. It is usually incompletely filled with cement and consequently becomes filled with decomposing food material and appears dark.[34] When the infundibulum is worn away, it leaves behind a small ring of infundibular enamel located on the lingual aspect of the tooth which is called the enamel spot (enamel ring or mark).[34] Due to the slower wear of enamel as compared to dentin, the enamel spot becomes elevated above the occlusal surface. The dental star represents exposure of secondary dentin that has been deposited within a former pulp cavity on the occlusal surface of incisor teeth. It appears sequentially in the central, middle and corner incisors (see Chapter 3). It first appears as a dark yellow transverse line on the labial aspect of the infundibulum. With further tooth wear it gradually becomes oval in shape and moves toward the center of occlusal surface.

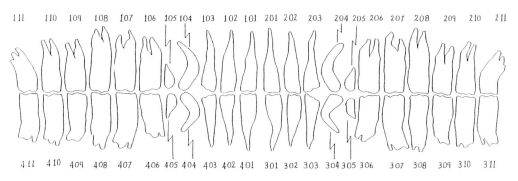

**Figure 1.19.** The Triadan Figure.

Galvayne's groove is a longitudinal groove that appears on the labial aspect of the upper corner (103, 203 – Triadan) incisors. A hook (localized dental overgrowth) is often recognized at the caudolabial aspect of the occlusal surface of the upper corner incisors (103 and 203) after about 6 years of age due to incomplete occlusal contact between the upper and lower corner incisors. It is often termed a '7-year hook' because it was traditionally (but erroneously) believed to always appear at 7 years of age.[7,38] Variations in incisor teeth appearance can also be due to individual and breed variation, differences in diets, environmental conditions, eruption times, mineralization rates, depth of enamel infundibulum, amount of infundibular cement and the presence of certain stereotypic behaviors such as crib-biting and windsucking.[35,39,40] The occlusal surfaces of incisors are elliptical in recently erupted incisors, but with wear, they successively become round, triangular and then oval in shape. These changes are more apparent in the central (301 and 401) and intermediate (302 and 402) than in the corner (303 and 403) lower incisors.[35,36]

## CANINE TEETH

The deciduous canine teeth are vestigial spicule-like structures 0.5–1.0 cm long that do not erupt. The lower ones are situated behind the corner incisor.[33] Male horses normally have four permanent canine teeth (two maxillary and two mandibular) that erupt at 4 to 6 years of age in the interdental space.[36] They are simple teeth (i.e. contain no coronal cement or enamel folding) and are pointed with a caudal-facing curve. They are also convex on their buccal borders, and slightly concave on their medial (lingual and buccal) aspects. In the young adult thoroughbred, they are 5–7 cm long with most as unerupted reserve crown. The lower canines are more rostrally positioned than the upper and thus there is no occlusal contact between them. This is alleged to be a reason why canine teeth are prone to develop calculus. Canine teeth are usually absent or rudimentary in female horses with a reported incidence of 27.8 per cent.[41]

## CHEEK TEETH

The 12 temporary molars are erupted at birth or do so within a week or so. They are later replaced by the larger permanent premolars at about 2.5, 3 and 4 years of age for the first to third cheek teeth respectively. In contrast to brachydont teeth and to equine incisors where the deciduous teeth are much smaller than the permanent teeth, the transverse (cross-sectional) area of equine deciduous cheek teeth can be somewhat similar to those of adult teeth.[27] The three deciduous cheek teeth in each row have a distinct neck between the crown and roots, unlike their permanent successors.[42] Latterly these teeth erupt into the oral cavity due to pressure from the underlying permanent tooth. They are simultaneously resorbed at their apices until eventually just a thin plate ('cap') of the temporary tooth remains (Fig. 1.20).

An adult equine mouth normally contains 24 cheek teeth (PM 2–4 and M 1–3, the latter erupt at approximately 1, 2 and 3.5 years of age respectively), forming four rows of six teeth that are accommodated in the maxillary and mandibular bones (Figs 1.20 and 1.21). On transverse section, equine cheek teeth are rectangular shaped, except the first and last, i.e. PM 2 and M 3 which are somewhat triangular shaped (Figs 1.22 and 1.23). The maxillary cheek teeth are wider and squarer in comparison with the mandibular cheek teeth that are narrower and more rectangular in outline. The long axes of all cheek teeth are relatively straight, except the sixth and to a lesser and variable extent the fifth, that have a caudal curvature of their reserve crown (later, more so of their roots) (Fig. 1.24). The buccal aspect of the upper cheek teeth has two prominent longitudinal ridges (cingula, styles) rostrally and a less prominent caudal ridge with two deep grooves between them, except the first which can have three grooves and four (often slight) ridges. The palatal aspect of the upper, and both lingual and buccal aspects of the mandibular cheek teeth contain much less distinct grooves and ridges (Figs 1.8 and 1.9).

In younger horses, the permanent cheek teeth possess long crowns, most of which is unerupted

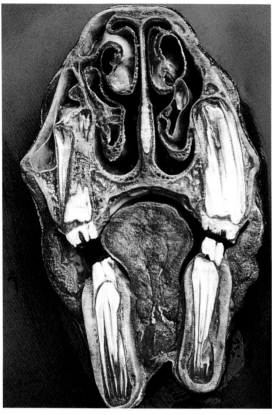

**Figure 1.20.** Oblique section of the skull of a 3.5-year-old horse at the level of the second maxillary cheek tooth (PM3) on right and between the second and third on the left, with part of the third in the rostral maxillary sinus. Note the remnants of the deciduous teeth ('caps'), the angulation of the occlusal surfaces and the anisognathia. There are wide common pulp chambers of the apices of the permanent teeth and absence of roots. The infundibula of the temporary maxillary teeth demonstrate cemental hypoplasia.

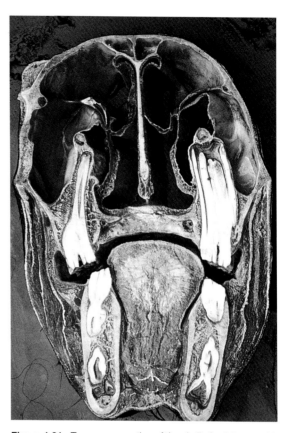

**Figure 1.21.** Transverse section of the skull of a 3.5-year-old horse at the level of the fifth maxillary cheek teeth that lie at the borders of the rostral and caudal maxillary sinuses. Due to their curvature, parts of the fifth and sixth mandibular cheek teeth are shown. The mandibular canal lies on the medial aspect of the mandible. The wide common pulp cavity of the left maxillary cheek tooth (with infraorbital canal above) has pulp horns that extend to within 1 cm of the occlusal surface.

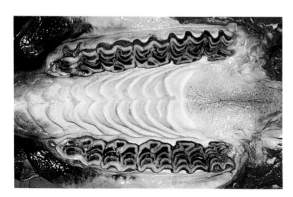

**Figure 1.22.** Occlusal view of the five maxillary cheek teeth of a 3-year-old horse. Note the absence of spaces between these teeth, the more pronounced ridges on the buccal aspects of these teeth and the triangular shape of the first tooth.

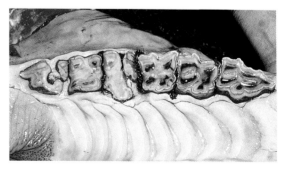

**Figure 1.23.** Occlusal view of a maxillary cheek teeth row of an aged horse. Just the roots (rostral roots separate) that have heavy peripheral cement deposits remain of the fourth and sixth. These remnants contain little enamel ('smooth mouth') and consequently will soon fully wear out. The infundibula of the remainder teeth have fully worn out and diastema is present between the rostral teeth.

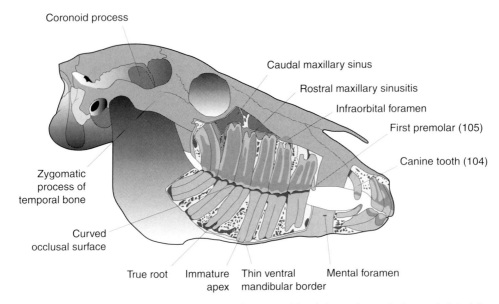

Coronoid process

Caudal maxillary sinus

Rostral maxillary sinusitis

Infraorbital foramen

First premolar (105)

Canine tooth (104)

Zygomatic process of temporal bone

Curved occlusal surface

True root     Immature apex     Thin ventral mandibular border     Mental foramen

**Figure 1.24.** Lateral view of a partially dissected skull of a 5-year-old male horse demonstrating ventral deviation of the mandible associated with eruption of the third cheek tooth. Note the shape and apposition of the incisors of this young horse. The angulation of the rostral and caudal cheek teeth and the curvature of the sixth tooth maintains tight apposition at the occlusal surface. The temporomandibular joint is 15 cm above the level of the occlusal surface. Note the small coronoid process and the area of mandibular muscle attachment.

reserve crown that is embedded in the deep alveoli (Figs 1.20 and 1.21). In thoroughbreds, the first cheek tooth is the shortest (about 5 cm maximum length), with the remaining cheek teeth up to 6–8 cm long before wear. Dental eruption proceeds throughout the life of equine teeth and normally the eruption rate corresponds with tooth wear (attrition) and has been calculated as 2–3 mm per year.[4,5] Therefore, since all equine permanent cheek teeth come into wear by 5 years of age, a 75 mm-long tooth should be fully worn by 30–35 years of age.[4]

The maxillary cheek teeth have five pulp compartments in contrast to their lower counterparts which contain two main pulp cavities with five to six subdivisions.[9,26] Once fully developed, the upper cheek teeth usually have three roots (two small lateral and a larger medial), but occasionally four[43] and the lower cheek teeth (except M3 which has three) possess two equally sized roots, one rostral and one caudal, that tend to become longer than those of their maxillary counterparts. One or both of the upper PM 1 and less commonly, the lower

PM 1 may also be present as the small, vestigial 'wolf teeth' with a reported incidence of 24.4 per cent in females and 14.9 per cent in males;[41] and in horses of both sexes, of 13 per cent[19] and 31.9 per cent.[44]

The alveoli of the first two cheek teeth and often the rostral aspect of the third, and usually all of this tooth in older horses[36] are embedded in the maxillary bone (Fig. 1.20), the caudal aspect of the third and the fourth lie in the rostral maxillary sinus and the fifth and sixth in the caudal maxillary sinus (Fig. 1.21). In young horses, the large reserve crowns occupy much of these sinuses, but with age and the subsequent eruption of their reserve crowns and retraction of their alveoli, the residual paranasal sinus cavities increase in volume. The apex of the curved sixth maxillary cheek tooth drifts rostrally from its site beneath the orbit in the young adult, to become sited rostral to the orbit in the aged horse. The intimate relation between the caudal cheek teeth and sinuses can allow periapical infections of the caudal four cheek teeth to cause maxillary sinus empyema.

The six maxillary cheek teeth form slightly curved rows, with their concavity toward the buccal and lingual aspects respectively.[36] The rows of mandibular cheek teeth form straight rows that match the angels of the mandibular rows. A common feature of all ungulates (mammals with hooves) including horses is the presence of an interdental space ('bars of mouth') between the incisors and the premolars, that may just be a side effect of the evolutionary increase in face length (dolicephalic) to allow these long-legged animals to graze more comfortably off the ground.[45] Its presence however necessitates the rostral cheek teeth to face caudally (distally) to help compress each row of cheek teeth (Fig. 1.24) (as they are not in an arc, the term row rather than arch is a better term for the six equine cheek teeth in each quadrant). In contrast, the complete arch of teeth of omnivores and many carnivores needs to be compressed in just a single direction with the rostrally (mesially) facing caudal teeth to promote this drifting of the teeth.[45]

The reserve crowns (and the roots once developed) of the first equine cheek teeth (PM 2) both upper and lower, are angled slightly rostrally (mesially) and therefore their clinical crowns are angled caudally (distally). The second, third and fourth cheek teeth are roughly perpendicular. The fifth and sixth cheek teeth have caudally facing reserve crowns with the sixth and to a lesser and variable extent the fifth also having caudal curvatures of their reserve crowns and roots. Consequently, their clinical crowns are angled rostrally. Pressure between the first and the caudal cheek teeth tightly compress the six cheek teeth together at their occlusal surface. This factor along with the continuing deposition of coronal cement (within the alveolus only) causes each row of six cheek teeth to act as a single functional unit (Figs 1.22 and 1.24). Continued eruption of the angulated cheek teeth usually maintains this tight occlusal contact until very late in life in normal horses, despite the fact that equine teeth slightly taper in toward their apex and with age, would otherwise develop spaces between the teeth (interproximally) that is termed diastema (Fig. 1.20).[46] Many very old horses (more than 20 years) do develop diastema between their incisors which is of little consequence in these teeth, unlike the situation with cheek teeth where diastema causes food to accumulate between the teeth and in the adjacent periodontal space.[46]

The occlusal surface of the rows of cheek teeth are not level in the longitudinal plane as occurs in some other species, but instead the surface of the caudal three cheek teeth curve upwards in the caudal direction that is termed the Curve of Spee.[6] This curvature is most marked in Arab-type breeds that often have a similar curvature on their (dished) facial bones, but can also be marked in other light breeds of horses.

In normal horses, the distance between the maxillary cheek teeth rows is wider (approximately 30 per cent) than that between the mandibular rows, which is termed anisognathia. This is in comparison to, for example, human teeth, that are equally spaced (isognathic). As noted, the maxillary cheek teeth are also wider than their lower counterparts. Consequently, when the mouth is closed, approximately one third of the occlusal surface of the upper cheek teeth are in contact with about half of the lower cheek teeth's occlusal surface. Additionally the occlusal surfaces of the cheek teeth are not level in the transverse (buccolingual) plane as is usually the case in brachydonts, but are angled at 10–15 degrees (angled from dorsal on their lingual (palatal) aspect to ventral on their buccal aspect) (Figs 1.20 and 1.21).

The terminology concerning the irregularities present on the occlusal surface of the cheek teeth can be confusing. A cusp is a pronounced elevation on the occlusal surface of a cheek tooth and is an area with thicker enamel. A ridge (or style) is a linear elevation on the surface (peripheral or occlusal) of a tooth and on the occlusal surface may be formed by connections between cusps. Because equine cusps contain sharp ridges of exposed occlusal enamel adjacent to craters of dentin (and cement at some sites) they are classified as lophs and thus the cusp pattern of equine teeth is termed lophodont. A fossa is a rounded depression and a fissure is a linear depression between cusps or ridges.[1,26] The opposing ridges and fissures of the upper and lower equine cheek teeth interdigitate when the mouth is shut. Each row of six cheek teeth contains of a total of ten to eleven ridges, two on the occlusal surface of each tooth, except the first and last which can contain one to three ridges. Other variations in cusp number, size and distribution are used for paleontological research and for taxonomic classification of different species.[2,26]

## NERVE SUPPLY OF TEETH

Because of its great importance in human dentistry, the innervation of teeth has been well studied in brachydont teeth. Pulpar nerves enter through the apical foramen and include sensory nerves derived from the trigeminal (5th cranial) nerve, that are most extensive in the coronal region of the pulp where they form the plexus of Raschkow,[12] and sympathetic fibers from the cervical ganglion which supply the vascular smooth muscles to regulate blood flow in the pulp.[23,47,48] The latter are also believed to control the differentiation and function of odontoblasts, including their circadian rhythm of activity.[23]

The type and duration of pain caused by stimulation of dentin are different from those of pulp. In brachydont teeth, dentin responds to various stimuli including excessive heat and cold and to therapeutic procedures such as drilling, with a sharp pain which stops when these stimuli cease. In contrast, stimulation of the pulpal nerves produces dull pain, which continues for some time after the stimulus is removed.[23] Nerves are present in the pulp of hypsodont teeth, although the role of sensory nerves is unclear, as these teeth have dentin constantly exposed on the occlusal surface, a situation that in some circumstances would cause marked pain in brachydont teeth.

## BLOOD SUPPLY OF TEETH

In brachydont teeth, the blood vessels enter the pulp through the apical foramen and form an extensive capillary network, particularly in the coronal region of the pulp.[23] These capillaries drain into an extensive venous network which has a more tortuous course than the arterioles and also exits via the apical foramen.[23] Due to

difficulties in distinguishing them microscopically from vascular capillaries it remains unclear if lymph vessels are actually present in pulp.[23] However, other authors believe that pulp tissues, like all other connective tissues, contain lymph vessels that in humans drain into the submandibular and deep cervical lymph nodes.

## SUPPORTING BONES AND MUSCLES OF PREHENSION AND MASTICATION

### ALVEOLAR BONE

Alveolar bone is very flexible and constantly remodels to accommodate the changing shape and size of the dental structures it contains. Alveolar bone can be divided into two main parts. First there is a thin layer of compact (radiodense) bone that lines the alveolus proper and in which Sharpey's fibers insert that is termed the lamina dura (lamina dura denta). This area is radiographically detectable as a thin radiodense line in brachydont teeth, but due to irregularities of the periphery of some normal equine cheek teeth, this radiographic feature is not always obvious on lateral radiographs. Second is the remaining alveolar bone surrounding the lamina, which cannot be morphologically differentiated from the remaining bone of the mandible or maxilla.[1] The most prominent aspect of the alveolar bone beneath the gingival margin is termed the alveolar crest (Fig. 1.3).

### MANDIBLE

The mandible, the largest bone of the equine face is composed of two components, hemimandibles, that fuse in the foal at 2 to 3 months of age.[33] It articulates with the squamous temporal bone at the temporomandibular joint. This bone contains the alveoli of the mandibular incisors and lower cheek teeth (and canines and PM 1 – if present). The ventral border of the horizontal ramus is wide and rounded in the young horse because of the deep reserve crowns it contains (Fig. 1.20). Some breeds, especially those that are descendants of the Arab horse (which in turn are descendants of *Equus cracoviensis* – Type IV horse) have shallow mandibles and maxillae and commensurately short reserve crowns, whereas most other breeds, for example those derived from *E. Muniensis* (Types I or mountain pony] or *E. mosbachensis* (Type III, forest or marshland horse) such as the North European draught and native British pony types (e.g. Exmoors) have deep alveoli and long reserve crowns[49] (AN Copeland, unpublished data, 1990).

It has been proposed that crosses between these two types of horses can develop pronounced ventral swellings under the developing apices of the second and third cheek teeth,[49] due to an imbalance between mandibular depth and tooth length. These mandibular 'eruption cysts' or 'osseous tubercles' (Fig. 1.24) usually occur at 3–5 years of age and unless they fistulate, they regress over the following 1 to 2 years.[27] Other authors suggest that some breeds of horses are predisposed to retention of deciduous cheek teeth which causes these mandibular swellings.[50] With age and continued eruption of the reserve crowns of the cheek teeth, the ventral mandibular border of lighter breeds often becomes thin and sharp, a feature formerly used by Arab horsemen to age horses.

The mental nerve (Vth) enters the mandibular foramen on the medial aspect of the vertical ramus, level with the occlusal surface of the cheek teeth and then continues along the mandibular canal. The mental nerve can be locally anesthetized at this site to facilitate painful dental procedures (e.g. oral extraction of a mandibular tooth) in the standing horse. The mandibular canal then passes to the ventral aspect of the mandible, below the apices of the teeth. However, in recently erupted teeth whose apices reach the ventral border of the mandible, the nerve usually lies on the medial aspect of the developing tooth (Fig. 1.20). The main part of the mental nerve emerges through the mental foramen on the rostrolateral aspect of the horizontal ramus, approximately halfway between the first cheek teeth and the incisors, while a smaller branch continues rostrally in a smaller canal along with the vasculature of the lower incisors.

Caudal to the alveolus of the sixth cheek tooth, the mandible becomes a very thin sheet of bone. This flattened area progressively increases in size with eruption of this tooth and contraction of its alveolus. At the angle of the jaw, this thin plate of bone expands medially and laterally into two wide lips that are roughened to allow muscle attachment (Fig. 1.24). These lips reduce in size toward the dorsal border of the vertical ramus. These normal roughened mandibular areas may be radiologically confused with pathological mandibular changes.

## THE TEMPOROMANDIBULAR JOINT AND MUSCLES OF MASTICATION

In contrast to carnivores that have a vertical power stroke, horses have a transverse power stroke in a lingual (medial) direction that is termed a lingual power stroke and consequently their masseter and medial pterygoid muscles are their most highly developed masticatory muscles. In horses, the temporomandibular joint is about 15 cm above the level of the occlusal surface and thus the movement arm of the masseter is longer. The articular extremity of the mandible is composed of the condyle caudally, and the coronoid process rostrally. The latter is poorly developed in the horse (Fig. 1.24) because it has smaller temporalis muscles in contrast to carnivores where the power stroke of the jaws is vertical and consequently both of these structures are larger. Between the articular surfaces of the mandible and the squamous temporal bone lies an articular disc that divides the joint cavity in two. The joint capsule is tight and reinforced by an indistinct lateral and an elastic posterior ligament.[33]

Although it allows just limited opening of the jaws, the equine temporomandibular joint has a wider range of lateral movements to permit the cheek teeth to effectively grind food, utilizing a side to side movement, that is combined with a slight rostrocaudal movement of the temporomandibular joint, with one side gliding rostrally and the other caudally (Chapter 2).

## MAXILLARY BONES

The upper jaws are largely formed by the maxillary bones that contain the alveoli of the upper cheek teeth (and PM 1 and canines if present). The first and second (and usually the rostral aspect of the third) cheek teeth are embedded in the rostral body of the maxillae. In younger horses, this rostral maxillary area may protrude laterally because of the presence of the underlying reserve crowns of these teeth. The overlying bone may even become thin and distended, with a temporary and focal loss of bone over the developing apices. Some 3 to 4-year-old animals develop marked bilateral firm swellings of the rostral maxillary bones during eruption of these teeth. These are the equivalent of the mandibular 'osseous tubercles' of this same age group.

The facial crest is a lateral protrusion of the maxilla that continues caudally as the zygomatic process. This joins the zygomatic parts of the malar and temporal bones to form the zygomatic arch (Fig. 1.24). After giving off a small branch that runs rostrally to innervate the maxillary incisor teeth, the infraorbital nerve (sensory, fifth) emerges through the infraorbital foramen, about 5 cm dorsal to the rostral aspect of the facial crest. Its point of exit is covered by the pencil-like levator labii superiorus muscle, that can be dorsally displaced to locally anesthetize this nerve. The dorsal and caudal borders of the maxillary bone are attached to the nasal and lacrimal bones respectively, while rostrally the maxillary is attached to the incisive bone. The thicker ventral border of each maxillary bone contains the alveoli. Each cheek tooth alveolus is fully separated by transverse interalveolar bony septa. The disposition of the cheek teeth in the various compartments of the maxilla have been previously discussed. The medial aspect of each maxillary bone forms a horizontal shelf (the palatine process) that join midline with their opposite counterpart to form the supporting bone of most of the hard palate, the remainder of which is formed caudally by the palatine and rostrally by the incisive bones.

## INCISIVE BONE

The paired incisive (premaxillary) bones form the rostral aspect of the upper jaw. The thick rostral aspects contain the alveoli of the incisors, while the thinner caudal aspects form the rostral aspect of the hard palate. The almost transverse caudal suture line between it and the maxillae is a common site for fractures. The canine teeth (if present) are on the maxillary side of this suture.

## ORAL MUCOSA

The mucosa of the gingiva and hard palate is a specialized masticatory mucosa. It can be keratinized, orthokeratinized or parakeratinized and has deep interdigitating rete pegs into the underlying vascular subcutaneous connective tissue that limits its mobility. Most of the gingiva is attached to the supporting bone, with a more mobile (usually non-keratinized) area termed the free (marginal) gingiva, which is the prominent area close to the tooth. Between the free gingiva and the tooth lies a depression termed the gingival sulcus that is lined by non-keratinized epithelium. In the deepest area of the gingival sulcus lies the junctional epithelium that is attached to the peripheral cement of the tooth, with the periodontal ligament lying directly below this layer. In the horse with its prolonged dental eruption, this area is constantly remodeling and reforming new periodontal ligaments and new gingival–dental attachments. In other species gingiva interdental papillae are present between teeth to prevent food trapping and subsequent periodontal disease but, as noted, most equine teeth are tightly compressed at the occlusual surface and have no interproximal spaces.

## THE SALIVARY GLANDS

The (paired) main equine salivary glands are the parotid, mandibular and sublingual glands. Minor salivary glandular tissue is also present in the lips, tongue, palate and buccal regions. The largest salivary gland is the parotid (which when stimulated may produce up to 50 mls of saliva/min) that lies behind the caudal aspect of the horizontal ramus of the mandible, ventral to the base of the ear, rostral to the wing of the atlas, extending ventrally to the tendon of origin of the sternomandibularis muscle.[5,33] Its lateral aspect is usually level with the masseter but in some horses, especially when turned out to grass, it may swell and protrude 1–3 cm above this level. Its dorsal aspect contains lymphatic tissue within its substance or lying on its medial aspect, that can become focally distended with purulent infections of that region, for example strangles. The parotid duct originates from its rostroventral aspect and lies on the medial aspect of the mandible, until it crosses the ventral aspect of the mandible behind the facial artery and vein. It then moves dorsally, perforating the cheek at the level of the third cheek tooth.[33]

The smaller, long and narrow mandibular gland curves around beneath the parotid salivary gland and mandible, extending from the base of the atlas as far as the basihyoid bone. Its duct arises on its concave aspect and travels almost the full length of the oral cavity in the sublingual fold, beside the sublingual salivary gland rostrally, and enters into the oral cavity on the lateral aspect of the sublingual caruncle.[5] The long thin sublingual salivary gland lies beneath the sublingual fold of the oral mucosa, between the tongue and mandible, extending from the mandibular symphysis to the fourth cheek tooth and drains through multiple small ducts into the oral cavity.

## REFERENCES

1. Berkovitz BKB and Moxham B (1981) Development of dentition: early stages of tooth development. In: *Dental Anatomy and Embryology*, ed. JW Osborn, Blackwell Scientific Publications, Oxford, pp. 166–174.
2. Bennet D (1992) The evolution of the horse. In: *Horse Breeding and Management*, ed. JW Evans, Elsevier, Amsterdam, pp. 1–29.
3. Butler P (1991) Dentition in function. In: *Dental Anatomy and Embryology*, ed. JW Osborn, Blackwell Scientific Publications, Oxford, p. 345.
4. Baker GJ (1985) Oral examination and diagnosis: management of oral diseases. In: *Veterinary Dentistry*, ed. CE Harvey, WB Saunders, Philadelphia, pp. 217–228.
5. Dyce KM, Sack WO and Wensing CJG (1987) *Textbook of Veterinary Anatomy*. WB Saunders, Philadelphia, pp. 473–477.
6. Easley J (1996) Equine dental development and anatomy. In: *In-depth Dentistry Seminar*, Proceedings of the American Association of Equine Practitioners, 42, 1–10.
7. DeLahunta A and Habel RE (1986) *Applied Veterinary Anatomy*. WB Saunders, Philadelphia, pp. 4–16.
8. Miles AEW and Grigson C (1990) *Colyer's Variations and Diseases of the Teeth of Animals* (revised edn). Cambridge University Press, Cambridge, pp. 2–15, 482.
9. Kirkland KD, Baker GJ, Marretta SM, Eurell JAC and Losonsky JM (1996) Effect of ageing on the endodontic system, reserve crown, and roots of equine mandibular cheek teeth. *American Journal of Veterinary Research*, 57, 31–38.
10. Warshawsky H (1983) The teeth. In: *Histology* (5th edn), ed. L Weiss, Macmillan Press, New York, pp. 609–655.
11. Fortelius M (1985) Ungulate cheek teeth: developmental, functional and evolutionary interrelations. *Acta Zoologica Fennica*, 180, 1–76.
12. Ten Cate AR (1994) Development of the tooth and its supporting tissues; hard tissue formation and its destruction; dentinogenesis. In: *Oral Histology* (4th edn), ed. AR Ten Cate, CV Mosby, St Louis, pp. 58–80, 111–119, 147–168.
13. Kollar EJ and Lumsden AGS (1979) Tooth morphology: The role of innervation during induction and pattern formation. *The Journal of Biological Buccale*, 7, 49–60.
14. Brescia NJ (1966) Development and growth of the teeth. In: *Orban's Oral Histology and Embryology* (6th edn), ed. H Sicker, CV Mosby, London, pp. 18–37.
15. Latshaw WK (1987) Face, mouth and pharynx. In: *Veterinary Developmental Anatomy – A Clinically Oriented Approach*, ed. WK Latshaw, BC Decker Inc., Toronto, pp. 95–100.
16. Ferguson M (1990) The dentition throughout life. In: *The Dentition and Dental Care*, vol 3, ed. RJ Elderton, Oxford Heinemann Medical Books, Oxford, pp. 1–18.
17. Suga SJ (1979) Comparative histology of progressive mineralisation patterns of developing incisor enamel of rodents. *The Journal of Dental Research*, 58, 1025–1026.
18. Eisenmann DR (1994) Amelogenesis; enamel structure. In: *Oral Histology* (4th edn), ed. AR Ten Cate, CV Mosby, St Louis, pp. 218–256.
19. Baker GJ (1979) *A study of dental disease in the horse*. PhD Thesis, Glasgow University, pp. 3–96.
20. Kilic S, Dixon PM and Kempson SA (1997) A light and ultrastructural examination of calcified dental tissues of horses: II Ultrastructural enamel findings. *Equine Veterinary Journal*, 29, 198–205.
21. Shellis P (1981) Dental tissue. In: *Dental Anatomy and Embryology*, ed. JW Osborn, Blackwell Scientific Publications, Oxford, pp. 193–209.
22. Stanley HR, White CL and McCray L (1966) The rate of tertiary (reparitive) dentine formation in the human tooth. *Oral Surgery, Oral Medicine and Oral Pathology*, 21, 180–189.
23. Jones SJ (1990) The pulp–dentine complex. In: *The Dentition and Dental Care*, vol 3, ed. RJ Elderton, Oxford Heinemann Medical Books, Oxford, pp. 1–18.

MORPHOLOGY

24. Fawcett DW (1987) *A Textbook of Histology*. WB Saunders, Philadelphia, pp. 603–618.

25. Kilic S, Dixon PM and Kempson SA (1997) A light and ultrastructural examination of calcified dental tissues of horses: III Dentine. *Equine Veterinary Journal*, 29, 206–212.

26. Kilic S (1995) *A light and electron microscopic study of the calcified dental tissues in normal horses*. PhD Thesis, University of Edinburgh.

27. Dixon PM and Copeland AN (1993) The radiological appearance of mandibular cheek teeth in ponies of different ages. *Equine Veterinary Education*, 5, 317–323.

28. Kilic S, Dixon PM and Kempson SA (1997) A light and ultrastructural examination of calcified dental tissues of horses: IV. Cement and the amelocemental surface. *Equine Veterinary Journal*, 29, 213–219.

29. Jones SJ (1981) Human tissue: Cement. In: *Dental Anatomy and Embryology*, ed. JW Osborn, Blackwell Scientific Publications, Oxford, pp. 193–209.

30. Kilic S, Dixon PM and Kempson SA (1997) A light and ultrastructural examination of calcified dental tissues of horses: I The occlusal surface and enamel thickness. *Equine Veterinary Journal*, 29, 191–197.

31. Capper SR (1992) *The effects of feed types on ingestive behaviour in different horse types*. BSc Thesis, University of Edinburgh, pp. 1–160.

32. Myers JS (1994) *The effects of body size, grass height and time of day on the foraging behaviour of horses*. MSc Thesis, Aberystwyth University, p. 56.

33. Sisson S and Grossman JD (1953) Splanchnology. In: *The Anatomy of the Domestic Animals* (4th edn), WB Saunders, Philadelphia, pp. 406–407.

34. Walmsley JP (1993) Some observations on the value of ageing 5–7-year-old horses by examination of their incisor teeth. *Equine Veterinary Education*, 5, 195–298.

35. Richardson JD, Lane JG and Waldron KR (1994) Is dentition an accurate indication of the age of a horse? *Veterinary Record* 137, 88–90.

36. St Clair LE (1975) Teeth. In: *Sisson and Grossman's the Anatomy of the Domestic Animals*, vol 1 (5th edn), ed. R. Getty, WB Saunders, Philadelphia, pp. 460–470.

37. Floyd MR (1991) The modified Triadan system of nomenclature for veterinary dentistry. *Journal of Veterinary Dentistry*, 8, 18–20.

38. Goody PC (1983) *Horse Anatomy*. JA Allen and Company Ltd. London, pp. 38–41.

39. Eisenmenger E and Zetner K (1985) *Veterinary Dentistry*. Lea and Febiger, Philadelphia, pp. 55–57, 153–157.

40. Mueller POE (1991) Equine dental disorders: cause, diagnosis, and treatment. *The Compendium of Continuing Education*, 13, 1451–1460.

41. Colyer JF (1906) Variations and diseases of teeth of horses. *Transactions of the Odontological Society of Great Britain*, New Series, 38, 47–74.

42. Huidekoper RS (1891) *Age of Domestic Animals*. FA Davis, Philadelphia and London, pp. 33–35.

43. Bradley OC (1923) *The Topographical Anatomy of the Head and Neck of the Horse*. W Green and Son, Edinburgh, pp. 85–92.

44. Wafa NSY (1988) *A study of dental disease in the horse*. MVM Thesis, University College Dublin, pp. 1–203.

45. Osborn H (1966) Cement. In: *Orban's Oral Histology and Embryology* (6th edn), ed. H Sicker, CV Mosby, London, pp. 155–212.

46. Dixon PM (1997) Dental extraction in horses: indications and preoperative evaluation. *Compendium of Continuing Education for the Equine Practitioner*, 19, 366–375.

47. Hayward AF (1981) Human tissue: pulp. In: *Dental Anatomy and Embryology*, ed. JW Osborn, Blackwell Scientific Publications, Oxford, pp. 187–190.

48. Torneck CD (1994) Dentine–pulp complex. In: *Oral Histology* (4th edn), ed. AR Ten Cate, CV Mosby, St Louis, pp. 169–213.

49. Speed JG (1951) Horses and their teeth. *The Journal of the Royal Army Veterinary Corp*, 22, 136–141.

50. Barrairon P, Blin PC and Moliner F (1980) Contribution a l'etude du mecanisme de formation de fistule des premolaires chez le jeune cheval. *Bulletin de l'Academie Veterinaire de France*, 53, 47–54.

# DENTAL PHYSIOLOGY

Gordon J Baker, BVSc, PhD., MRCVS, Diplomate ACVS, University of Illinois, College of Veterinary Medicine, Urbana, IL 61802

## INTRODUCTION

Following the chapter 1 description of the structure of the teeth of the horse, this chapter describes how the dental system functions to prepare ingesta for digestion. It has been said that dental function in mammals is still poorly understood and that, from a functional point of view, the teeth of herbivores have had limited study.[1] There has, however, been a great expansion of scientific interest in all aspects of mastication (chewing) in mammals since the pioneer studies in which serious examinations of the occlusal relationship during chewing between the upper and lower teeth were made.[2] Subsequently, other studies have been concerned with the patterns of jaw movements. It has been noted that these patterns are a reflection of the complex relationship between muscle activity, forces exerted on food, and the relationship between food consistency, particle size and the nervous control of mastication.[3] In comparison to the highly complex appendicular skeleton and its movement, the skeletal components of mastication are simple and consist of just a few joints with muscles.

## FUNCTIONAL MORPHOLOGY

The Eocene ancestor of the family equidae (Hyracotherium or Eohippus) was a small (26–inch), three-toed animal with a series of low-crowned (brachydont) cheek teeth, made up of four premolars and three molars. All of the teeth had simple crown patterns and chewing mainly depended on the three molar teeth. Subsequent changes in the environment during the later Miocene period produced a rapid change in the Eocene teeth. These favorable mutations were a modification of the crown pattern, an increase in the height of the crown (i.e. reserve crown development) and the development of cement. What once had been two open valleys on the teeth had now become deep, closed pits and numerous wrinkles and spurs appeared on the side of the main crest. These changes were similar in both upper and lower jaws, but the changes were less extreme in the lower teeth.[4]

The process whereby the premolar teeth became anatomically similar to the molar teeth is described as molarization. The formation of high-crowned cheek teeth of the Merychippus in the late Miocene period was accompanied by the development of cementum. This substance appeared on the outside of the enamel crown and developed to fill all its valleys, and in so doing protected the brittle enamel from cracking. In this way, a permanently erupting cheek tooth was formed with a crown height (including reserve height) of at least twice its width. Such a tooth erupts at a rate equal to the rate of the wear of the crown by attrition.

It is known that as animals get bigger there is a cube factor relationship between size and food requirement between animals of different sizes. A doubling of height requires eight times the food intake. It is logical to suggest that as the equid species doubled in size, and almost trebled its height, that the dental changes are a result of favorable adaptions to accommodate the requirement for increased food intake. Under free-range conditions modern-day equids spend up to 14 hours a day feeding. The complete arcade of cheek teeth in Eohippus was no more than 10 cm in mesial–distal length – essentially the same as the mesial–distal length of two cheek teeth of *Equus caballus*.

From the viewpoint of dental function, diseases and treatment we can view the head of the horse as the body of the food processor, it houses the teeth – the blades of the food-processing machine. Molarization of the cheek teeth of the horse, and most herbivores, forms a continuous row of teeth that function as a single unit. The lips, cheeks, palate, muscles, temporo-mandibular joints and bones maintain the position of the teeth, and the tongue, the lips and salivary glands facilitate the process of food prehension and mastication. The muscles of mastication are all supplied by the 5th cranial nerve. They are primarily the paired lateral muscles from the maxilla and cranium to the mandible, these are the masseter and temporalis muscles that close the jaw and pull to the acting side. The medial pterygoideus muscles also close the jaw.

In comparison to the large bulk of jaw closure muscles, the bulk of the mandible depressor muscles is small. Jaw opening results from the contraction of the anterior belly of digastricus combined with the contraction of geniohydeus, and the inferior fibers of genioglossus coupled with the sternohyoideus and omohyoideus. In many mammals, particularly carnivores, jaw opening is aided by elevation of the head. This component is not, however, as important in most herbivores.

The disproportionate muscle mass between the jaw elevators and depressors is easily understood when the nature of jaw movements in feeding is studied. The jaws close against resistance whereas opening is a free movement synergized by gravity. Food breakdown is accomplished during jaw closure and requires forces that exceed the requirements of simply elevating the mass of the mandibular structures. Jaw muscles have faster contraction rates

than most other striated muscles, with a total cycle contraction rate that ranges from 333 to 500 cycles/min in the pygmy goat.[5]

The muscles of the cheeks and lips are supplied by the 7th cranial nerve and consist of the levator and depressor labii maxillaris and mandibularis, the orbicularis oris, the incisivus mandibularis and maxillaris, the buccinator and zygomaticus muscles. These muscles control the functions of lip closure, elevation, retraction and depression as well as the flattening of the cheeks.

The arrangement of the teeth within the upper and lower arcades is such that the curve of the upper dental arcade is not fully accommodated by the conformation of the lower arcade, i.e. the lower arcade is straighter and the distance between the left and right arcades is less in the mandible than in the upper jaw (anisognathism). At the same time the cheeks of the horse are, compared to other species, relatively tight fitting. The temporomandibular joint is large and has a thick meniscus.

Examination of the occlusal surfaces of the cheek teeth of horses reveals a complete system of folded enamel (lophs). The arrangement of lophs in the maxillary arcade is matched (mirrored) by their occlusal counterparts in the mandibular arcade (Fig. 2.1). It is interesting to note that in a study on food processing and digestibility in horses, measurements were made of total cheek teeth enamel ridge perimeter and it was found that there was only 7 cm more in the total enamel perimeter measurement in a 1000 kg horse when compared to a 350 kg pony.[6]

The design, angles of attack and composition of horse tooth structure is ideally suited, when aided by the process of mastication, to produce shear forces on food substances that fracture stalks, leaves and grains. How these forces are created and applied may be understood from analyses of jaw movements.

## MASTICATION – THE CHEWING CYCLE

Chewing is based upon the repetition of a cyclical movement that results from controlled rhythmic contraction of all the muscle groups

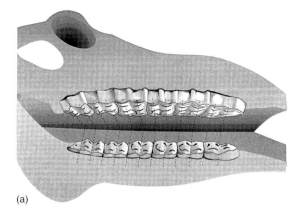

(a)

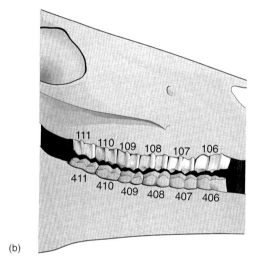

(b)

**Figure 2.1.** (a) Occlusal surfaces of maxillary and mandibular cheek teeth with architectural points documented. (b) Lateral view of occlusal waves.

Recent video analysis of horses feeding and observations of masticatory movements have yielded interesting data. The masticatory movements of horses fit the general masticatory cycle of herbivorous mammals. They have been described as having a masticatory cycle of three phases: the opening stroke (0), the closing stroke (C) and the power stroke (P).[6] It is the relative displacement of the mandible that defines the phases.[8] Figure 2.2 represents isolated frames from a video recording of equine mastication. Figure 2.3 shows the positional changes of the mandible. Note that frames 1–4 represent the opening stroke, frames 5–6 represent the closing stroke and frames 7–10 represent the power stroke. It may be observed that this analysis of

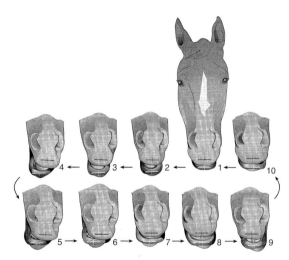

**Figure 2.2.** Reproduction from video recordings of chewing cycles of the horse (note in this reproduction, 'frame' relates to individually frozen time sections).

associated with the opening (depression) and closing (elevation) of the jaws. In studies of the chewing cycle in many species it was found that, with the exception of man, mammals have consistent chewing patterns – consistent both individually and specifically within species. There is, however, no 'standard pattern'. What happens to the food and how it is broken down depends on the form of the cheek teeth. The literature may be confusing because of the absence of a standard start point of the chewing cycle. In this description of the chewing cycle of the horse, the start point will be assigned to incisor contact. Other conventions use maximum incisor gap as the start point.

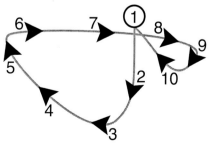

**Figure 2.3.** Frontal view of mandible during the chewing cycle – compare to Figure 2.2 and Figure 2.4.

31

the horse suggests in fact a fourth stroke – a post power 'recovery' stroke.

It has been observed for sometime that horses appear to be either right sided or left sided chewers. This observation is not strictly accurate even though some horses consistently demonstrate major lateral mandibular excursion to one side only. The masticatory movements of 400 horses in a veterinary medical teaching hospital with a variety of feeds including fresh grass, grass hay, alfalfa hay, oats and various sweet feeds and proprietary horse diets were documented. The observations were made on a wide range of horse ages, breeds and a considerable range of medical and surgical disorders. Incomplete observations were made in 63 horses (16 per cent), 45 horses (11 per cent) were seen to chew both to the left and to the right, 163 horses (41 per cent) moved the mandible to the right (i.e. clockwise as viewed from the front) and 131 (32 per cent) chewed counter clockwise (i.e. mandibular movement to the left).

It has been suggested that during the power stroke there is only contact with one side of the arcade at a time.[1,9] However, the measured extent of anisognathism negates this observation, i.e. there has to be some contact with both sides. It is however true that major pressure is first applied to one side and then, as the surfaces slide across each other, is transferred to the other side (frames 5–10, Fig. 2.4). It might be concluded from these observations that there is a tendency for unequal attrition as a result of the variation in masticatory physiology. However this cannot be confirmed by examination of the wear of occlusal surfaces at necropsy.

When eating, the horse uses its upper and lower lips as instruments to select, 'test' and

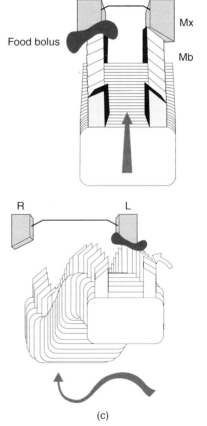

**Figure 2.4.** Representation of the power stroke component of the chewing cycle (from Tremaine,[9] 1997, with permission of the editor of *In Practice*).

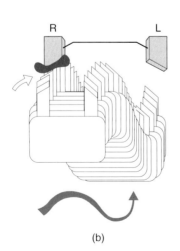

pull food into the mouth between the incisor teeth. Short sliding strokes of the incisors cut or grasp the food material. This process continues until the rostral portion of the mouth is filled with food material and cheek-tooth grinding of food is initiated. Just as the food-processor analogy of mastication is valid, the 'auger' analogy may be applied to the process of the movement of food across the mouth from each arcade and distally within the oral cavity. The tight-fitting cheeks contain the feed material within the intradental oral cavity (IDOC).

The loph basins of the cheek teeth (the food channels across the occlusal surfaces) direct food as it is crushed into the IDOC. Collinson's (1994) study of molar function in horses describes how cheek teeth occlusal shape facilitates this process.[6] In that the canal of the entoflecid and the tray of the metaconid of the mandibular teeth directs food into the parastyle of the maxillary teeth (the terms entoflecid and metaconid refer to the specific slopes of the occlusal surfaces) (Fig. 2.5). Subsequent masticatory cycles crush and move food into the IDOC. The auger analogy is continued by examination of the morphology of the palatine ridges. There are a

total of 18 pairs of palatine ridges. Each ridge is curved from lateral to midline and is incomplete and offset in the midline. Food material is squashed into the IDOC and pressed against the palatine ridges by the tongue. The rotatory action of mastication and tongue and cheek compression moves the food caudally in a spiral fashion (Fig. 2.5).

As boluses of food collect in the oropharynx, pharyngeal constriction, elevation of the soft palate, epiglottic retraction and laryngeal contraction result in movement of food through the lateral food channels and around the larynx into the esophagus and this constitutes swallowing.

The rotatory auger analysis concept has been confirmed by observations of food-bolus shape in toothless horses. Horses without teeth can survive on special feeds – crushed and soaked feeds for example. If however they try and feed on grass or hays they produce long, spiral boluses of a rope-like consistency that may lead to esophageal obstruction.

Factors that influence masticatory movements include fiber and moisture content of the diet. Chew rates have been calculated from electromyographic data (Table 1).[7] It was noted that horses were capable of attaining higher than 11 per second chew rates, particularly at the onset of feeding. The data in Table 1 were recorded over a 10 minute period. This study, however, did not confirm earlier observations that higher fiber content and lower moisture content reduces the extent of excursion of the mandible.[10]

The video analysis studies reported here did, in fact, confirm the observation that food type influences chewing pattern. The molar teeth initiate triturations ('grinding to powder') with a series of chopping actions, similar to the puncture/crushing portions of the power strokes in other species. Once the IDOC has filled with a critical mass, a 'mouthful', further lip and incisor function is limited and true arcade 'sliding' takes over, resulting in complete breakdown of food materials. It can be seen that there is greater lateral excursion with lush feeds – the drier the feed the less the lateral excursion.

Observations also suggest that there is rostral movement of one side at a time of the lower jaw during the masticatory cycle. This is achieved

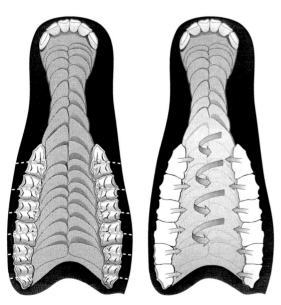

**Figure 2.5.** Representation of food 'channels' across the occlusal surface of maxillary cheek teeth and their relationship to palatine ridges.

**Table 1.** Mean (± SD) values for mastication parameters for the four horses used in the food-processing experiment (From Collinson, 1994,[6] with permission).

| Mastication parameter | Fiber diet | | |
| --- | --- | --- | --- |
| | Low | Medium | High |
| gm/'mouthful' | 12.1 ± 2.1 | 9.5 ± 2.4 | 8.1 ± 1.3 |
| chew rate/10 s | 11.6 ± 0.6 | 11.5 ± 0.2 | 11.4 ± 0.2 |
| energy/g/chew | $9.4 ± 4.8 \times 10^{-3}$ | $8.9 ± 6.4 \times 10^{-3}$ | $1.4 ± 1.4 \times 10^{-2}$ |
| duration of grind (s) | 0.51 ± 0.08 | 0.53 ± 0.03 | 0.55 ± 0.02 |
| incisor displacement (cm) | 4.4 ± 0.6 | 4.5 ± 0.6 | 4.4 ± 0.3 |
| premolar 4 velocity (cm.s$^{-1}$) | 10.4 ± 1.8 | 9.7 ± 2.4 | 8.5 ± 0.4 |

by the configuration of the temporomandibular joint and the contraction and relaxation of the masseter and medial pterygoid muscles. These movements result in oblique contacts with the upper and lower dental arcades.

## SUMMARY

Horses have an elegantly designed and functioning masticatory apparatus that prepares feed materials for digestion. The hypsodont tooth structure and continuous eruption of reserve crown matches tooth loss from attrition caused by occlusal contact. The chewing cycle is a repetitive pattern of mandibular movement with three components – an opening stroke, a closing stroke and the power stroke. During the power stroke the exposed enamel components of the dental arcades crush and fragment feed materials. Caudal movement of feed material within the IDOC is facilitated by the valley of the cheek teeth, by the contour and angles of the palatine ridges and by the lifting and pressing actions of the tongue (Fig. 2.4).

After trituration food is moved as an augered spiral and forms a caudal oropharyngeal bolus, that is swallowed.

## REFERENCES

1. Forteluis M (1982) Ecological aspects of dental functional morphology in the Pleistocene rhinoceroses of Europe. In: *Teeth, Form, Function and Evolution*, ed. B Kirsten, Columbia University Press, New York, pp. 163–181.
2. Butler PM (1952) The milk-molars of Perissodactyla with nematodes on molar occlusion. *Proceedings of the Zoological Society of London*, 121, 777–817.
3. Hiiemae KM (1978) Mammalian mastication: a review of the activity of the jaw muscles and the movements they produce in chewing. In: *Development, Function and Evolution of Teeth*, eds PM Butler and KA Joysey. Academic Press, London, pp. 359–398.
4. Simpson GG (1951) *Horses*. Oxford University Press, Oxford, pp. 106–108.
5. Gans C and DeVree F (1974) Correlation of accelerometers with electromyograph in the mastication of pygmy goats (*Capra hircus.*) *Anat Rec*, 306, (Abstract), pp. 1342–1343.
6. Collinson M (1994) *Food processing and digestibility in horses* (Equus caballus). BSc dissertation, Monash University, pp. 36–42.
7. Weijs WA and Dantuma R (1975) Electromyography and mechanics of mastication in the albino rat. *Journal of Morphology* 146, 1–34.
8. Fortelius M (1985) Ungulate cheek teeth: developmental, functional and evolutionary interrelations. *Acta Zoologia Fennica* (Helsinki), 180, 78.
9. Tremaine H (1997) Dental care in horses. *In Practice Journal of Veterinary Postgrad Clin Study*, 19, 186–199.
10. Leue G (1941) *Beziehungen zwischen Zahnanomalien und Verdauungsstörungen beim Pferde unter Heranziehung von Kaubildern*. Veterinary Medicine Dissertation, Hanover, pp. 170–174.

# 3

# AGING

Sofie Muylle, DVM, Department of Morphology, Faculty of Veterinary Medicine, University of Ghent, Salisburylaan 133, B-9820 Merelbeke, Belgium

## INTRODUCTION

The age of a horse can be an important consideration when forecasting its useful working life, when purchasing the animal, for insurance policies and for the prognosis of diseases. Furthermore, as long as no indelible identification methods for horses are imposed, age evaluation contributes to the identification of an animal.

Throughout the life of a horse specific changes occur to the appearance of its teeth. Dental examination therefore provides the most convenient means of age determination. Age-related dental changes of equine teeth were documented as long ago as 600 BC by the Chinese and by the ancient Greeks and Romans,[1] and many manuals and articles have been published ever since.[2–12]

The most appropriate teeth for aging horses are the (lower) incisors. The localization of premolars and molars interferes with a comfortable inspection. Canines are not well fitted for age determination; because contact between upper and lower canines is seldom made, canines do not wear down in a regular way and have no age related occlusal surface. When determining a horse's age by its incisors, the eruption dates and the changes in appearance of the occlusal surfaces are the main criteria. Neither is wholly dependable but the first is the more reliable, although limited in application to younger animals. The second may be used throughout the life span but becomes increasingly inaccurate with age.[13] Incisival characteristics that are frequently used for dental aging in horses are summarized below.

## ERUPTION

In this context gingival emergence is used as the reference point for eruption.

### ERUPTION OF THE DECIDUOUS INCISORS (Fig. 3.1)

The deciduous incisors are smaller than the permanent ones. The surface of their crown is white and presents several small longitudinal ridges and grooves. The occlusal tables of deciduous incisors are oval in mesiodistal direction.

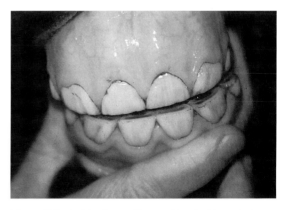

**Figure 3.1.** Arabian horse, 2 years. The deciduous incisors have small ridges and grooves on their labial surface.

## ERUPTION OF THE PERMANENT INCISORS
(Figs 3.2 and 3.3)

Permanent incisor teeth are larger and more rectangular in shape than the deciduous incisors. Their crown surface is largely covered with cement and has a yellowish appearance. The upper incisors generally present two distinct longitudinal grooves on their labial surface, the lower incisors have only one clearly visible groove.

## CHANGES OF THE OCCLUSAL SURFACE
(Fig. 3.4a)

### APPEARANCE OF THE DENTAL STAR

The dental star is a yellow-brown structure on the occlusal surface which becomes apparent

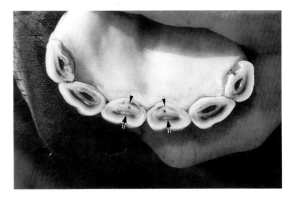

**Figure 3.4a.** Standardbred horse, 8 years. Dark-colored dental stars are present in all lower incisors. The characteristic white spot in the center of the dental star appears in the centrals (arrows). Cups have disappeared from the central incisors. The remaining marks are oval (arrowheads). Deep cups are still present on the middle and corner incisors.

with wear. In young animals it is linear and situated labial to the dental cup. With age it becomes oval and then round, moving toward the center of the table. The dental star consists of secondary dentin that occludes the pulpal chamber when the latter risks being exposed by wear. The dental star is distinguishable from primary dentin by its darker color. Because horses without access to pasture or grass-fodder usually have pale, yellowish dental stars in contrast to horses at pasture which have brown colored dental stars, the dark color is probably caused by an impregnation of plant pigments. When equine incisor teeth are sectioned longitudinally one can observe that the dark color of the dental star extends only a few millimeters beneath the occlusal surface and that the color-intensity is higher near the occlusal surface and fades toward the pulpal chamber. When incisors with pale dental stars are put in a mush of crushed grasses, dental stars obtain a darker color after a few days, and when they are put in a buffered (pH 6.8) solution of various diphenols (caffeic acid; 3,4-dihydroxybenzoic acid and 3,4-dihydroxyphenylalanine (10 mmol/L) dental stars obtain a deep brown color after 72 hours.

With age a characteristic white spot appears in the center of the dental star. The exact nature of this uncolored zone is still unknown but its

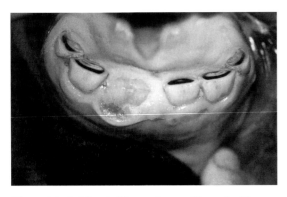

**Figure 3.2.** Belgian draft horse, 2 years 10 months. The right permanent central incisor is emerging through the gums. All other incisors are deciduous.

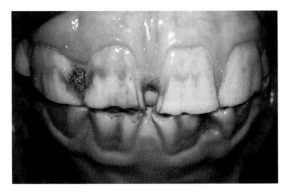

**Figure 3.3.** Belgian draft horse, 5 years 7 months. All incisors are permanent and have a yellowish appearance.

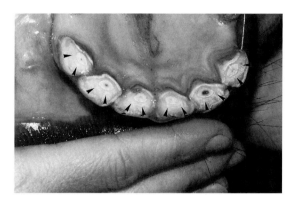

**Figure 3.4b.** Standardbred horse, 12 years, deprived of fresh grass. Dental stars are yellowish (arrowheads). It is difficult to distinguish the white spot in the center of the stars.

# CHANGES IN SHAPE OF THE INCISORS

## CHANGES IN SHAPE OF THE OCCLUSAL SURFACES (Fig. 3.5)

Due to extensive wear, the sequential shapes of the occlusal tables represent the cross-sections of the incisor teeth at various levels. The sequence of shapes ranges from oval in mesiodistal direction, to trapezoid and triangular, and finally to oval in labiolingual direction.

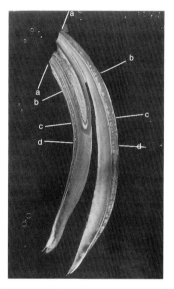

**Figure 3.5a.** Longitudinal section of the lower central incisor of a standardbred horse (4 years).

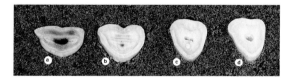

**Figure 3.5b.** Lower central incisor of a 5-year-old standardbred horse. Cross sections at various levels as indicated in Fig. 3.5a. In (c) and (d) the pulpal cavity is open.

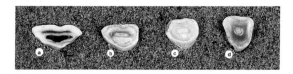

**Figure 3.5c.** Occlusal tables of the lower central incisor of standardbreds (a) aged 5 years, (b) 8 years, (c) 14 years and (d) 20 years. In the occlusal tables (c) and (d) the pulpal cavity is occluded by secondary dentin.

appearance is age related. In horses that do not get access to pasture or that are deprived of fresh grass, dental stars have a pale yellowish color. In these cases it is difficult to distinguish the white spot in the center of the star (Fig. 3.4b).

## DISAPPEARANCE OF THE CUPS

The infundibulum is an enamel infolding in the occlusal surface of the equine incisor. The superficial half of the infundibulum is empty or filled with food particles. This part is called the cup. The bottom of the infundibulum is filled with cement. When wear has brought this infundibular cement layer into the occlusal surface, the cup is filled in or has disappeared. The exposed cement core and the surrounding enamel ring are called the mark.

## DISAPPEARANCE OF THE MARKS

The shape of the mark generally corresponds with the contour of the occlusal table of the incisor. In young horses marks are oval in mesiodistal direction. When wear progresses, marks become smaller and rounder and move caudally (lingually) on the occlusal surface. With age the cement of the infundibular bottom wears away and eventually the remaining enamel spot disappears from the occlusal surface.

## DIRECTION OF UPPER AND LOWER INCISORS
(Fig. 3.6)

When incisors are viewed in profile, the angle between the upper and lower incisors changes with age. In young horses the upper and lower incisors are positioned in a straight line (angle ± 180°) with each other. With age, the angle between upper and lower incisors becomes increasingly acute. The lower incisors are the first to obtain an oblique position followed later by the upper incisor teeth.

## THE HOOK ON THE UPPER CORNER INCISOR
(Fig. 3.6a)

The caudal edge of the upper corner incisor sometimes exceeds the occlusal surface of the lower corner, especially when the lower incisors have acquired their oblique position. If the caudolateral portion of the upper corner incisor does not contact its lower counterpart any more, it wears more slowly, forming a notch in the occlusal surface. Later, when the upper incisors obtain their oblique position and the caudal edge of the upper corner incisor contacts its lower counterpart again, this notch can disappear.

## THE GALVAYNE'S GROOVE
(Fig. 3.6b)

The Galvayne's groove is a shallow longitudinal groove on the labial surface of the upper corner incisor. In the unworn tooth it starts halfway from the occlusal surface to the apex and continues three fourths of the distance to the apex. The groove is buried within the alveolus when the tooth first comes into wear.[14] With age, and due to the prolonged eruption of the tooth, the Galvayne's groove first appears at the gumline. In time it reaches the occlusal edge and then starts to disappear at the gumline and finally varnishes completely. The appearance of the groove and its usefulness in aging horses was mentioned for the first time in the early 1880's by an American horsetamer called Sample. Later, his theory was adopted by Sidney Galvayne, an Australian horseman.[15] It was in his first work *'Horse Dentition: Showing how to*

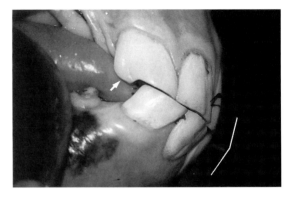

**Figure 3.6a.** Belgian draft horse, 6 years. The upper and lower incisors are positioned in a straight line with each other. Notice the presence of a hook on the upper corner (arrow).

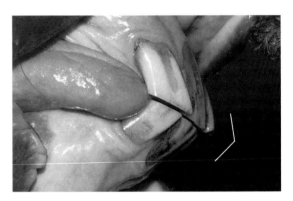

**Figure 3.6b.** Standardbred horse, 16 years. The angle between upper and lower incisors is more acute. The upper corner presents a Galvayne's groove over the entire length of its labial surface.

*tell exactly the age of a horse up to thirty years'* (published prior to March 1886) that Galvayne described the groove, which now bears his name, on the vestibular surface of the permanent upper corner incisor.[16] The presence and length of the Galvayne's groove as an accurate guide to the age of the older horse became known throughout the English-speaking world. However, it was not until World War I when several investigations were undertaken to 'validate' his theory.[15] Contrary to Galvayne's statements, these investigations showed that the groove may be absent in more than 50 per cent of the horses between the ages of 10 to 30 years.

# DENTAL AGING IN DIFFERENT HORSE BREEDS

Many standard textbooks dealing with aging of horses suggest that the characteristics discussed here give an accurate indication of a horse's true age. However, some reports are inconsistent in their guidelines and show large discrepancies in the dental features described at specific ages. A possible explanation for the non-uniformity of existing guidelines is the lack of evidence that any system was used to validate an author's recommendations for aging.[17-18] A recent study performed by Richardson *et al.* (1995) cast serious doubts on the belief that the age of a horse can be determined accurately from an examination of its teeth. In that study[19] a large group of horses with documented evidence of birth was examined and age was estimated both by experienced clinicians and by a computer model. There was little difference between the accuracy of the computer model and the clinical observers, but neither method was accurate when compared with the actual age. In older horses there was much greater variability between the dental age and the actual age. It is indeed a fact that the accuracy of dental aging of horses declines markedly with increasing age. Most standard texts do not provide exact data concerning breed, sex and nutrition of the examined horses. However, anatomical, physiological, environmental and behavioral differences between individuals ensure differences in rate of equine dental wear.[20] The concealment of these data may explain the discrepancies between different reports. Inaccuracies in the dental aging system of horses may also result from differences between breed and type of horse involved. Eisenmenger and Zetner (1985) stated that the teeth of thoroughbreds erupt earlier than those of Lipizzaners and coldblood horses. Teeth of ponies may also have rates of eruption and wear that differ from the teeth of horses.[21] As for donkeys, both ancient literature data[22] and recent investigations[23] have suggested that their degree of dental attrition in donkeys is slower than in horses.

Based on the suggestion that the degree of attritional dental wear is correlated with the breed of horse,[17] four unrelated horse breeds have recently been subjected to a comparative study.[24-26] However, the nature of diet can also play a part in the abrasion of horse incisors. Dental wear is caused not only by grinding of opposing crowns against one another, but also by contact of abrasive particles in food such as silicate phytoliths which form part of the skeleton of grasses. Other plant-borne abrasives include cellulose and lignin.[16] In order to preclude the influence of the quality of nutrition on the rate of dental wear, it is necessary that the horses being examined for breed variability are raised and kept under similar environmental and nutritional conditions. All horses examined in the study discussed here were raised in western Europe, were given access to daily pasture and were fed concentrates and hay. None of the horses were crib biters nor suffered from other vices which could influence dental wear. The incisor teeth had not been rasped in any individual. It is evident that in practice one has to be vigilant for these considerations. Factors that are difficult to control and that could not be taken into consideration were the horses' individual chewing habits and the amount of food ingested.

A critical evaluation of the dental aging technique revealed that the rate of attritional dental wear is different in different horse breeds. Indentation hardness-tests, performed with a Knoop diamond indenter, showed slight breed-differences in the hardness of equine enamel and dentin. These different micro-hardness values seem to contribute to the differences in the rate of attritional dental wear.[27] The following text describes the appearance of lower incisor teeth at various ages as generally seen in the standardbred horse, the Belgian draft horse, the Arabian horse and the mini-Shetland pony population of western Europe. It must be emphasized that this text is not a truism. When determining a horse's age one must register all dental features together and take account of clinical factors that may have influenced the aspect of the horse's teeth. The following descriptions will therefore be accurate in many cases, but may be incorrect for any individual.

## ERUPTION OF THE DECIDUOUS INCISORS

The central incisors generally erupt during the first week of life. The middle incisors emerge through the gums at 4 to 6 weeks and the corners erupt between the sixth and the ninth month of life. In the mini-Shetland pony eruption of the middle and the corner incisors is retarded. The middle incisor starts erupting at the age of 4 months whereas the corner incisor breaks through the gums between 12 and 18 months of age.

## ERUPTION OF THE PERMANENT INCISORS

The upper and lower permanent incisors erupt almost simultaneously. In some horses shedding begins with the maxillary, in others with the mandibular incisor teeth. Arabian horses shed their central, middle and corner incisors at 2.5, 3.5 and 4.5 years of age, respectively. In standardbreds and in Belgian draft horses shedding generally occurs later, namely at nearly 3, nearly 4 and nearly 5 years of age (Fig. 3.7). In mini-Shetland ponies eruption of the permanent incisors is still further delayed by 2 to 3 months. In male animals the canines erupt at about 4.5 to 5 years of age. Generally, these teeth are absent or rudimentary in mares.

## APPEARANCE OF THE DENTAL STAR

Dental stars appear sequentially in the central, the middle and the corner incisors. In standardbreds and in Arabian horses they appear on the centrals at 5 years, on the middles at 6 years and on the corners at 7 to 8 years. In Belgian draft horses and mini-Shetland ponies stars appear somewhat earlier, i.e. on the centrals at 4.5 years, on the middles at 5.5 years and on the corners at 6.5 to 7 years (Fig. 3.7). With age the characteristic white spot becomes visible inthe center of the dental star (Figs 3.8–3.10). In standardbreds and in Arabian horses this white spot appears on the central incisors from the age of 7 to 8 years onwards, and on the middle incisors from the age of 9 to 11 years onwards. In Belgian draft horses and in mini-Shetland ponies the white spot

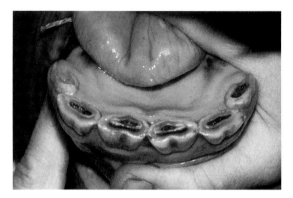

**Figure 3.7a.** Standardbred horse, 5 years. The permanent central and middle incisors are in place, the corner incisor is emerging through the gums. The dental star is present on the centrals, absent on the middles and the corners. All lower incisors have deep cups.

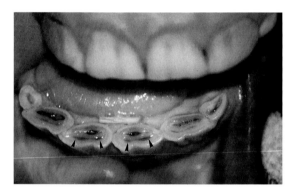

**Figure 3.7b.** Belgian draft horse, 4 years 8 months. The permanent central and middle incisors are in place. The corner incisors are still deciduous. Dental stars are present on the centrals (arrowheads) and appear also on the middles. Cups are present in the central and middle incisors.

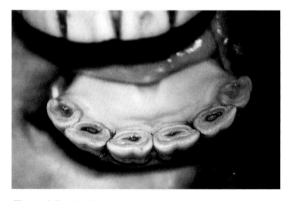

**Figure 3.7c.** Arabian horse, 5 years. All lower incisors are permanent, the corners are not yet fully in wear. There are no obvious dental stars. Deep cups are present on all lower incisors.

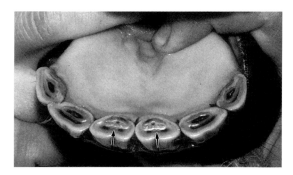

**Figure 3.8a.** Standardbred horse, 8 years. Dental stars are present on all incisors. In the central incisor the white spot in the dental star becomes apparent (arrows). Cups are filled-in on the centrals. On the middles and the corners cups are still present. The occlusal tables of the central incisors are becoming trapezoid, those of the middles and the corners are still oval.

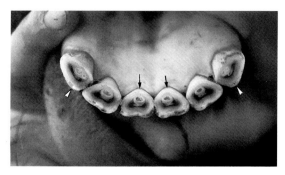

**Figure 3.9a.** Standardbred horse, 12 years. Dental stars, consisting of a white spot and a dark periphery, are present on all lower incisors. Cups have disappeared and the marks are small oval to rounded. The occlusal tables of the central and the middle incisors are trapezoid. On the central incisor the lingual apex is visible (arrows). The corner incisors have an apex on the labial side (arrowheads).

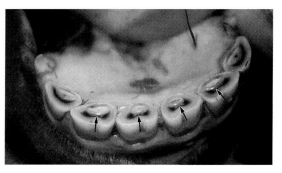

**Figure 3.8b.** Belgian draft horse, 8 years 6 months. Dental stars are present on all incisors. In the central and the middle incisors the white spot in the dental star becomes apparent (arrows). Cups are filled-in on all lower incisors. The remaining marks are oval. The occlusal tables of the centrals and the middles are becoming trapezoid.

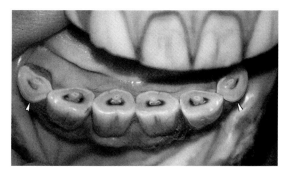

**Figure 3.9b.** Belgian draft horse, 12 years. Dental stars, consisting of a white spot and a dark periphery, are present on all lower incisors. Marks are rounded and on the central incisors they have almost disappeared. The occlusal tables of the centrals and middles are trapezoid. On the corner incisors the labial apex is obvious (arrowheads).

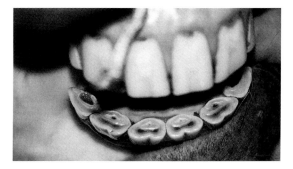

**Figure 3.8c.** Arabian horse, 8 years 6 months. Dental stars are present on the central and middle incisors. The white spot in the dental star is appearing in the central incisor. Cups on the centrals and the middles have nearly disappeared, the remaining marks are oval (middles) to triangular-shaped (centrals). Deep cups are still present on the corner incisors. The occlusal tables of the centrals have become trapezoid.

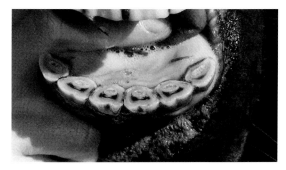

**Figure 3.9c.** Arabian horse, 12 years. Dental stars are present on all lower incisors. On the central and middle incisors the white spot in the dental star is visible. Cups have disappeared. The remaining marks are oval and still clearly visible. The occlusal tables of the centrals and the middles are trapezoid. The corner incisor presents a labial apex.

41

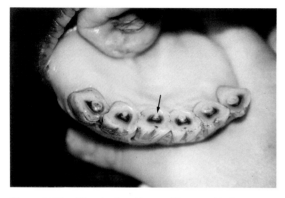

**Figure 3.10a.** Standardbred horse, 18 years. Marks are small and rounded. On the central incisors they have almost disappeared (arrow). The occlusal tables of the centrals and the middles are trapezoid, those of the corner incisors are triangular with an apex to the labial side.

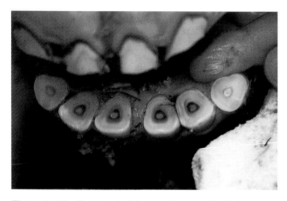

**Figure 3.10b.** Belgian draft horse, 18 years. Marks have disappeared from all lower incisors. The occlusal surfaces are triangular. Those of the central and middle incisors have a lingual apex, those of the corners have a labial apex.

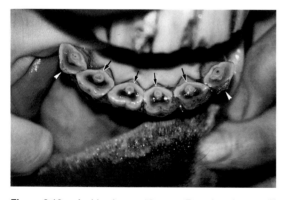

**Figure 3.10c.** Arabian horse, 18 years. Round marks are still clearly visible on all lower incisors. The occlusal surfaces of the centrals and the middles are trapezoid with a lingual apex (arrows), those of the corner incisors are oval with a labial apex (arrowheads).

becomes visible on the centrals at the age of 6 to 7 years and on the middles at the age of 8. In all breeds, the appearance of the white spot in the dental star of the corner incisors is variable and occurs between 9 and 15 years.

## DISAPPEARANCE OF THE CUPS

The disappearance of the cups is an unreliable feature for age determination because it does not occur between narrow age limits. In all breeds cups on the central incisors disappear at the age of 6 to 8 years, whereas cups on the middle incisors disappear variably between 7 and 11 years and those on the corner incisors between 9 and 15 years.

The variations in the age at which the cups disappear may be due to a difference in the depth of the cup. The accumulation of cement in the infundibulum is variable, i.e. superabundant in some individuals and almost non-existent in others.

## CHANGES IN SHAPE OF THE MARKS

On the central incisors big oval marks are visible until the age of 6 to 7. These marks become oval to triangular from the age of 7 to 8 years onwards in Belgian draft horses, from the age of 8 to 10 years onwards in standardbreds and Arabian horses, and from the age of 10 years onwards in mini-Shetlands. Round marks on the central incisors are visible at 9 to 10 years in Belgian draft horses, at 13 to 14 years in standardbreds and mini-Shetlands and at 15 to 17 years in Arabian horses.

## DISAPPEARANCE OF THE MARKS

From all age-related dental characteristics, the disappearance of the marks is the one with the highest variability between breeds. In draft horses marks on the central incisors disappear from the age of 12 to 15 years and those on the middle and corner incisors from 14 to 15 years onwards. In mini-Shetland ponies marks on the central, middle and corner incisors disappear at the age of 15, 16 and 17 years respectively. In standardbred horses marks disappear some years later, on the centrals they disappear in 18-year-old horses and on the middle and corner incisors in 19- to 20-year-olds. In Arabian horses marks on the lower incisors may persist for a very long time. They start disappearing at the age of 20 but with considerable individual variations (Fig. 3.10).

## CHANGES IN SHAPE OF THE OCCLUSAL SURFACES

Changes in shape of the occlusal surfaces of the lower incisors are useful but inaccurate indicators of age. The changes are difficult to judge objectively because successive shapes shade off into one another and are hardly distinguishable. The sequential shapes of the tables of the central and middle incisors are oval, trapezoid, triangular with the apex pointing to the lingual side and biangular. A survey of the most important changes is given in Tables 3.1–3.4. It is striking that the shape of the lower corner incisors does not conform to the sequential changes described above. The lower corner incisors remain oval for a long time and gradually develop an apex at the labial side. In Belgian draft horses and mini-Shetland ponies the labial apex appears at the

age of 9 years, and in standardbreds at 11 years. In Arabian horses the apex is a constant characteristic in individuals aged over 12 years (Figs 3.9 and 3.10).

## DIRECTION OF UPPER AND LOWER INCISORS

The arch formed by the incisors of the opposing jaws as they meet when viewed in profile, changes as the teeth advance from their alveoli and undergo attrition (Fig. 3.6). In young horses the upper and lower incisors are positioned in a straight line ($\pm 180°$). From the age of approximately 10 years onwards, the angle between upper and lower incisors becomes more acute. Because exact measurements of the age-related incisival angle are not available, the evaluation of the angle provides only a rough estimate of an animal's age.

The same applies for the curvature of the dental arch formed by the lower incisive tables. In young horses this arch is a semi-circle whereas in older individuals it forms a straight line. In view of the gradual character of this change it is impossible to determine the exact age at which it occurs.

**Table 3.1.** Aging Belgian draft horses

|  | I1 (central incisors) | I2 (middle incisors) | I3 (corner incisors) |
|---|---|---|---|
| **Shedding** | ± 3y | ± 4y | ± 5y |
| **Appearance of the dental star** | 4.5y | 5.5y | 6.5y–7y |
| **Appearance of the white spot in the dental star** | 6y–7y | 7y–8y | 11y–13y |
| **Disappearance of the cup** | 5y–8y | 7y–11y | 9y–15y |
| **Shape of the mark** | | | |
| oval | until 6y | | |
| oval–triangular | ≥ 7y–8y | | |
| round | ≥ 9y–10y | | |
| **Disappearance of the mark** | 12y–15y | 14y–15y | 14y –15y |
| **Shape of the occlusal table** | | | |
| oval | until 6y | until 7y | until 10y |
| trapezoid | ≥ 7y | ≥ 8y–9y | – |
| trapezoid with lingual apex | ≥ 7y | ≥ 9y | – |
| labial apex on 303 or 403 | – | – | ≥ 9y–10y |
| **Hook on 103 or 203** | | | variable |
| **Galvayne's groove** | | | variable |

MORPHOLOGY

**Table 3.2.** Aging Standardbred horses

| | I1 (central incisors) | I2 (middle incisors) | I3 (corner incisors) |
|---|---|---|---|
| Shedding | ± 3y | ± 4y | ± 5y |
| Appearance of the dental star | 5y | 6y | 7y–8y |
| Appearance of the white spot in the dental star | 7y–8y | 9y–11y | 11y–13y |
| Disappearance of the cup | 6y–7y | 7y–11y | 9y–15y |
| Shape of the mark | | | |
|   oval | until 6y | | |
|   oval–triangular | 8y–10y | | |
|   round | ≥ 13y | ≥ 14y | |
| Disappearance of the mark | 18y | 19y–20y | 19y–20y |
| Shape of the occlusal table | | | |
|   oval | until 6y | until 7y | until 12y |
|   trapezoid | ≥ 7y | ≥ 8y–9y | – |
|   trapezoid with lingual apex | ≥ 9y | ≥ 10y | – |
|   labial apex on 303 or 403 | – | – | ≥ 10y–11y |
| Hook on 102 or 203 | | | variable |
| Galvayne's groove | | | variable |

**Table 3.3.** Aging Arabian horses

| | I1 (central incisors) | I2 (middle incisors) | I3 (corner incisors) |
|---|---|---|---|
| Shedding | ± 2.5y | ± 3.5y | ± 4.5y |
| Appearance of the dental star | 5y | 6y | 7y–8y |
| Appearance of the white spot in the dental star | 7y–8y | 9y–11y | 13y–15y |
| Disappearance of the cup | 7y | 7y–11y | 9y–15y |
| Shape of the mark | | | |
|   oval | until 7y | | |
|   oval–triangular | ≥ 8y–10y | | |
|   round | ≥ 15y–17y | | |
| Disappearance of the mark | ≥ 20y | ≥ 20y | ≥ 20y |
| Shape of the occlusal table | | | |
|   oval | until 6y | until 7y | until 12y |
|   trapezoid | ≥ 8y–9y | ≥ 9y–11y | – |
|   trapezoid with lingual apex | ≥ 10y –11y | ≥ 14y | – |
|   labial apex on 303 or 403 | – | – | ≥ 12y |
| Hook on 103 or 203 | | | variable |
| Galvayne's groove | | | variable |

## THE HOOK ON THE UPPER CORNER INCISOR

The hook on the caudal edge of the upper corner incisor has long been considered as the typical characteristic for a 7- or 13-year-old horse. However, hooks on the upper corner, 103 and 203, are seen in a minority of horses and at practically any age over 5 years. Only 13 per cent of all 7-year-olds and 8 per cent of all 13-year-olds that were examined for this study presented a hook on one upper corner. On the other hand,

**Table 3.4.** Aging mini-Shetland ponies

| | I1 (central incisors) | I2 (middle incisors) | I3 (corner incisors) |
|---|---|---|---|
| **Shedding** | ≥ 3y | ± 4y | ± 5y |
| **Appearance of the dental star** | 4.5y | 5.5y | 6.5y–7y |
| **Appearance of the white spot in the dental star** | 6y–7y | 8y | 10y–12y |
| **Disappearance of the cup** | 7y–8y | 8y–12y | 9y–13y |
| **Shape of the mark** oval oval–triangular round | until 8y ≥ 10y ≥ 13y | | |
| **Disappearance of the mark** | 15y | 16y | 17y |
| **Shape of the occlusal table** oval trapezoid trapezoid with lingual apex labial apex on 303 or 403 | until 6y ≥ 7y ≥ 11y–12y – | until 7y ≥ 8y–9y ≥ 14y – | until 10y – – ≥ 9y–10y |
| **Hook on 103 or 203** | | | variable |
| **Galvayne's groove** | | | variable |

hooks were seen in 14 per cent of the 5- and 6-year-old horses, in 22 per cent of the horses aged between 8 and 12, and in 13 per cent of all horses aged over 13 years. As the presence of hooks on 103 and 203 cannot be related to any specific age category it is considered irrelevant for the estimation of age in horses.

## THE GALVAYNE'S GROOVE

The Galvayne's groove is a feature that is most often observed in horses aged over 11 years. However, as its presence, length and bilateral symmetry are variable and inconsistent, the groove is considered to be of little value for age determination in horses.

## CONCLUSION

Age determination in horses based upon the inspection of the incisor teeth can only provide an approximate guess rather than an exact evaluation. In older horses most of the so-called characteristic features can only be judged subjectively. It is therefore obvious that the accuracy of the dental-age determination declines markedly with age.

An important factor interfering with a faultless dental-age determination in horses is the breed dependence of the attritional dental wear. A comparison of the dental criteria in different breeds reveals that, in general, the incisor teeth of draft horses and mini-Shetland ponies are more liable to attrition than standardbreds' incisors, whereas the incisors of Arabian horses wear more slowly than those of standardbred horses.

### REFERENCES

1. Kertesz P (1993) In search of Mr Bishop. *Veterinary Record*, 133, 608.
2. Zipperlen W (1871) Over de ouderdomskennis van het paard of de tandleer. In: *Geïllustreerd veeartsenijkundig handboek*, B Dekema, Utrecht, p. 171.
3. Dupont M (1901) *L'âge du cheval*, Librairie J.B. Baillière, Paris, pp. 1–187.
4. Frateur JL (1922) *De ouderdomsbepaling van het paard door het gebit*. E Marette, Brussel, pp. 1–47.
5. American Association of Equine Practitioners (1966) *Official guide for determining the age of the horse* (1st edn). Fort Dodge Laboratories, Fort Dodge, IA pp. 1–36.
6. Barone R (1997) 'Dents'. In: *Anatomie comparée des mammifères domestiques* (3rd edn). Vigot, Paris, p 91.
7. Dyce KM and Wensing CJ (1980) *Anatomie van het paard*. Scheltema-Holkema, Utrecht, p. 14.

8. Willems A (1980) *Ouderdomsbepaling van het paard* (5th edn). D Van de Sompele, Oud-Heverlee, p. 14.

9. Habermehl KH (1981) Wie sicher ist die Altersbestimmung beim Pferd? *Berliner und Münchener Tierärztliche Wochenschrift*, 94, 167.

10. McMullan WC (1983) Dental criteria for estimating age in the horse. *Equine Practice*, 5, 10, 36.

11. Walmsley JP (1993) Some observations on the value of ageing 5–7-year-old horses by examination of their incisor teeth. *Equine Veterinary Education*, 5, 295.

12. Sack WO (1994) *Rooney's Guide to the Dissection of the Horse* (6th edn). Veterinary Textbooks, Ithaca, p. 182.

13. Dyce KM, Sack WO and Wensing CJ (1996) *Textbook of Veterinary Anatomy* (2nd edn). WB Saunders, Philadelphia, p. 491.

14. St Clair LE (1975) *Sisson and Grossman's The Anatomy of the Domestic Animals* (5th edn). WB Saunders, Philadelphia, p. 460.

15. McCarthy PH (1987) Galvayne: the mystery surrounding the man and the eponym. *Anat. Histol. Embryol*, 16, 330.

16. Galvayne S (1886) *Horse Dentition: Showing how to tell exactly the age of a horse up to thirty years.* Thomas Murray and Son, Glasgow.

17. Richardson JD, Cripps PJ, Hillyer MH, O'Brien JK, Pinsent PJN and Lane JG (1995) An evaluation of the accuracy of ageing horses by their dentition: a matter of experience? *Veterinary Record*, 137, 88.

18. Richardson JD, Lane JG and Waldron KR (1994) Is dentition an accurate indication of the age of the horse? *Veterinary Record*, 135, 31.

19. Richardson JD, Cripps PJ and Lane JG (1995) An evaluation of the accuracy of ageing horses by their dentition: can a computer model be accurate? *Veterinary Record*, 137, 139.

20. Hillson S (1986) *Teeth*. Cambridge University Press, Cambridge, p. 183.

21. Eisenmenger E and Zetner K (1985) *Veterinary Dentistry*. Lea and Febiger, Philadelphia, p. 25.

22. Marcq J and LaHaye J (1943) *Extérieur du cheval*, ed. J Duculot, Gembloux, p. 11.

23. Misk NA (1997) Radiographic studies on the development of incisors and canine teeth in Donkeys. *Equine Practice*, 19, 230.

24. Muylle S, Simoens P and Lauwers H (1996) Ageing horses by an examination of their incisor teeth: an (im)possible task? *Veterinary Record*, 138, 295.

25. Muylle S, Simoens P, Lauwers H and Van Loon G (1997) Ageing draft and trotter horses by their dentition. *Veterinary Record*, 141, 17.

26. Muylle S, Simoens P, Lauwers H and Van Loon G (1998) Ageing Arab horses by their dentition. *Veterinary Record*, 142, 659.

27. Muylle S, Simoens P, Vorbreak R, Ysebaert M and Lauwers H (1998) Dental wear related to the micro-hardness of enamel and dentine. *Veterinary Record*, (in press).

# DENTAL DISEASE AND PATHOLOGY

# 4

# ABNORMALITIES OF DEVELOPMENT AND ERUPTION

Gordon J Baker, BVSc, PhD., MRCVS, Diplomate ACVS, University of Illinois, College of Veterinary Medicine, Urbana, IL61802

## INTRODUCTION

The essentials of the development and embryonic origins of the teeth have been reviewed in Chapter 1. The impact of both genetic and environmental factors may result in the abnormal development of teeth as well as contribute to maleruptions.

The essential forces which result in the penetration of the gum by teeth have been the subject of much theory and experimentation. Physiologic tooth movement may be described in general terms under three headings: (a) pre-eruptive tooth movement made by both deciduous and permanent tooth germs within the tissue of the jaw before they begin to erupt, (b) eruptive tooth movement made by a tooth to move from its position within the bone of the jaw to its functional position in occlusion and (c) post-eruptive tooth movement which maintains the position of the erupted tooth in occlusion while the bones of the jaw and head continue to grow, and also movements that compensate for occlusal wear.[1]

We can recognize the results of pathological changes associated with all three of these physiological categories in foals, in adult horses and in ponies.

## PHYSIOLOGY OF DENTAL ERUPTION AND MATURATION

Radiographic evidence of enamel formation (secretion by ameloblasts in the tooth bud) within the deciduous check teeth can be seen as early as 112 days of fetal life. The ultimate shape of any tooth is orchestrated by the foldings that occur within the ameloblast layer and the subsequent deposition of enamel and contacting dentinal tubules produced by the odontoblasts (Fig. 4.1). During this process there is a large increase in the size of the developing tooth and induced changes within the surrounding tissues to accommodate this increase and the changes in shape. By this process, what will eventually be recognized as the alveolar (tooth) socket, assumes its unique profile, a profile that matches the complexity of the folds of the enamel and eventually the reserve crown and tooth roots.[2] Nutrition of all the tissues of the developing tooth is afforded by vessels in the apical 'pulp' and in the maxillary teeth and the incisors from vessels that descend from the coronal surface

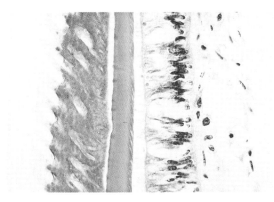

**Figure 4.1.** Predentin separating odontoblast and ameloblast layers (hematoxylin-eosin, magnification × 950).

49

DENTAL DISEASE AND PATHOLOGY

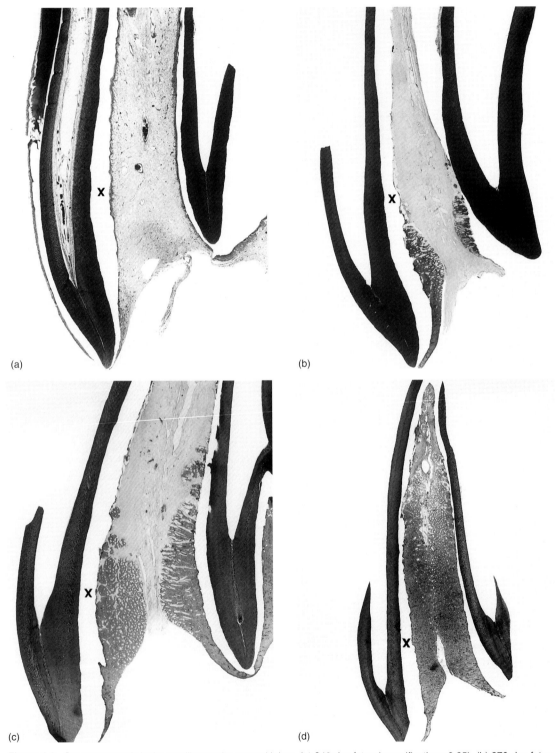

(a)

(b)

(c)

(d)

**Figure 4.2.** Cementogenesis in the maxillary molar enamel lakes, (a) 240-day fetus (magnification ×8.25), (b) 270-day fetus (magnification ×8.25), (c) 300-day fetus (magnification ×8.25), (d) 49-day neonate (magnification ×4.25). X = enamel lost by decalcification.

into the enamel invaginations that are designated enamel (cement) lakes and infundibulae (cups) respectively (Fig. 4.2).

There are profound differences between the physiological movements of simple (brachydont) and complex (hypsodont) teeth. In both, however, it should be noted that root formation and maturation continues long after there is penetration of the gum by the erupting tooth. Four possible mechanisms have been described to explain the process of tooth eruption. These mechanisms are (a) root growth, (b) hydrostatic pressure, (c) selected deposition and resorption of bone and (d) the pulling of the periodontal ligament.[1] These four mechanisms require further evaluation for hypsodont (continuously erupting) teeth. Experiments on the continuously erupting incisors of rodents suggest that the forces for eruptive tooth movement reside in the periodontal ligament.[3] The complete absence of true root formation at the time of eruption of a horse's teeth would confirm that root growth, i.e. a 'pushing' of the tooth toward the gum, is the least significant of these four mechanisms in this species. All horse owners and veterinarians are familiar with the mandibular and maxillary changes that occur in young horses and which reflect both the vascular and bone remodeling changes that accompany tooth eruption. They have been referred to as teething bumps or pseudocysts (Figs 4.3 and 4.4).[4] In most cases, such swellings are benign and resolve as the musculoskeletal components of the head enlarge and mature. In some instances however, there may be internal nasal swellings that cause respiratory obstruction or there may be true dental impactions and subsequent periapical pathology (see pp. 79–81).

## DEVELOPMENTAL ABNORMALITIES

### HYPOPLASIA OF CEMENTUM

Cemental hypoplasia is seen in all incisors and maxillary cheek teeth. There is no evidence that it is pathological in incisors, but it may predispose some cheek teeth to endodontic disease (see Chapter 7). It is unusual to see defects of peripheral coronal or reserve crown and root

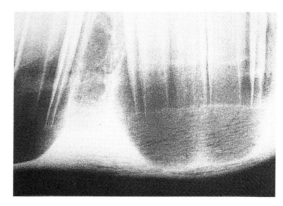

**Figure 4.3.** Radiograph of erupting 308 illustrating hydrostatic and vascular changes associated with tooth eruption in the horse (eruption cyst).

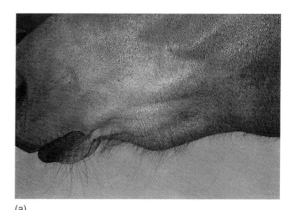

(a)

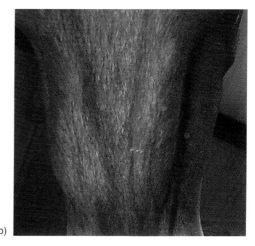

(b)

**Figure 4.4.** (a) and (b) Mandibular swellings associated with eruptions of permanent cheek teeth (from Tremaine, 1997, with permission of the editor of *In Practice*).

cement although inflammatory disease associated with periodontal disease may result in lysis of cementum, hyperplasia of cement and the formation of nodules of cement.[5]

The process of cementogenesis within the enamel invaginations of the maxillary cheek teeth can be recognized histologically at least 160 days prior to eruption. These cementoblasts originate from the mesenchymal cells of the dental papilla and they break through the epithelial sheath and come to rest beneath the ameloblast layer. In this way, a collar of cementoblasts forms within the enamel invagination (Fig. 4.2). At first the cement that is formed is sponge- or coral-like in appearance but it continues to mature becoming more dense as long as the tissues receive a vascular supply. Once the tooth erupts however, this vascular supply is broken and cement formation in this locus stops.

It has been seen that although all maxillary teeth show some degree of cemental hypoplasia, the 'severity' of the condition cannot be ascertained by studying the occlusal surfaces of the maxillary cheek teeth.[5] Vertical sections of cheek teeth through the enamel lakes demonstrate the true extent of hypoplasia of cementum.[6]

Prior to the detailing of maxillary cementogenesis[6] the condition of cemental hypoplasia had been misnamed as caries[7,8,9] and infundibular necrosis.[4] The significance of hypoplastic cement within the enamel lakes of the maxillary cheek teeth has been reviewed by a number of authors. In summary it can be said that in most cases the condition is benign. In many cases it can be seen that during mastication, food material can become pressed into the depths of the hypoplastic tissue via the previous vascular pathways (Fig. 4.5). Subsequent microbial fermentation and dissolution of existing cement – caries of cement is possible. Such a relationship was recognized in some of the earlier German studies of equine dental disease.[10]

Teeth with extensive occlusal exposure of lake cement hypoplasia, may exhibit abnormal wear and subsequent 'cupping out' that is a concavity of the occlusal surface. Such changes can, if uncorrected, initiate 'wave-mouth' formation. In turn, changes in shape of the occlusal surface may result in stress concentra-

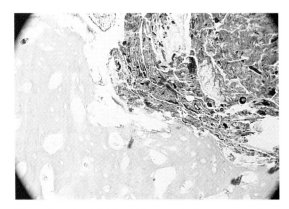

**Figure 4.5**. Food debris within hypoplastic cementum of maxillary tooth enamel lake (decalcified hematoxylin-eosin, magnification ×350).

tion during mastication and the creation of shear forces that lead to fracture of the affected tooth.

As has been stated, for the most part, hypoplasia of cement is benign and the pulp is protected as the occlusal surface is worn away and deeper areas of hypoplasia are exposed. Ultimately the enamel invaginations and the contained cement are worn away (Fig. 4.6).

## OLIGODONTIA

The absence of a tooth or teeth (oligodontia) is seen frequently in many abattoir specimens. Tooth absence is usually either the result or the

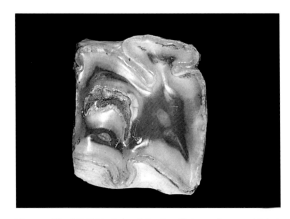

**Figure 4.6.** Attrition of cheek tooth with loss of enamel lakes – note distal lake replaced by dentin at the bottom of the infundibulum.

sequel of periodontal or dental disease. In some cases, however, a developmental abnormality may have occurred that resulted in the failure of the formation of a tooth bud, hence no tooth forms. When a single tooth is missing there will be movement of adjacent teeth so that the result will be a shortening of the mesial–distal length of the arcade rather than a gap in the dentition. Such a shortening will cause abnormal occlusion and changes in wear across the teeth. Some cases may require extraction of the 'extra' tooth or teeth in the normal arcade or, in the case of incisor teeth, attention will need to be given to the bite alignment of the incisor arcades (Fig. 4.7).

The complete dental complement for the horse is 44 teeth. We recognize that canine teeth are absent in females and that 305 and 405 (mandibular wolf teeth) are rarely seen. Such oligodontics are normal in the horse.

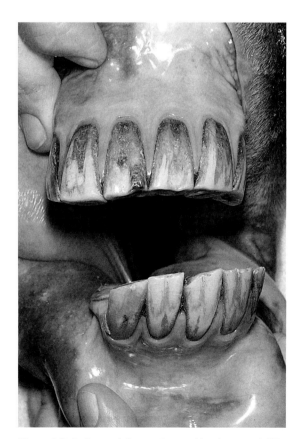

**Figure 4.7.** Incisor malalignment caused by absence of 403.

## POLYODONTIA

Polyodontia, or extra teeth, may be the result of the splitting of developing tooth buds from trauma, for example fractures, tooth avulsions or as a result of a developmental abnormality in which extra tooth germs are budded from the dental lamina. Traumatic division of tooth buds leads to the formation of misshapen, malformed and often misplaced, malerupted teeth or tooth components. These are treated by extraction.

Single extra teeth, for example seven incisors or seven cheek teeth in a single dental arcade will result in occlusal abnormalities similar to those that are seen in cases of oligodontia.

Cases have been described, however, in which there is true duplication of all teeth in an arcade, for example upper or lower incisors or permanent molars. Such conditions usually result in malocclusions, periodontal disease and difficulty in chewing. Early extraction of extra teeth may restore normal occlusal contact but, in fact, most cases of true polyodontia have been recorded from terminal subjects or from specimens that have been collected and for which no clinical information was available.

## ENAMEL HYPOPLASIA

Failure of enamel formation is a factor in numerous dental tumors. Partial failure, enamel hypoplasia, may be the result of the impact of teratogenic drugs or may be idiopathic.

In appearance, there are defects in the teeth in which not only is enamel absent, but there is a defect in coronal cementum. The condition is not of any clinical significance.

## BRACHYGNATHIA (PARROT MOUTH)

The lower jaw is shorter than the upper jaw leading to an overjet or overbite (depending on severity). In most cases, the defect is limited to incisor malocclusions, that is the defect is a shortening of the rostral component of the mandible, a shortening of the interdental space and there is often only a minor malocclusion of the cheek teeth (Fig. 4.8). The condition has been the subject of much discussion as to its etiology,

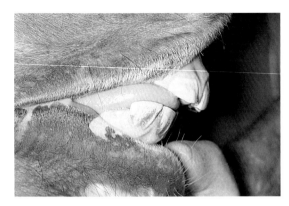

**Figure 4.8.** Parrot mouth in a 4-year-old thoroughbred.

for example is there genetic control? In some countries and in some breeds there are restrictions on the use of stallions for breeding (e.g.

thoroughbreds in the UK and quarter horses in the USA). Many people are familiar with particular stallions who appear to throw a high number of 'parrot-mouthed' offspring (see Chapter 14).

It is unusual for parrot-mouthed individuals to have difficulty feeding or grazing except for those cases in which the lower incisors impact and start to lacerate the palatine mucosa. Parrot-mouthed horses tend to develop incisor-related periodontal disease and an exaggeration of rostral hooks on 106 and 206 and caudal hooks on 311 and 411. In recent years, techniques have been described to limit the extent of this congenital and developmental condition. These may use orthodontic devices to inhibit growth of the premaxilla or bite-plane devices to both inhibit premaxillary extension and encourage mandibular extension (see Chapter 14).

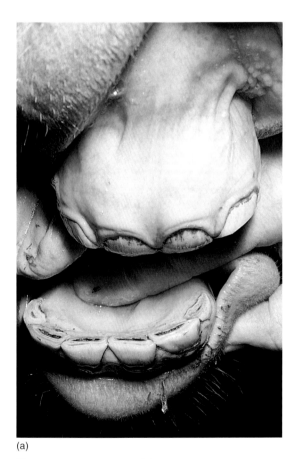

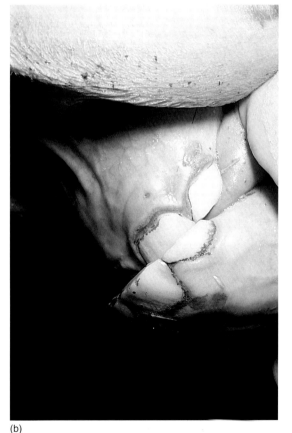

(a)

(b)

**Figure 4.9.** Monkey mouth, (a) rostral and (b) lateral views.

## PROGNATHIA (SOW MOUTH, MONKEY MOUTH)

This condition is seen less commonly than parrot mouth. Small horse breeds, ponies and miniature horses form the group in which moderate to severe underbites may be seen (Fig. 4.9).

In severe cases there may be nasal or nostril deformity as a result of shortening of the pre-maxilla and maxillary bones. Consequently nostril collapse, obstruction and stertorus breathing may occur.

Owners should be advised to change breeding strategies if their programs result in a number of foals with underbites. As with parrot-mouthed animals, individual cases will require regular attention to incisor alignment and incisor (upper) reduction to avoid mucosal pressure sores on the mandibular diastema.

## CAMPYLORRHINUS LATERALIS (WRY NOSE)

This is a condition in which there is a major developmental (and congenital) deformity of one side of the rostral region of the face (Fig. 4.10). There is a dysplasia of one side of the maxilla and premaxilla so that there is lateral deviation of the nose – to the dysplastic side. Close examination will often also show an enhanced concavity of the palate in the area rostral to the cheek teeth. The deformity also affects the congruity of the nostrils and the nasal septum with, in some cases, severe nasal obstruction as a result, caused by septal deviation.

The condition occurs occasionally in all breeds and may be related to fetal malpositioning. There seems to be a higher incidence in the Arabian breed and it is suggested that in this breed at least there may be a genetic cause.

The condition can be treated by facial reconstruction involving a frontal plane division of the face at a line from the first cheek tooth. Incisions are made to elevate the palatine mucosa, periosteum and the palatine arteries. The palatine maxillary bones and nasal septum are then divided. The nose may then be re-aligned and stabilized with external fixators (Fig. 4.11a, b, c and d). Post-operatively, a tracheostomy is essential and follow-up rhino-

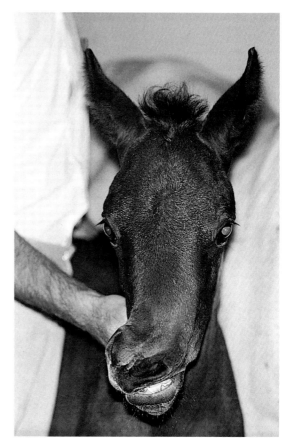

**Figure 4.10.** Wry nose in a 3-week-old Arabian foal.

plasty procedures may be required to alleviate residual nasal obstruction.

## RUDIMENTARY TEETH

Teeth that do not assume normal maturity and shape are defined as being rudimentary. In mares canine teeth are usually absent; this is a sex-linked genetic control. In some cases, however, there is partial formation of a simple structured tooth or teeth – a single or pair of rudimentary canines. They are usually small, from 2–6 mm in circumference and some 3–8 mm in length. They are sometimes unerupted and may only be detected by palpation through the overlying mucosa.

It is a common custom for maxillary wolf teeth (105 and 205) to be extracted. Consequently,

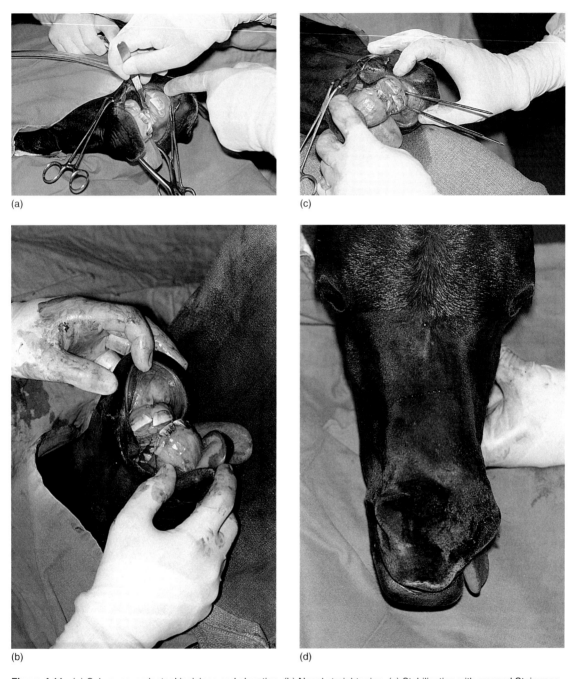

**Figure 4.11.** (a) Sub muco-periosteal incisions and elevation, (b) Nasal straightening, (c) Stabilization with crossed Steimman pins. (d) Post operation wry nose.

data relating to the prevalence of the rudimentary first cheek teeth, gathered from the examination of necropsy specimens, is likely to give a false incidence (13 per cent).[6] An examination of thoroughbred fetal skulls demonstrated that only 20 per cent contained wolf teeth.[6] Examination of yearling standardbreds revealed an incidence of 60 per cent. No explanation can

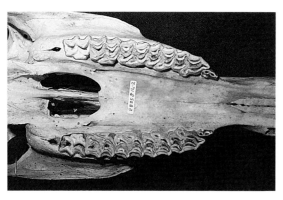

**Figure 4.12.** 'Molarized' wolf teeth in a zebra (from WR Cook with permission).

be afforded for these differences. In other equine species (e.g. the plains zebra), the incidence is nearly 100 per cent (WR Cook, personal communication, 1974). In the plains zebra it is not uncommon to find that the maxillary wolf teeth are large and often make occlusal contact with the first mandibular cheek teeth (306 and 406) and so are still functional in mastication (Fig. 4.12). Mandibular wolf teeth occur only rarely in *Equus caballus* and are also rare in other equid animals (e.g. zebras).

## ABNORMALITIES OF ERUPTION

The essential forces which result in the penetration of gums by teeth may be described in six anatomical stages.[10]

Stage   I:  preparatory stage (opening of the bony crypt)
Stage  II:  migration of the tooth toward the oral epithelium
Stage III:  emergence of crown tip into the oral cavity (beginning of clinical eruption)
Stage IV:  first occlusal contact
Stage  V:  full occlusal contact
Stage VI:  continuous eruption and movement.

The mechanism for tooth eruption in the horse has been reviewed and those components based on the selected deposition and resorption of bone, the involvement of vascular and intraosseous hydrostatic pressure changes, and the pulling of the periodontal ligament are the most important.[3] Abnormalities of eruption

may occur at any stage and may be traumatic, genetic, viral or teratogenic.

Trauma to developing teeth and surrounding bones may lead to malorientation of the tooth bud and subsequent misplacement or maleruptions (Fig. 4.13). Whenever possible, care should be taken when repairing fractures or avulsions that involve teeth to try and avoid damage to the developing permanent dentition when placing the transfixing pins of external fixators or other osteosynthetic devices.

Reference has already been made to the vascular and hydrostatic forces that accompany tooth eruptions. The general pattern of the sequence of eruption of mammalian teeth is based on a mesial to distal progression (Table 4.1). This sequence applies to both deciduous and permanent teeth, but it can be seen that

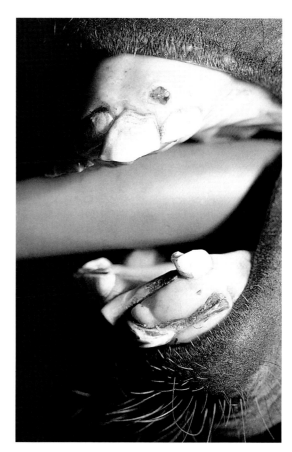

**Figure 4.13.** Incisor maleruption and malposition subsequent to mandibular symphyseal fracture and fracture repair.

**DENTAL DISEASE AND PATHOLOGY**

**Table 4.1.** Eruption sequence of cheek teeth

| Cheek tooth number | Mammalian eruption sequence | *Equus caballus* |
|---|---|---|
| (100, 200, 300, 400) | | |
| 06 | 4 | 3 |
| 07 | 5 | 4 |
| 08 | 6 | 6 |
| 09 | 1 | 1 |
| 10 | 2 | 2 |
| 11 | 3 | 5 |

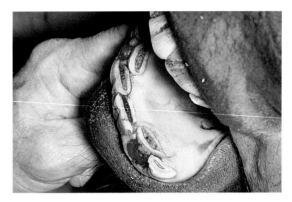

**Figure 4.14.** A common form of incisor maleruption in a 2.5-year-old standardbred horse.

an overlap in the time sequence so that permanent teeth 108, 208, 308 and 408 (premolar 4s or third cheek teeth) have a tendency to be crowded because they erupt into a potentially crowded space that is made by the 07 and 09 teeth (premolar 4's and first molars).

## DENTAL IMPACTIONS

It should be appreciated that the sequencing of the anatomical stages of eruption – particularly stages II–IV are mutually dependent. In which case if the eruption pathway is not complete, if there is a minor change in position of the erupting permanent tooth in replacing its deciduous predecessor or if the space is too small then there is the possibility of disease processes resulting from this impaction.

In the case of incisor teeth, caudal eruptions of permanent incisors are seen quite commonly (Fig. 4.14). In most cases these positional changes are corrected spontaneously when the deciduous tooth is shed. In other cases the displacement may be severe enough to warrant extraction of the deciduous incisor (seen particularly with 302 and 402) and even grinding down the mesial and distal margins of the adjacent teeth.

In horses (stallions and geldings) there is often a 6 to 8 month delay between the eruption of the first and of the second of a pair of canine teeth. This may result in the formation of an inflammatory fibrous reaction over the unerupted crown of the impacted tooth. These swellings may be painful on palpation or cause abnormal reactions to bit contact. The clinician has two options to relieve the problem of an impacted

canine. Under sedation and local analgesia the overlying tissue should be divided in a cruciate pattern, using a scalpel and an elevator, thus enhancing the eruption pathway and enabling entry of the tooth into the mouth. If there is continued failure to erupt the second choice is to extract the tooth (see Chapter 15).

Similar local reaction is seen occasionally over the crown of an impacted or misplaced wolf tooth. In these cases extraction of the tooth is the recommended course of treatment.

The most frequent sites of cheek teeth impaction are seen associated with the eruptions of the 8s (i.e. 108, 208, 308 or 408). The result is an expansion of the 'eruption cyst' and, in many cases, a break out of the inflammatory process to periapical structures. This may result in dental fistula formation, periradicular disease or sinusitis depending upon the location of the tooth involved.

Impaction of 108 and/or 208 may result in palatal displacement of the affected permanent tooth or teeth (Fig. 4.15). This will result in an irregular arcade and the formation of a buccal cheek pocket or pouch. As food is chewed it will spill laterally into this space and there will be local periodontal disease. Treatment is based on amelioration of the pocketing. It can be accomplished by grinding or sloping the distal margins of 107 or 207 and the mesial margins of 109 or 209. In this way, the shape of the pocket is changed and food accumulation is avoided. It may, in some cases, be necessary to extract the misplaced tooth (108 or 208)

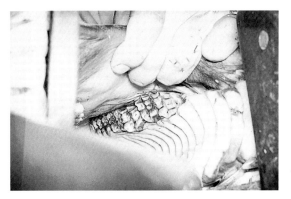

**Figure 4.15.** Palatal displacement of 108.

The most frequently seen disease associated with dental impactions is, as has been stated, the effect of impacted 8s. It is the author's opinion that this problem is the single most important cause of apical osteitis and the subsequent development of mandibular dental fistula formation (see Chapter 7).

## DECIDUOUS CAPS

As the deciduous teeth are worn away and permanent teeth erupt to replace them, the occlusal remnants of the deciduous teeth are referred to as deciduous caps (Fig. 4.16).

The caps are normally shed as part of the eruptive process and do not cause problems. In

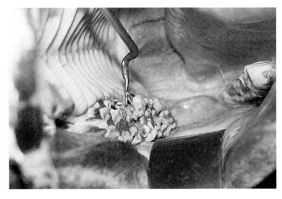

**Figure 4.16.** Dental caps on right maxillary arcade.

some cases, however, they may become unstable, change position and result in oral or buccal discomfort. Loose caps and displaced or rotated caps should be removed. They may be elevated with an elevator, or even the end of a screwdriver, and removed. It is important to keep in mind that early removal of caps will stop cementogenesis within the enamel lakes of the maxillary cheek teeth and thereby enhance hypoplasia of cementum at these sites.

## SUMMARY

Abnormalities of dental development and eruptions occur quite commonly in the horse and result in a wide range of clinical signs and symptoms.

### REFERENCES

1. Ten Cate AR (1989) Physiologic tooth movement, eruption and shedding. In: *Oral Histology, Development, Structure and Function* (3rd edn) ed. AR Ten Cate, CV Mosby, St Louis, pp. 275–298.
2. Kupfer M (1937) *Tooth Structure in Donkeys and Horses*, Gustav Fischer, Jena, pp. 1–103.
3. Berkovitz BKB (1975) Mechanisms of tooth eruption. In: *Applied Physiology of the Mouth*, ed. CLB Lavelle (1st edn) J Wright, Bristol, pp. 53–72.
4. Baker GJ (1971) Some aspects of dental radiology. *Equine Veterinary Journal*, 3, 46–51.
5. Baker GJ (1970) Some aspects of equine dental disease. *Equine Veterinary Journal*, 2, 105–110.
6. Baker GJ (1979) *A study of equine dental disease*. PhD Thesis. University of Glasgow, pp. 36–38.
7. Colyer F (1931) *Abnormal conditions of the teeth of animals in their relationship to similar conditions in man*. London, The Dental Board of the United Kingdom, pp. 36–38.
8. Hofmeyer CFB (1960) Comparative dental pathology (with particular reference to caries and paradontal disease in the horse and dog). *Journal of South African Veterinary Medical Association* 29, 471–480.
9. Honma K, Yamakawa M, Yamouchi S and Hosoya S (1962) Statistical study on the occurrence of dental caries in domestic animals. 1. Horse. *Japanese Journal of Veterinary Research* 10, 31–36.
10. Becher E (1939) *Treatment of Dental Disease in the Horse*. Deutche Tierarztt, 6, 29–31.

# 5

# ORAL AND DENTAL TRAUMA

TRC Greet, BVMS MVM CertEO DESTS DipECVS FRCVS, Beaufort Cottage Equine Hospital, Cotton End Road, Exning, Newmarket, Suffolk CB8 7NN

## ORAL ANATOMY

The mouth is the most rostral portion of the alimentary canal. It is bounded laterally by the cheeks, dorsally by the hard and soft palates and ventrally by the mandible, tongue and mylohyoid muscles. It is a long cylindrical cavity and, when closed, is almost entirely filled by the tongue and teeth. The oral cavity communicates caudally with the oropharynx through the isthmus faucium.

The mucous membrane of the mouth is continuous at the margin of the lips with the skin and caudally with the mucosa of the oropharynx. It is of squamous type with multiple small papillae which are the openings of the ducts of the labial glands. The lips are muscular folds surrounding the orifice of the mouth. The angles of their union are called the commissures and are situated at the level of the first premolar cheek teeth.

The cheeks are muscular in nature and the gums are composed of dense fibrous tissue intimately united with the periosteum of the mandible and the dental structures which it surrounds.[1] Motor innervation of the cheeks and lips is provided by the seventh and oral sensation by the fifth cranial nerves.

The hard palate is bounded rostrally and laterally by the dental arcades. Although its mucous membrane is smooth there are eighteen transverse curved ridges along its length.[1] The blood supply to the mouth is well developed and formed from the facial and buccinator arteries.

There is a rich venous plexus beneath the mucosa of the hard palate supplied by the palatine arteries and veins.

The tongue is a muscular structure situated in the floor of the mouth between the horizontal rami of the mandibles and supported by a muscular sling formed by the mylohyoid muscles. Caudally it is attached to the hyoid apparatus. It is covered with a squamous epithelium and the dorsal surface is covered with a variety of papillae. On either side of its root sits a dense aggregate of lymphoid tissue – the lingual tonsils. The blood supplied to the tongue is provided by the lingual and sublingual branches of the external maxillary artery and its corresponding veins. Motor supply to the tongue is provided by the 12th cranial nerves. Sensation to the rostral two thirds is provided by the 5th and the 7th cranial nerves. Sensation to the caudal one third comes from the lingual branch of the 9th cranial nerve.[1]

There are three pairs of salivary glands which have ducts entering the oral cavity. The parotid ducts enter the mouth via papillae situated approximately at the level of the fourth upper premolar teeth. The mandibular ducts open into the floor of the mouth at the level of the lower canine teeth via flattened papillae – the sublingual caruncles. The sublingual glands enter the oral cavity by a series of approximately 30 ducts in the sublingual fold. Other smaller salivary glands are found throughout the mouth.[1]

## ORAL EXAMINATION

Injuries to the oral cavity can be assessed by visual inspection of the mouth. Obvious external injuries to the lips and cheeks may be readily assessed, however lesions within the oral cavity can be more difficult to evaluate. Examining the mouth can usually be performed by gently grasping the tongue and rotating it within the mouth at the level of the interdental space.[2] Great caution should be observed if there is any possibility of a pre-existing lingual injury. A pen torch may be used to examine the oral cavity although a good head lamp may be better as it allows freedom to use both hands enabling careful palpation of the molar arcades, tongue, gums and other oral structures. Great caution should always be observed when inserting a hand into a horse's mouth as serious injury to the examiner may result from the teeth. The safer option may be the use of an oral speculum such as a Hausmann's gag. There are other similar types of speculum available. This apparatus should be used with the horse heavily sedated as there is risk of injury to the examiner from such a heavy metal object. In the presence of oral injury and consequent pain even the use of a full mouth speculum may be precluded and general anaesthetic will be required. A speculum provides a secure means of examination of even the most caudal structures within the oral cavity.

An endoscopic examination of the nasal passages and nasopharynx may be useful in assessing defects of the hard and soft palate and may allow identification of some oropharyngeal foreign bodies which protrude through the intrapharyngeal ostium. An endoscopic examination of the oral cavity may be carried out in the sedated horse with a speculum, but there is a risk of instrument damage and so extensive oral endoscopy should be done under general anesthesia. The endoscopic light not only allows means of inspecting the oral cavity but illuminates the cavity to allow lavaging and surgical repair of some more inaccessible wounds.

Radiographic views of the head are helpful in assessing the extent of oral injuries when damage to bones or teeth is suspected. Lateral views or oblique views taken with the horse in the standing position are helpful. Intra-oral occlusal views of the mandibular or maxillary incisor arcade may also be of great value in demonstrating injuries to these areas. Such views require the horse to be sedated heavily and it may be preferable to have the horse under general anesthesia. The use of oral barium sulfate may permit identification of an oronasal fistula and plain radiographic views may allow identification of metallic foreign bodies within the tongue, cheeks or gums. It should be remembered that artefactual shadows can be created by restraining devices such as headcollars. A rope halter is probably the most satisfactory means of restraining a horse for radiography of the head. Assessing functional disturbances of swallowing is best achieved using image intensification and fluoroscopy. Barium sulfate suspension either on its own or mixed with food material can be used as a contrast agent.

## ORAL TRAUMA

A variety of injuries affecting the oral cavity are commonly encountered in horses. Lacerations of the lips may be associated with wire or bit injuries and are occasionally caused by kicks or other forms of direct trauma (Fig. 5.1). Horses are prone to grasping fixed objects such as doors, mangers or buckets and this may lead to fractures of the mandible or maxilla usually associated with avulsion of the incisor teeth. Occasionally the incisor teeth may be damaged without significant injury to the surrounding bone and this is particularly likely when deciduous teeth are involved in such injuries.

Injuries may occur to the interdental space where the bit sits. The injury may result from over zealous handling by a rider or the use of restraining devices such as a chiffney. There is often ulceration just rostral to the premolar teeth and in some cases damage to the underlying bone may produce sequestra. More severe fractures of the mandibles or maxillae may also occur at this level usually as the result of direct trauma.

Injuries to the tongue are less common but may also, be associated with over zealous restraint using a chiffney. Severe laceration and even transection of the tongue is not unknown

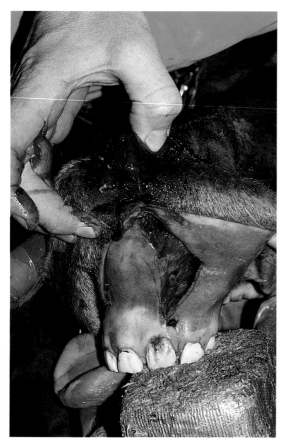

**Figure 5.1.** A severe laceration to the upper lip that extends into the oral cavity. This a full thickness laceration which should be repaired in layers.

under such circumstances. Less severe injuries can be caused by stable hooks or clips, twisted loose deciduous molar caps or foreign bodies in the feed. Grasping the tongue while examining the mouth of a horse may also predispose it to oral injury. There was one famous account of a farrier who literally pulled a horse's tongue out of its mouth while restraining the horse for shoeing. More commonly grasping the tongue with excessive force results in tearing of the lingual frenulum.[6]

Injuries to the hard and soft palate are less common but may follow the incorrect or careless use of dental instruments, for example during the removal of wolf teeth. Iatrogenic damage to the soft palate may follow surgery for laryngopalatal dislocation or epiglottal entrapment.

Injuries to the salivary glands are rare.[3] However lacerations or other injuries to the face may involve the parotid salivary duct producing a salivary facial fistula.

## ORAL ENVIRONMENT AND HEALING OF ORAL INJURIES

The oral cavity is exposed to the external environment and is bathed in a solution of saliva. Saliva is composed of mucus and serous fluids containing electrolytes and proteinaceous enzymes, for example amylase. It facilitates mastication and deglutition. Saliva also contains glycosaminoglycans and glycoproteins which are responsible for its lubricant characteristics. Saliva is secreted in large volumes (50 ml/min from a single parotid gland) as a result of mastication and its production is controlled by the autonomic nervous system.[3] The mouth is frequently in contact with food material and subjected to the movements of mastication. There are large numbers of bacteria within the oral cavity, many of which are anerobic. All these factors have a considerable bearing on the effects of injury to the mouth and to the methods of management of oral trauma.

Many minor lacerations to the lips cheek and tongue will heal by second intention without the need for surgical reconstruction because of the excellent oral blood supply. However in certain situations surgical reconstruction of oral structures is indicated.[4,5,6] Typically injuries involving complete laceration of the cheeks, lips or tongue are candidates for surgical repair. Management of such injuries should involve careful wound preparation with particular attention given to the removal of foreign material. In most cases oral lacerations quickly become filled with food as well as clotted blood. Localized infections may subsequently produce necrosis at the site and in some cases bony fragments may become sequestrated. Careful debridement of the wound must be performed. If the wound is extensive or inaccessible in the standing horse, a general anesthetic should be administered to ensure that appropriate wound assessment and management can be carried out. Removal of all necrotic material and debris is essential, producing healthy tissue margins which bleed freely. When significant injury occurs to the lips or cheeks the wound should be closed in layers.[5,6] At the very least, separate skin and mucosal closure is required. In most cases, a third layer which incorporates the muscular tissue and fascia should also be repaired using absorbable suture material. The tissues should be reconstructed with accurate apposition of the layers and it is preferable to use non-absorbable suture material or stainless steel staples for the skin.

Following repair care must be observed in preventing self-mutilation by the horse. While most horses seem unbothered by sutured facial wounds others seem to find such wounds irritating. In these circumstances the use of long-term sedation, muzzling or cross-tying the horse can be helpful in preventing failure of the repair or worsening of the original damage.

## TREATMENT OF SPECIFIC SOFT TISSUE INJURIES

### THE LIPS AND CHEEKS

Injuries to the lips and cheeks are readily treated by suturing after preparation of the wound. If the wounds are extensive and involve all the layers of the lips the horse should either be heavily sedated or given a general anesthetic and the wounds repaired in layers (Figs 5.2–5.5). It is preferable to repair the oral mucosa first and this should be done with simple interrupted sutures or continuous appositional sutures of absorbable material such as polyglactin 910 or polydioxanone. Knots can be tied within the oral cavity. In most cases a second layer which should incorporate the muscular and fascial tissue should be carried out using the same material. Lavage of the incision with polyionic fluid containing soluble penicillin at this stage will assist in minimizing the risk of wound infections. The skin of the lips can then be repaired using a non-absorbable suture material such as monofilament nylon, sheathed polyamide or stainless steel skin staples. In small lesions the use of simple interrupted sutures is preferable. However with more extensive lesions simple interrupted sutures can be alter-

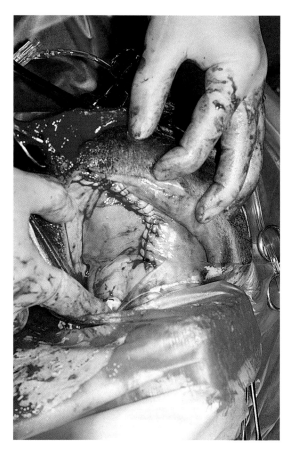

**Figure 5.2.** Repair of the oral cavity using a continuous suture of 4 metric polydioxanone, same case as in Fig. 5.1.

nated with vertical mattress sutures to assist in spreading the tension of the wound therefore reducing the risk of subsequent dehiscence. If extensive cheek lacerations are encountered great care must be taken to assess whether the parotid salivary duct has been involved. If this has been damaged its wall should be repaired to prevent subsequent development of a facial salivary fistula (see pp. 67–68). Similarly extensive lesions may involve injury to branches of the facial nerve. Major facial nerve injuries have a poor prognosis and may result in permanent disability.

When the edge of the lip is involved care should be taken to restore complete function by repair of the orbicularis oris muscle. The close proximity of the skin, mucosa and musculature at this site potentially creates excessive

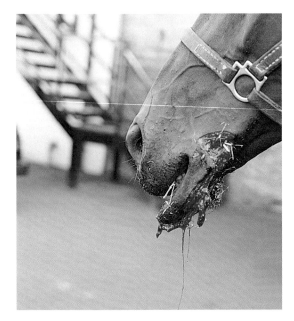

**Figure 5.3.** Separating the skin from the underlying musculature.

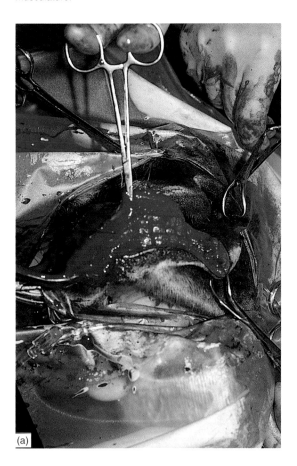

(a)

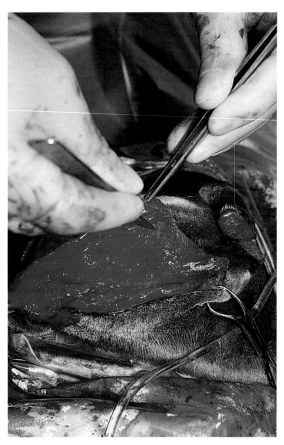

**Figure 5.4.** Repair of facial musculature using a continuous suture of 4 metric polydioxanone.

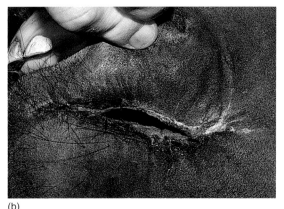

(b)

**Figure 5.5.** (a) Shows an extensive laceration of the lower lip which also has a full thickness defect through the left cheek into the mouth. This lesion was repaired in layers but partial wound dehiscence resulted in an orofacial fistula (b) that was subsequently repaired successfully.

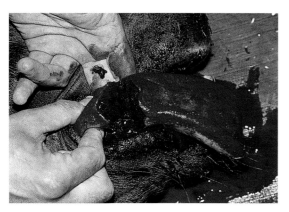

**Figure 5.6.** This is a severe laceration of the tongue which is severed almost completely. This injury was repaired using simple interrupted sutures of polydioxanone alternated with vertical mattress sutures of the same material.

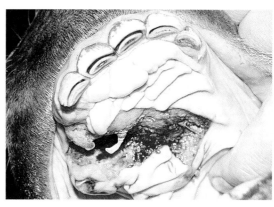

**Figure 5.7.** This horse sustained severe trauma to the maxilla which resulted in a fracture of the premaxillary bone and laceration of the hard palate. There was direct continuity between the mouth and the nasal passages.

movement at the suture line particularly during prehension. To minimize this the skin and mucosa should be separated from the adjacent musculature at the edges of the wound.[5,6] This facilitates closure in layers and reduces the incidence of dehiscence. The wound edges should be aligned accurately to ensure healing is satisfactory and to minimize the risk of subsequent wound dehiscence and disfigurement which might affect function.

Should the repair of a lip or cheek laceration subsequently dehisce, the wound may be left to heal by second intention. However if extensive lesions are involved an attempt should be made to carry out secondary repair of the wound. It may be necessary to use tension relieving devices such as a quill of polythene tubing from a giving set for fluid administration. These are incorporated into vertical mattress sutures to protect the wound from dehiscence. When carrying out secondary repair it is of paramount importance to carry out radical debridement of necrotic material down to healthy bleeding tissue. In general the prognosis for the healing of lacerations to the lips and cheeks is very good. However in those cases where secondary or tertiary repair is attempted there will often be a cosmetic blemish particularly at the margin of the lips. Occasionally an orofacial fistula may remain (Fig. 5.5).

## THE TONGUE AND OROPHARYNX

Injuries to the tongue mostly involve lacerations caused by damage from bits or restraining devices such as a chiffney. Minor splits to the tongue will heal readily without need for repair. Even more severe injuries may heal without need for repair. Occasionally a horse is examined which has previously sustained a severe laceration of the tongue which has healed without complication leaving a large defect in its lateral border. Lacerations of the lingual frenulum which usually occur due to excessive traction on the tongue, need not be repaired and usually heal without complication. However most severe lacerations involving the body of the tongue are best managed surgically.[6]

The horse should be given a general anesthetic and the wound assessed carefully to ensure tongue viability. A gauze bandage may be used as an effective tourniquet when applied caudal to the wound. The bandage also provides good exposure to the injury when gentle traction is applied to it. Glossectomy may be necessary if the tongue tip is unviable and removal of tissue up to the level of the attachment of the frenulum is unlikely to affect function.[6] Intravenous administration of sodium fluorescein has been recommended as an aid to assessing lingual viability, the tongue can be examined using a Woods lamp 5 min after injection of 4 or 5 g of the compound.[6] Oversewing the body of the tongue with simple interrupted or a continuous suture of polyglactin 910 or polydioxanone should be attempted after removal of the necrotic tip. In severe lacerations the tongue is repaired using simple interrupted and interrupted vertical mattress sutures (Fig. 5.6). The latter should incorporate a significant bulk of lingual musculature to take up some of the tension and to ensure more satisfactory healing. All dead space should be obliterated if possible. Multiple layer closure may be required. It should be remembered that the tongue is very mobile and the risk of wound dehiscence is significant unless care is taken to align the tongue correctly and to repair the injury accurately. If the injury is not dealt with in the acute situation, a degree of necrosis and contamination of the wound may occur. In these circumstances devitalized tissue must be carefully debrided to reduce the risk of wound dehiscence. When placing vertical mattress tension sutures care must be taken not to interfere with the blood supply to the tongue. Although this is very good, vascular compromise may result in necrosis of the tongue. This applies particularly if the tip is involved. The dorsum of the tongue has a much stronger mucosal covering than the ventral region and suture retention is better in this site. Tension sutures are therefore best applied in this area.[4]

Lesions to the base of the tongue and the oropharynx are more difficult to evaluate and certainly more difficult to repair due to their inaccessibility. However in most circumstances inaccessible wounds will heal well without need for repair. Daily lavage of the oral cavity with a saline solution may be of value in reducing the contamination of such wounds with food material.

Rarely, horses are encountered which have developed sub-epiglottal infections or granulomatous abscesses. These presumably are the result of earlier mucosal penetration or an injury which has been undetected. Surgical removal of granulomatous swellings at this site is difficult but may be achieved via an oral approach or through a ventral midline pharyngotomy. This

site is also prone to damage by ingested foreign bodies which are usually twigs or pieces of wood. In most circumstances affected horses show oral discomfort, dysphagia, hyperptyalism and occasionally epistaxis. Foreign bodies in the oropharynx can often be visualized by nasopharyngeal endoscopy as they frequently protrude through the intrapharyngeal ostium. Foreign bodies are usually retrieved manually with the horse under heavy sedation or general anesthesia. No repair of the mucosal injury is usually necessary. Parenteral antibiotics and non-steroidal anti-inflammatory medication should be administered for several days following removal of foreign bodies from this region.

## THE HARD AND SOFT PALATES

Injuries to the hard palate are rare but may accompany severe trauma to the head. (Fig. 5.7). In some circumstances there may be an underlying fracture of the palate which usually involves the palatine processes of the premaxilla and/or the maxilla. In most circumstances these can be left as open wounds to heal by second intention. However an oronasal fistula should be repaired surgically. A suspected oronasal fistula may be confirmed by a combination of a thorough clinical and endoscopic examination and radiography after oral administration of barium sulfate suspension. While such a fistula may resolve by second intention healing, surgical repair should be attempted if the site is accessible. It may be possible to repair the injury simply by suturing the palatal mucosa with interrupted sutures of polydioxanone (Fig. 5.8). If the mucosal defect can not adequately be repaired it may be possible to close the defect by creating a mucoperiosteal flap or by producing tension-relieving incisions in adjacent portions of the palate. Care should be taken to avoid damage to the palatal blood supply.[4]

Post-repair feeding should be carried out by nasogastric intubation for the first 4 or 5 days to reduce the risk of suture-line dehiscence.

If the rostral portion of the skull is grossly unstable following a maxillary or premaxillary injury the fractures may require surgical repair (see Chapter 17). Congenital defects of the hard

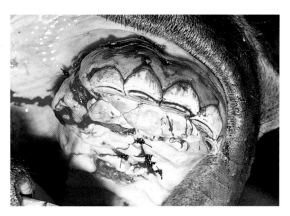

**Figure 5.8.** This is the surgical repair of the injury illustrated in Figure 5.7. The fracture has been reduced with cerclage wire after radical debridement of the site and the palate has been repaired partially using simple interrupted and vertical mattress sutures of 4 metric polydioxanone.

palate are uncommon and in the authors opinion surgical repair is not indicated.

Injuries to the hard palate and more specifically the palatine artery may follow removal of a wolf tooth or repulsion of cheek teeth. In such cases moderately severe hemorrhage may occur. Control of the hemorrhage by pressure is usually effective. If there is a large enough defect it may be possible to insert some gauze bandage packing.

Injuries to the soft palate are uncommon but may occur following attempted surgical treatment of the soft palate or other adjacent structures such as epiglottal entrapment. Full thickness injuries to the soft palate almost inevitably result in the development of an oronasal fistula because of contamination by food material and saliva. Surgical repair of such injuries should therefore be attempted as soon as possible after the injury has been identified. Access for surgical repair is very difficult. The horse should be given a general anesthetic and the mouth opened maximally using an oral speculum. Good lighting should be provided and the area may be examined by a fiberoptic or videoendoscope to assess the extent of the injury. Long handled retractors should be used to depress the tongue and retract the cheeks in order to help in assessing the injury and its subsequent repair. Long handled needle holders,

forceps and scissors are also of great help when it comes to repair. Separation of the oropharyngeal mucosa from the overlying musculature will facilitate closure.

If possible the soft palate should be repaired in at least two layers. The muscular tissue and nasopharyngeal mucosa may be repaired together with an absorbable suture material. The author prefers to use polydioxanone as a simple, continuous suture. A similar suture is used in the oral mucosa.

Even though such defects may be closed satisfactorily, dehiscence of the wound is common. This is because of the highly mobile nature of the palate during mastication and the presence of food material and saliva within the oral cavity. It is common for second or even third attempts at repair of full thickness palatal defects to fail. However, small fistulae may heal spontaneously. As described above feeding post-repair should be by nasogastric intubation to reduce the risk of dehiscence of the suture line.

Clefts of the soft palate are more common than those of the hard palate but in the author's opinion these should not be repaired surgically. The affected animal should be destroyed if the degree of disability (dysphagia or exercise intolerance) is more than slight.

## INJURIES TO THE SALIVARY DUCTS

Injuries to the salivary glands may occur as a result of direct trauma. The parotid is the most vulnerable because of its size and situation behind the angle of the jaw. Such injuries can usually be repaired simply by wound debridement, cleansing and closure of the skin. Salivary cutaneous fistulae are rare after this sort of injury.[3]

Injuries to the parotid duct are more common and may be associated with direct trauma to the ventral border of the mandible at which point the duct crosses before entering the oral cavity. In some cases there may be little evidence of an injury to the duct and it may heal without need for treatment. However in a proportion of cases there is direct continuity between the duct and the skin wound and this often results in the development of a salivary facial fistula. Such injuries are often quite dramatic as there may be a profuse discharge of saliva during eating and mastication. While the nature of saliva tends to discourage closure of the fistula most cases will eventually heal if given adequate time. Those cases in which healing has not occurred can be repaired by surgical closure. The duct should be dissected from the edge of the fistula and closed with a simple interrupted sutures of 2 metric polyglactin 910. Insertion of a catheter into the parotid duct may facilitate suturing. The catheter demarcates the walls of the duct making accurate repair easier.

Injury to the parotid salivary duct may occur inadvertently during facial or dental surgery, or transection of the duct may be carried out electively in performing buccostomy techniques for removal of mandibular or maxillary cheek teeth. In these cases, end to end anastomosis of the duct can be carried out using simple interrupted sutures of 2 metric polyglactin 910. A parotid duct fistula may occur following repair of the surgical incision use to remove sialoliths which are encountered occasionally in older horses. Secondary closure of these incisions may be effective or alternatively the incision may be left to heal by second intention.

Injuries to the mandibular or sublingual salivary ducts are rare. The author has encountered one horse with a ranula associated with a sublingual salivary duct. This was managed successfully by oral marsupialization of the ranula.

## TREATMENT OF INJURIES INVOLVING TOOTH AND BONE

### DENTAL TRAUMA

Teeth may become fractured as a result of a direct blow to the mouth. If the pulp cavity is exposed ascending infection may result in periapical sepsis and the tooth may need to be removed. However in a number of instances secondary dentine may be laid down and periapical inflammation may be avoided. In evaluating a horse with a dental fracture a thorough clinical and radiographic assessment should be made of the injury. Unless the tooth is severely

injured it is better to opt for a conservative policy initially (see Chapter 16). The horse should be treated with antibiotic medication usually penicillin and the mouth lavaged frequently with a saline solution. Loose dental fragments may be removed and a complete recovery can be expected in a significant proportion of cases.

If a dental injury is severe it may be possible to remove the tooth with the horse sedated. However this is usually achieved more easily with the horse under general anesthesia.

A dental fracture may be associated with injury to the surrounding alveolus or supporting bone. The injury should be assessed by radiography and by a thorough clinical examination. In a proportion of cases the tooth may become avulsed with its surrounding bone and a decision must be made whether to repair the injury or to remove the tooth and the surrounding bone. This decision is based upon the size of the fragment, its integrity and also on economics. Sometimes dental injury may occur associated with a more complex comminuted fracture of the mandible or maxilla. In most circumstances it is preferable to treat the acute injury in a conservative manner, that is by the administration of antibiotics and non-steroidal anti-inflammatory medication. This should be allied with lavage of the area with saline. In many instances a conservative approach will result in healing of the injury. If the injury does not heal completely it may heal to a significant extent allowing a less radical procedure to remove sequestra or dental fragments at a later date, 4 to 6 weeks post-injury. If such injuries are associated with extensive soft tissue lacerations attention should be paid to the soft tissue laceration and the underlying osseous or dental lesion may be left for assessment at a later date. Postoperative antibiotic and non-steroidal anti-inflammatory medication is usual following these injuries.

### INJURY TO THE BONES OF THE UPPER OR LOWER JAW

Fractures of the mandible just rostral to the molar arcade are quite commonly seen associated with over zealous use of restraining devices such as a chiffney or as a bit injury in riding horses. In most cases there is a non-healing ulcer at the typical site (Fig. 5.9) and radiographic views of the mandible will usually identify a small fragment of bone. In most cases this can be removed either with the horse standing or under general anesthesia. Following gentle curettage of the underlying bone and lavage most horses go on to make an uneventful recovery.

Unilateral fractures of the horizontal ramus of the mandible can be treated conservatively as the contralateral mandible provides very good stability. Repair of the soft tissue injury is not usually required although lavage of the open wound will minimize the risk of contamination and secondary infection. Antimicrobial medication is also indicated. If both horizontal rami are fractured, instability of the mandible occurs and the injury should be treated by external fixation. Such a device can usually be created with the use of Steinmann bone pins inserted across both horizontal rami of the mandibles and fixed to a metal bar or a plastic tube. The latter is filled with methyl methacrylate. Alternatively a dynamic compression plate could be used either attached to the bone itself or to the cheek teeth and incisor arcade.

Maxillary fractures are almost always managed without fracture fixation. There is often a debate about whether to repair the oral mucosa when a severe laceration is related to a fracture of the jaw. After careful cleansing and debridement of food material and other debris, primary closure may be carried out if the surrounding tissue can be closed easily and has suitable strength for suture holding. In all other circumstances the wound may be left open to heal by second intention and the owner instructed on carrying out frequent lavage with saline to minimize the risk of food contamination and possible secondary infection. The administration of prophylactic antimicrobial cover is sensible but not essential in every case. Serious wound infections which result in delay or prevention of fracture healing are almost unknown in injuries affecting the mouth unless foreign material or a sequestrum are involved.

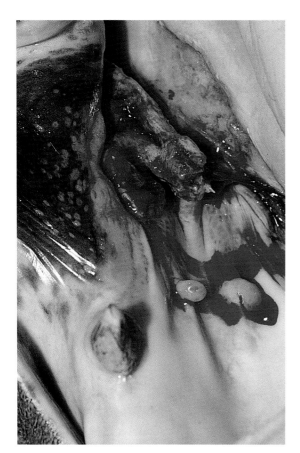

**Figure 5.9.** This is an oral ulcer in the interdental space of the right mandible of a horse which suffered an injury following restraint using a chiffney. A large sequestrum can be seen which was removed. The horse made a complete recovery.

### REFERENCES

1. Anon (1975) Equine digestive system. Ed. R Getty, WB Saunders, Philadelphia.
2. Baker GJ (1985) Oral examination and diagnosis: management of oral diseases. In: *Veterinary Dentistry*, ed. CE Harvey, WB Saunders, Philadelphia, pp. 217–234.
3. Auer JA (ed.) (1992) *Equine Surgery.* WB Saunders, Philadelphia, pp. 306–308.
4. Scott EA (1982) Surgery of the oral cavity. *Veterinary Clinics of North America Large Animal Practice*, 4, 3–31.
5. Howard RD and Stashak TS (1993) Reconstructive surgery of selected injuries of the head. *Veterinary Clinics of North America Large Animal Practice*, 9, 185–198.
6. Robinson NE (ed.) (1997) *Current Therapy in Equine Medicine*, 4. WB Saunders, Philadelphia, pp. 148–149.

# ABNORMALITIES OF WEAR AND PERIODONTAL DISEASE

Gordon J Baker, BVSc, PhD., MRCVS, Diplomate ACVS, University of Illinois, College of Veterinary Medicine, Urbana, IL 61802

## INTRODUCTION

In reviewing the chewing cycle of the horse, it was shown that the structure and function of the teeth, support structures, bones, joints and muscles produce a coordinated, efficient 'machine' that initiates the digestive process. It was also suggested that the efficiency of this process could be changed by minor alterations in occlusal contact pattern and thereby reduce the efficiency. In this chapter the recognition of occlusal surface abnormalities, the induced pathological changes and their clinical effects and management will be described.

## DEFINITIONS

A range of descriptive and architectural terms are used to describe occlusal surface irregularities that develop in horses teeth as a sequel to abnormalities of wear. It is clear that any irregularities that develop will progress, i.e. become worse, as the teeth continue to erupt.

Incisor teeth irregularities result in changes of the 'bite plane' – the normal horizontal plane that is made by contact of the upper and lower incisors. In parrot-mouthed and monkey-mouthed horses, the overjet/overbite or underjet/underbite there may be no incisor contact and so the bite plane, in its definitive sense, does not exist. A subject that has arisen in recent discussions on dental prophylactic techniques in the horse has been the exact relationship, from an etiological point of view,

between incisor and cheek teeth contact. It has been suggested that as horses age and the frontal plane of incisor contact becomes more horizontal, there arises a condition in which the incisors may 'lock up' and thereby change cheek teeth occlusal contact patterns. More data and studies are required to evaluate this suggested hypothesis, i.e. what is the chicken and what is the egg? Contact irregularities will be discussed further in this chapter.

When viewed from the side, the cheek teeth arcades conform to a series of interlocking, regular irregularities. These surfaces afford a completely efficient machine to chew food. It must be noted that the cheek teeth erupt in a series of arcs – they can be seen radiating in a series from the temporomandibular joint. In general as horses age, and to some extent depending upon the nature of the feeds consumed, these occlusal surfaces 'blades' are maintained throughout life. It is normal for the edges to be slightly reduced, i.e. the surface gets a little smoother, with age. There are some breed differences that are seen in the plane of the cheek teeth arcades. Smaller breeds of horses, ponies and miniature horses have cheek teeth arcades that are not truly horizontal and this slight dishing, i.e. more crown rostrally and caudally, becomes more obvious with age.

In a study of age-related morphology of equine mandibular cheek teeth,[1] it was shown that even though erupted crown is lost constantly as a result of masticatory wear, an overall increase in tooth length occurred during the first year following eruption, with no change in length from 1–2 years following eruption (Fig. 6.1). This apparent discrepancy is caused by the rate of increase in root length during the first 2 years following tooth eruption exceeding the rate of loss of erupted crown (Fig. 6.2). This resulted in an overall increase in the first year and lack of change in the second year in overall tooth length, even though occlusal loss due to wear was occurring. Three years following eruption the loss of erupted crown due to wear exceeded root length formation and a net loss of overall tooth length occurred (Fig. 6.3).

While the crown and reserve crown length decreased each year from 0 to 8 years following eruption, the rate of tooth loss was not constant. The rate of crown loss increased each year from 0 to 5 years and then decreased from 5 to 7 years following eruption. Similarly, the rate of root formation was highest from the time of eruption until 5 years after eruption and then decreased from 5 to 7 years of tooth age (Fig. 6.2). These results suggest that equine cheek teeth undergo an increased rate of attrition, an increased rate of eruption or both during the period of rapid root formation in the first 5 years following eruption. The results of this investigation indicated that crown loss due to masticatory wear was not constant, as has previously been reported, but was variable. This variable rate of crown loss may be influenced by the rate of root formation, the rate of eruption of reserve crown, a variance in tooth hardness or the amount of chewing.

The increased rate of control of coronal loss in cheek teeth during the first 5 years post eruption may contribute to the rapid reformation of enamel points following removal. Due to the staggered eruption times of the cheek teeth of the horse, individual horses from 1 to 9 years of age possess cheek teeth that are, in the first 5 years, relatively longer following eruption. Horses under the age of 9 years may, therefore, require more frequent oral examinations and dental flotations to remove enamel points.

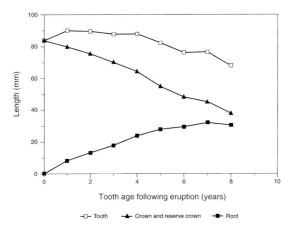

**Figure 6.1.** Mean tooth, crown and reserve crown, and root length (From Kirkland 1994, with permission).

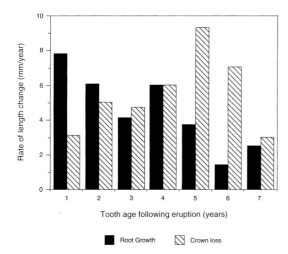

**Figure 6.2.** Rate of root formation and crown loss (From Kirkland 1994, with permission).

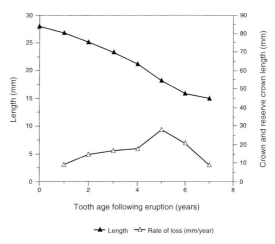

**Figure 6.3.** Crown length and rate of crown loss (From Kirkland 1994, with permission).

Mean occlusal length decreased at a constant rate in cheek teeth from 0 to 8 years of age (Fig. 6.4). This trend corresponds with the shape of equine cheek teeth which taper in circumference from the crown to the tooth end. As occlusal crown is lost due to wear, the tooth erupts a narrower reserve crown. This decrease in crown length over time shortens the mesial to distal length of the cheek teeth arcade and results in a shortened masticatory surface. This decreased surface area may be an important factor to consider in geriatric patients suffering weight loss and/or poor thrift. The eruption of intermittently narrower cheek tooth crowns may also be a factor in the increased incidence of periodontal disease in older horses.[2] As teeth of variable mesial to distal crown lengths make up the cheek tooth arcade of older horses, the integrity of the once tightly packed battery of teeth may be lost. The interproximal spaces, the space between two adjacent teeth, increase in size and may allow the areas to trap food and predispose the cheek teeth to gingivitis and periodontal disease.

Specific irregularities that are frequently seen include: rostral hooks (106 and 206) and caudal hooks (311 and 411) – these beak-like occlusal overgrowths develop as a result of incomplete occlusal contact (Fig. 6.5).[3] Hooks 106 and 206 may cause oral pain, bit-pressure points and buccal-surface calluses or ulcers. They are easily diagnosed and corrected by grinding or floating. Enamel points (enamel edges) – the folding

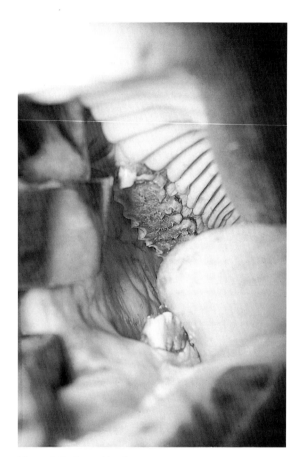

**Figure 6.5.** Rostral hook 106.

of the enamel organ and subsequent secretion of enamel in the unique pattern of the maxillary and mandibular teeth results in the appearance of enamel points on the buccal edges of the maxillary (Fig. 6.6) and the lingual edges of the mandibular cheek teeth. Incomplete full occlusal contact tends to exacerbate these points and, in turn, contact with the oral mucosa may lead to ulcers and callus formation (Fig. 6.7). Such areas may be sensitive to cheek pressure on palpation and on mouth opening and may subsequently lead to further abnormalities in chewing patterns and hence a compounding of the tooth-surface irregularities. Step mouth – absent teeth lead to mesial and distal movement of adjacent teeth and consequently changes in the conformation of the occlusal surfaces. Such overgrowth and points may result in bizarre occlusal patterns (Fig. 6.8). Large hooks on 311 and 411

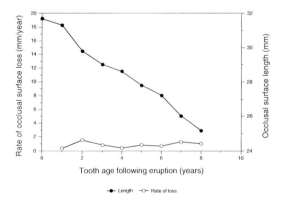

**Figure 6.4.** Occlusal length (308 mesial to distal) and rate of reduction post eruption (From Kirkland 1994 with permission).

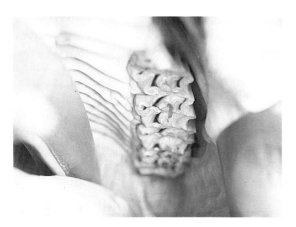

**Figure 6.6.** Enamel points, buccal margins of left maxillary arcade, Rostrol hook 206.

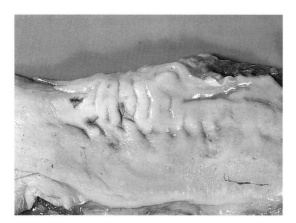

**Figure 6.7.** Buccal trauma resulting from presence of enamel points.

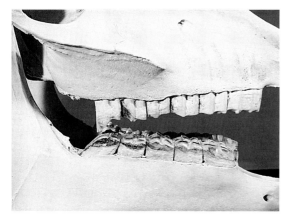

**Figure 6.8.** Irregular dental arcades following loss of 411.

may cause penetration of the palatine mucosa, ulcer formation and even, in rare cases, laceration of the palatine artery. If the occlusal defects persist, there may be rotation of adjacent or opposing teeth and an arcade alignment that will defy therapy short of exodontia. Wave mouth – this is the term that is used to describe a series of convex and concave changes of the teeth crowns and occlusal surfaces – usually with reciprocal concave and convex changes on the opposing arcade that may occur over time. It results in an inefficient grinding surface with a tendency for the slopes to become rather smooth. The severity, and perhaps irregularity, of the waves may be influenced by concomitant dental pathology – maleruptions, impactions or missing teeth – and also by the shape and size of the horse's head. Those animals that have a marked caudal slope along their mandibular arcades as a result of head shape will exacerbate the waves (e.g. ponies). Another contributing factor to wave formation is the presence of enamel lake cemental hypoplasia on 109 and 209 and from this, a tendency for the forces of attrition to cause these teeth to cup out. Ramps – this is the presence of more crown in a rising 'ramp' on 309–311 and 409–411. Both waves and ramps require careful evaluation and appropriate floating and grinding to correct the defects. In cases of abnormal wear, it may not be possible to decide the precise process that has resulted in some teeth becoming completely worn away and the opposing tooth overgrown. Does it indicate that there are changes in density or hardness of odd teeth so that a particularly 'soft' tooth is worn away while its opposing number super erupts (Fig. 6.9)? This is unlikely but it does show that the pathophysiology of chewing is complex and that irregularities of wear have a multifactorial etiopathogenesis. Shear mouth – this is an extreme form of cheek tooth malocclusion with reduction of the lingual surfaces of the maxillary teeth and buccal surfaces of the mandibular teeth. There is complimentary overgrowth of the buccal surfaces of the maxillary teeth and lingual surfaces of the mandibular teeth. The result is an extreme malalignment of the cheek teeth surfaces and extremely sharp and ineffective edges. This

73

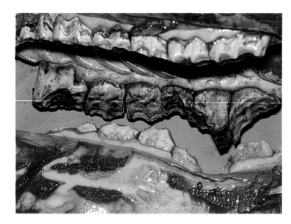

**Figure 6.9.** Gross irregularities of wear and associated periodontal pathology.

condition results in profound chewing dysfunction, loss of body condition and may lead to death. Management is not easy and requires multiple re-alignment and tooth reduction procedures as well as special diets.

It is frequently noted that there is very little accumulation of dental plaque and dental calculus on normal teeth of horses.[2,3] The exception to this observation is the presence of both plaque and calculus on the canine teeth. It is concluded that the normal frictional forces of chewing are extremely effective in keeping the surrounding tissues of the teeth of the horse healthy. Invariably, abnormal occlusal contact results in the formation of dental plaque and calculus.

## PERIODONTAL DISEASE

Periodontal disease is the presence of disease and loss of tissue in those structures that surround the tooth or teeth. Periodontium means around the tooth and in that sense is confined to the bony socket. In clinical practice the periodontium includes the alveolus (bony socket) cement, periodontal ligament and the gingivae. Diseases of the periodontal structures have been known since antiquity. Skulls of some ancient cave dwellers show evidence of chronic periodontal disease. An acute form, now known in man as acute necrotizing gingivitis or Vincent's infection, was reported at least as early as 400 BC in soldiers of the Greek army of Xenophon.[4]

Clarification of various periodontal diseases is difficult as nearly every case begins as a minor localized disturbance which, unless adequately treated, gradually worsens until the alveolar bone is resorbed and the tooth is exfoliated. This means that a variety of etiological stimuli may produce similar end-stage pathology and so the true etiopathogenesis may not be defined. In human medicine the descriptive pathological reports of John Hunter were the basis of all subsequent analyses of periodontal disease.[5]

The term parodontal disease was used in human dental pathology[5] and introduced into veterinary literature to describe gingival and dental disease processes in dogs and horses in 1939 and continued in 1948 and 1960.[6,7,8] It was subsequently concluded, after reviewing the literature and referring to the classifications of periodontal disease in man that the generic term periodontal disease is the most suitable term to use in veterinary dental pathology and clinics.[9]

Pathology of the periodontium may be grouped in four categories (American Academy of Periodontology, 1957)

1. inflammation (gingivitis, periodontitis)
2. dystrophy (gingivosis, periodontosis)
3. neoplastic
4. anomalies.

All four categories are known to occur in the horse, but most information is available for category 1, inflammatory periodontal disease. Periodontal inflammation has been recognized for years as being important in the horse. It was suggested that 'quidding' was a pathognomatic sign of periodontal disease or alveolar periostitis.[10] In those observations, it was noted that the lesions start primarily in the interproximal areas of the teeth and the caudal mandibular spaces were most affected. In an examination of 50 equine skulls in the 1930s, 30 per cent were found to be affected with periodontal disease.[5] In that study it was concluded that the disease was initiated by gingival trauma caused by the feeding of coarse chaff. Repeated observations in the 1970s and 1990s in the UK and USA have shown similar high prevalence levels of the disease.[3,9] It was found that in an examination of the teeth and gums of 218 and 446 skulls, the incidence of periodontal disease changed with age. There was a 40 per cent prevalence in horses 3–5 years of age, this fell in horses 5–10 years of age, and then increased to 60 per cent in horses over the age of 15 years (Fig. 6.10).

Work in other species, dogs in particular, has shown that dental work is necessary for the maintenance of the health of the gingival mucosa. Studies in ferrets[11] and dogs[12,13] concluded that the frictional forces associated with chewing hard substances was sufficient to keep the teeth free of dental scale and the gums in a healthy state.

The physiological process of eruption of the permanent dentition is responsible for the frequency of periodontal disease seen in younger horses. It suggests that at least some levels of periodontal pathology will resolve once normal occlusion is achieved by the permanent dentition. Thereby reinforcing the concept that the detection and correction of abnormalities of wear is a key factor in the prevention of periodontal disease.

In man at least there is an increasing body of evidence linking the presence of periodontal disease to numerous other serious diseases. In the UK it was found that there was an association between poor oral health and overall mortality in that there was an increase in risk (mortality) of 2.6 in patients with poor oral

health (periodontal disease) when compared to those with good oral health.[14] Consequently, it is common in periodontic practice in man to supplement antibiotic coverage as a prophylaxis against cerebral and myocardial infarctions during periodontal treatment and periodontal surgery.[14]

Numerous studies have attempted to show similar correlations in other animals without definitive proof. One study involving blood cultures in horses undergoing tooth extractions and periodontal curettage failed to prove that periodontal surgery resulted in bacteremias.[3]

## PERIODONTAL ANATOMY AND FUNCTION

Each tooth is independently and firmly attached to the bony structure (alveolus) within the bones of the head. The teeth are attached by bundles of connective tissue fibers referred to as the periodontal membrane or ligament (Figs 6.11a and b).

The arrangement of fibers in the periodontal ligament is complex. Dense bundles of collagen run in various directions from the bone of the socket wall to the cement covering the reserve crowns and the tooth roots. The embedded portions of the collagen bundles are referred to as Sharpeys fibers. In general, the fibers are arranged in such a fashion that occlusal forces, pressures, are translated into longitudinal forces on the fibers to provide resistance. The periodontal ligament contains blood vessels and nerves. The arrangement of the collagen fibers protects the vessels from occlusal pressure that might result in ischemia. In this way the tooth is suspended firmly within the alveolus and at the same time it is permitted some slight movement.

The gingiva have a mucous membrane surface with dense internal fibrous attachment to the periosteum. Extending from the epithelial attachment of the gum to the crown of the tooth is a free margin of gum enclosing the gingival margin of the gum, the gingival sulcus (crevice). The interdental gingival tissue is referred to as the col. The col is covered with a non-keratinized epithelium. The free gingiva 'sticks'

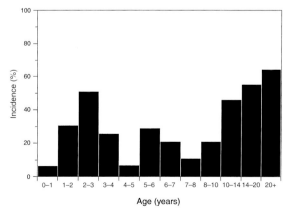

**Figure 6.10.** Prevalence of periodontal disease in 416 skulls related to age.

**DENTAL DISEASE AND PATHOLOGY**

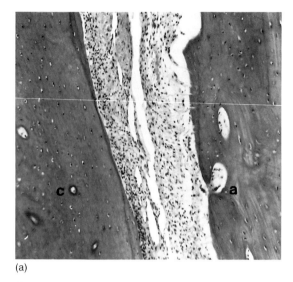

(a)

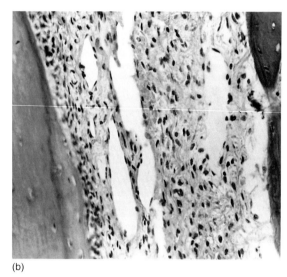

(b)

**Figure 6.11.** (a) Periodontal ligament: c = cementum, a = alveolar bone, decalcified H and E ×110. (b) Periodontal ligament, H and E ×250.

to the crown of the tooth by surface tension. It is customary to use the terms sub- and supragingival to refer to the locations below and above the gum line. If and when the gingival sulcus deepens in periodontal disease, it is referred to as a periodontal pocket (perio pocket). In examining and charting oral and dental disease, it is common practice to measure the depths of these pockets in millimeters.

## CLINICAL SIGNS OF PERIODONTAL DISEASE IN THE HORSE

Gingival hyperemia, edema, ulceration, deepening periodontal pockets and packing of feed material into these spaces are the classic pictures of periodontal disease (Figs 6.12, 6.13, 6.14). It is necessary, of course, to carry out a thorough examination of the mouth to detect such conditions (see Chapter 9). There will be both supra- and subgingival plaque and calculus deposits associated with these lesions. Periodontal disease in the horse has been divided into four categories[3] based on evaluation of the severity of the lesion:

1  local gingivitis with hyperemia and edema
2  erosion of gingival margin 5 mm and periodontal pocket

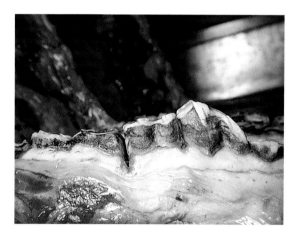

**Figure 6.12.** Gingival hyperemia and edema.

3  periodontitis with loss of gum
4  gross periodontal pocketing, lysis of alveolar bone, loosening of bone support (Fig. 6.15)

Horses with grades 1 and 2 periodontal disease may not show overt signs of oral discomfort. The careful owner may notice some excess salivation and a sensitivity to cold water. Halitosis is the pathognomic sign for severe periodontal disease in the horse and for this reason the use of disposable gloves is recommended when examining the oral cavity of the horse.

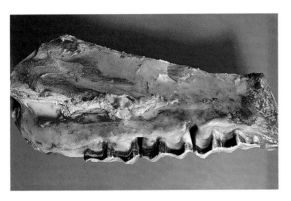

**Figure 6.13.** Periodontal pocketing.

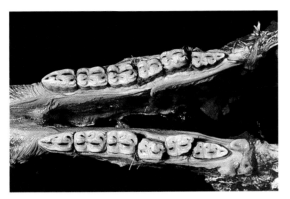

**Figure 6.14.** Gross pocketing with food impactions.

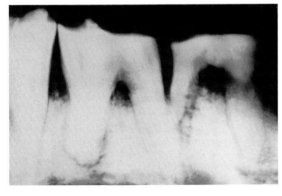

**Figure 6.15.** Grade IV periodontitis with loss of alveolar bone – radiological appearance.

## ETIOLOGY OF PERIODONTAL DISEASE

The role of normal dental work in maintaining the health of periodontal structures has been documented in most mammals. It therefore is

not surprising that abnormalities of wear associated with tooth eruptions in young horses and arcade irregularities in older horses are the most common initiating factors in the pathogenesis of periodontal disease in the horse.

Other factors influence the development and progression of periodontal disease and it is commonly described as being a multifactorial infection.[15] Some of these factors include plaque, oral microflora and calculus, as well as age, general health, chewing patterns, breed, immune status and local irritants (e.g. grass awns).

Plaque is an organic matrix made up of salivary glycoproteins and contains oral bacteria as well as inorganic material derived from feed materials. Bacterial fermentation within this layer releases free radicals and material that results in injury to the gingiva and within the gingival sulcus. Aerobic bacteria are more prevalent in supragingival plaque and facultative anaerobes live in the sulcus. Bacterial numbers and types change in the presence of initial gingival inflammation and the 'domino' cycle of

inflammation → plaque build up → hyperemia

↑

loss of tooth                                    ↓

↑

bone loss   ←   loss of support   ←   edema
                                        tissue

is initiated.

In advanced disease, there is significant loss of alveolar bone. Periodontal inflammation may result in attempted repair with the production of excess cementum over the surface of the reserve crown – in some cases this may progress to a form of hypercementosis and the production of nodules of cementum.

## TREATMENT

The horse is no exception to the general rule of periodontologists that states that prevention is better than treatment. Once gum recession and loss has occurred, it is not possible to undertake a treatment regime that will result in re-attachment of gum and a reduction of gingival pocket size in the horse. Consequently, the

DENTAL DISEASE AND PATHOLOGY

equine clinicians role is to eliminate irregularities of wear, oral ulcers and other conditions that may initiate the progressive process of periodontal pathology (see Chapter 13).

In horses with major irregularities of wear and advanced periodontal pocketing treatment is aimed at restoring, as closely as possible, normal or near normal occlusion. Loose teeth should be extracted, periodontal pockets irrigated and opened where possible, i.e. enlarged so as to discourage food impactions in these areas.

## SUMMARY

Irregularities of wear and periodontal disease have been described as the scourge of the horse in the era of horse transport and farming.[5] These observations of the early nineteenth century have been re-examined and it is clear that although there has been an improvement in the general health of the horse in the past 60 years, irregularities of wear and periodontal disease are still extremely common.

### REFERENCES

1. Kirkland KD (1994) *The morphology of the endodontic system reserve crown and roots of equine mandibular cheek teeth*. MS Thesis, University of Illinois, pp. 24–102.
2. Baker GJ (1979) *A study of dental disease in the horse*. PhD Thesis, University of Glasgow, pp. 42–56.
3. Becker E (1962) Dental disease in the horse. In: *Handbook of Special Pathology of Domestic Animals*, ed. Joest, Paul Parey, Berlin, pp. 642–651.
4. Shafer WG, Hine MK and Levy BM (1963) *A Textbook of Oral Pathology* (2nd edn). WB Saunders, Philadelphia.
5. Colyer F (1931) Abnormal conditions of the teeth of animals in their relationship to similar conditions in man. The Dental Board of the United Kingdom, London, pp. 38–43.
6. Wright JG (1939) Some observations on dental disease in the dog. *Veterinary Record*, 51, 409–421.
7. Shuttleworth AC (1948) Dental disease of horses. *Veterinary Record*, 60, 563–567.
8. Hofmeyer CFB (1960) Comparative dental pathology (with particular reference to caries and parodontal disease in the horse and dog). *Journal of the South African Veterinary Medical Association* 29, 417–480.
9. Baker GJ (1970) Some aspects of dental disease. *Equine Veterinary Journal*, 2, 105–110.
10. Little WM (1913) Periodontal disease in the horse. *Journal of Comparative Pathology and Therapeutics*, 24, 240–249.
11. King JD (1947) Experimental investigations of parodontal disease. *British Dental Journal*, 82, 61–69.
12. Brown MG and Park JF (1968) Control of dental calculus in experimental beagles. *Laboratory Animal Care*, 18, 527–535.
13. Lindhe J, Hamp SE and Loe H (1973) Experimental periodontitis in the beagle dog. *Journal of Periodontal Research*, 3, 1.
14. DeStefano F, Andra RF, Kahn HS *et al.* (1993) Dental disease and risk of coronary heart disease and mortality. *British Medicine*, 306, 688.
15. Wiggs RB and Lobrise HB (1997) Periodontology. In: *Veterinary Dentistry Principles and Practice*, eds, RB Wiggs and HB Lobrise, Lippincott-Raven, Philadelphia.

# DENTAL DECAY AND ENDODONTIC DISEASE

Gordon J Baker, BVSc, PhD., MRCVS, Diplomate ACVS, University of Illinois, College of Veterinary Medicine, Urbana, IL 61802

## INTRODUCTION

In many species and particularly in man dental caries is the most common cause of dental decay. Caries is a disease of the calcified tissues of the teeth characterized by a demineralization of the inorganic, and a destruction of the organic, substance of the tooth. In ancient times, dental caries was associated with the idea of worms in or around the teeth. It was believed that the gastric juice from a pig would expel worms – as large as earthworms – from a decayed tooth. Gallen believed that dental caries was produced by an abnormal condition of the blood that affected the internal structure of the tooth.[1]

Dental caries does occur in the horse, but the term has been subjected to various interpretations based on etiopathogenesis.[2–10] In this chapter dental decay, as it occurs in the horse, will be reviewed and the pathophysiology of endodontic disease (e.g. pulpitis) illustrated and analyzed.

## DENTAL CARIES

Working in Koch's laboratory in 1889, Miller found that organisms from carious dentin produced lactic acid when cultured with starch or with sugar.[11] From these observations, he formulated the 'chemico-parasitic' theory of dental caries:

> Dental decay is a chemico-parasitic process consisting of two stages, the decalcification of enamel, which results in its total destruction, and the decalcification of dentin as a prelim-inary stage, followed by dissolution of the softened residue. The acid which affects this primary decalcification is derived from the fermentation of starches and sugar lodged in the retaining centers of the teeth.
>
> (Miller, 1889, p. 72)

In the past 100 years, many, many studies have detailed this process giving us the role of specific bacteria, the microscopic, transmission and electron microscopic appearance and the prophylaxis of dental caries in man.[12]

The bulk of scientific evidence does implicate carbohydrates, oral micro-organisms and acids in dental caries. A proven relationship was made in human caries between prevalence and the acid-producing bacterium *Lactobacillus acidophilus*.[13] Under laboratory conditions, dental caries in hamsters and rats was considered to be an infectious and transmissible disease. Pure cultures of streptococci isolated from hamster caries would induce the typical picture of active caries in other hamsters.[14] The transmissible and infectious nature was confirmed in gnotobiotic rats. In a study in which gnotobiotic rats were fed on a coarse-particle, high-sugar diet which would produce dental caries in normal animals, the subjects (gnotobiotes) did not develop caries. However, a single strain of oral streptococcus isolated from a control rat on the same diet and introduced into the gnotobiotic animals resulted in caries development.[15]

Cariogenic acid is produced beneath the macrobacterial layer which forms on the surface of the tooth, plaque. There is a significant difference in the pH of plaque in carious teeth and non-carious teeth (5.5 and 7.1 respectively).[16] It has been proposed that there may be two forms of caries pathogenesis. In one type, micro-organisms invade the enamel lamellae, attach to the enamel and involve the dentin before there is clinical evidence of caries. In the other, bacteria in the dental plaque form acids which decalcify the enamel prior to invasion by micro-organisms.

In apparent conflict with acid production and lowering of pH, it was also noted that by proteolysis-chelation, demineralization of enamel could occur at a neutral or even alkaline pH.[17] This process is brought about by an initial breakdown of the protein and other components of the enamel, chiefly keratin by keratinolytic micro-organisms. In this way, soluble chelates are formed with the mineralized component of the tooth and decalcification results. It can, therefore, be concluded that it is possible for the initial attack to be on both the organic and inorganic portions of the tooth simultaneously.

Horse caries (dissolution of the calcified tissues of the teeth) occurs under a number of circumstances. In some environments, and under some feeding programs, foods that are cariogenic (i.e. caries forming) may adhere to the tooth crowns. The use of sweet foods, the high sugar content of molasses or the by-products of sweet-potato-processing plants produce a cariogenic diet. Consequently there is surface erosion – particularly of the incisor teeth labial surfaces – that is directly caused by bacterial fermentation and acid production (below 7.1 pH) within the adherent dental plaque. The surfaces become mottled and may be discolored with exposed dentin (Fig. 7.1).

In other sections of this textbook, the process of cement formation – both peripheral and within the incisor and maxillary cheek teeth infundibula have been discussed (Chapter 4). It has been frequently misinterpreted that infundibular cemental hypoplasia is in fact caries. Histopathological examination, however, reveals that this is not the case. It has been suggested that 'an open infundibulum' is the cause of the dental decay.[18] Clearly this concept is at fault in

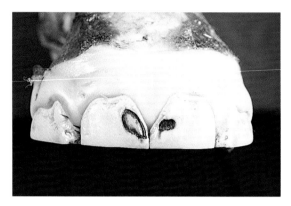

**Figure 7.1.** Carious lesions of deciduous incisors.

that all maxillary and incisor teeth have open infundibula – the channel that represents the vascular pathway to cementogenesis. The belief that cemental hypoplasia is of major pathological significance has even encouraged people to 'fill' these defects.[19] Despite the confusion over the incidence and significance of maxillary cheek teeth cemental hypoplasia, there is no doubt that the presence of feed material impacted into areas of hypoplastic cement does create the potential for bacterial fermentation, acid production and caries of cement to be initiated. No data are available as to the prevalence of caries of cement as distinct from cemental hypoplasia in the horse. Perhaps the interesting question is why we do not see a greater incidence of carious pathology associated with cemental hypoplasia in the horse. It has been suggested that although conditions exist for acid production at this location, it may not occur because of the hostile microclimate that exists in this region during life.[5] More research work needs to be directed toward this problem.

The complexities of pathologic bacterial fermentation within the periodontal structures of horses with periodontal disease may result in dental caries. This analysis leads to the concept of four forms of dental caries in the horse:

1 caries of cement from the occlusal surface
2 caries of peripheral cement
3 caries of root cement originating from purulent periodontitis
4 caries from an open pulp cavity.[5]

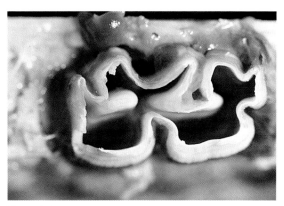

**Figure 7.2**

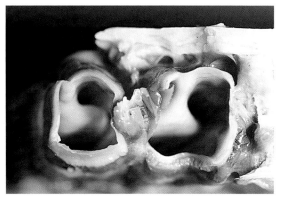

**Figure 7.3**

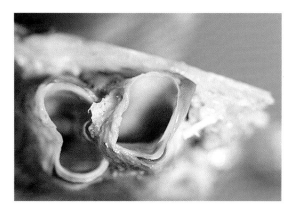

**Figure 7.4**

**Figure 7.2, 7.3, 7.4.** Developing root ends over two years. Note changes in pulp chamber shape and root formation.

It is also clear that conditions that interfere with the normal 'cleansing' action of the frictional forces of the chewing cycle will create tooth surface conditions that predispose to carious

demineralization. It is, therefore, not surprising that there is a complex and interdependent relationship between dental and oral pathology in the horse, for example, malformation, maleruption, fracture, irregularities of wear, periodontal disease and dental decay.

## ENDODONTIC DISEASE

The pulp cavities of teeth have a multicellular morphology and a vital role in the formation of the teeth and the maintenance of the health of the teeth. Dental pulp is seen to develop as a condensation of connective tissues under the inner enamel epithelium at the bell stage of tooth embryology (dental papilla). At an extremely early stage, odontoblasts are differentiated from cells in the pulp and they, in turn, begin to secrete a collagenous matrix. This matrix is known as predentin or uncalcified dentin or dentinoid and represents the beginning of hard tissue formation of the tooth.[20] Tissues within the dental papilla continue to elaborate and the definitive structure of the dental pulp is established. The dental pulp contains odontoblasts, collagen and elastic fibers, and as they form, nerve tissue and vascular channels. Fibroblasts, histiocytes, mast cells, polymorphonuclear leukocytes, lymphocytes, plasma cells and eosinophils are also found in dental pulp – the majority of these latter cells are present under conditions of inflammation. It appears that a low-grade inflammatory response is a normal histologic feature of dental pulp and reflects the physiologic response of dental tissues.

The pulp chambers change in size and shape with age and also in response to crown attrition and tooth root formation.[21] In the incisors and canines, the pulp chamber is a simple cone with a single root apex. Mandibular and maxillary teeth have more complex pulp chamber shapes. Mandibular teeth have, initially, a common pulp chamber with five coronal extensions and two large root openings. As the horse ages there is, eventually, separation of the two root systems, but it is not yet defined how consistent these separations are related to age. One study suggests that for at least 3 years post eruption, there is still a connection between the pulp chamber as related to the mesial and distal roots.[21] Transverse sections of the reserve crowns of the maxillary cheek teeth also show five coronal extensions of the pulp chamber. When casts of the pulp chamber are made, these coronal extensions give the appearance of tentacles arising from a pre-root common chamber and the apical extensions of the true roots (Figs 7.2, 7.3, 7.4 and 7.5). Maxillary teeth have three roots. Details of root apex structure are not available for the horse. In most species, the pulp chamber within the root apices is complex and is referred to as the apical delta. Standard patterns include two or three side branches to give the appearance of a branching river delta.

As horses age, we recognize a number of changes within the pulp chamber. These can be summarized as a decrease in the cellular components, a tendency for dentinal sclerosis and a decrease in the number and quality of blood vessels and nerves. The most important change, however, is a reduction in size and volume of the pulp chamber as a result of the deposition of secondary, and in some cases reparative, dentin. In hypsodont teeth, where there is a pattern of occlusal attrition and, under normal conditions, a matching continuous eruption of reserve crown, it should be clear that without formation of secondary tissue there would be exposure of the pulp cavity. This tissue is secondary dentin and it is formed circumferentially throughout the life of a vital tooth. The mechanism that results in the formation of secondary dentin is complex and its production is initiated by signals transmitted to the pulp through the dentinal tubules. Dentinal sclerosis occurs when the tubules become filled with mineral deposits.[22] This is part of the aging process of the tooth and explains why rates of tooth attrition (the 'wear away' rate) decrease with age, i.e. teeth become more dense with age. Signals that stimulate physiologic secondary dentin production include pressure, temperature and chemical signals.

In the presence of inflammation, the pulp defense mechanism includes the mobilization of histiocytes and their conversion to defensive macrophages. Inflammatory changes result in the release of agents that change capillary and venule blood flow within the pulp. There may be an increase in arteriovenous anastomosis blood flow so that pulp ischemic changes develop, i.e. there appears to be an increase of blood flow within the tooth but the flow bypasses vital tissues of the pulp and ischemia and pulp necrosis results.[23] Because the pulp has no collateral circulation it is particularly vulnerable to this type of injury – as are the lamellae of the foot and hoof. Under such conditions there is again stimulation of pulp odontoblasts, and as a result the production of reparative dentin (this may, in some teeth, be referred to as secondary dentin, irritation dentin or tertiary dentin). Reparative dentin has a variable quality depending on the severity of the inflammatory insult.

Pulpitis in the horse may be caused by a number of factors. Trauma to the mouth and teeth may result in overt and covert tooth fractures which in turn will create periodontal lysis and periapical pathology. Tooth crown fractures and dental procedures, such as the cutting of overgrown teeth, may also penetrate the pulp chambers. It can be stated that under normal occlusal contact and wear, the pulp chambers of the horse do not reach above the gum line. However, care must be taken when working on overgrown teeth because there is a reduction in the rate of production of secondary dentin and consequently accidental pulp exposure can be a problem. When acute pulp exposure happens, particular techniques are needed to retain pulp vitality (see Chapter 6). It is also clear that other

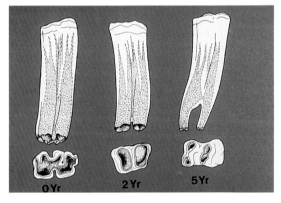

**Figure 7.5.** Representation of the maturation changes that occur in mandibular pulp chambers.

forms of dental work effect the dental pulp. It has been suggested that some human dental procedures are in fact 'cooking the pulp in its own juices'.[23] In recent years there has been an increase in the development and availability of power tools for dental work in the horse. It is important that we recognize the consequences of the thermal effects of power equipment. It should always be accompanied by the use of some coolant, for example an attached, continuous water spray. It is interesting to note that in those species in which pulp responses to thermal effects have been documented there is no safe speed and, in fact, at low rpm rates (under 50 000) there are major changes in odontoblastic effect.

Figure 7.6 is a schematic representation of the possible sequelae of pulpitis in the horse.[5] It can be appreciated that the end result of pulpitis for example dental fistula, facial swelling and sinus empyema, is based not on the specifics of the pulp disease, but more on the location of the tooth. It is then the local response to the periapical disease that results in the specifics of individual cases and the particular clinical signs that are seen. A constant feature of pulpitis is dental pain. Pain receptors in the pulp are stimulated either directly when exposed, or indirectly via the odontoblast process. Pain is reduced in chronic disease such that in teeth affected by

pulpitis, apical osteitis and draining mandibular fistulae may not demonstrate a painful reaction when stimulated.

In case studies on dental extractions for dental decay, it is noted that the teeth most frequently affected are the 8's (i.e. 108, 208, 308, 408).[5] It has been inferred that the effect of delayed and impacted eruptions accounts for major vascular changes in the pulp and subsequent anachoretic pulpitis.[24] In this condition, bacteria are attracted to the inflamed pulp through the dentinal tubules.

Diagnosis of pulpitis in the horse is relatively simple when there is traumatic exposure of the pulp. In most cases, however, the veterinarian does not see the horse until there are fairly advanced clinical signs such as facial or mandibular swelling, fistula formation and loosening of teeth. Radiology is of major importance in documenting the presence of pathological changes resulting from pulpitis and periradicular (around the root) disease (see Chapter 11). The clinician may, however, be misled in the appearance of certain radiographic phenomena in that they are susceptible to multiple interpretations including apical radiolucency. In one study, three endodontists made radiographic interpretations of some 250 films and re-examined the same films 6 to 8 weeks later. They agreed with their own interpretation only 72 per cent of the time.[25] In an earlier study, six endodontists agreed with each other less than 50 per cent of the time.[26]

Techniques that are available in other species to test for pulp sensitivity and viability such as thermal (hot and cold) pressure and electrical testing have not been used in the horse. There are, however, some indications that these tests will be used in the future as endodontic therapies become more widely adopted.

## SUMMARY

Dental decay in the horse is a consequence of the loss of pulpal blood supply, either from direct trauma, usually acute, or from the inflammatory disease processes associated with pulpitis. The clinical signs depend upon both the chronicity of the disease process and the

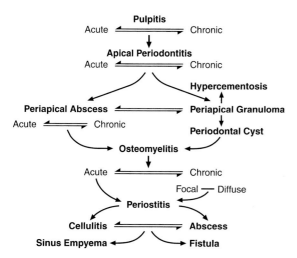

**Figure 7.6.** Representation of the potential sequelae of pulpitis in the horse.

location of the tooth. In teeth with reserve crowns and roots that are not within the maxillary sinuses the signs relate to apical osteitis and drainage through the surrounding bone and skin e.g. teeth 308 and 408 and the development of mandibular dental fistulae. In some cases there may also be drainage into the oral cavity. Commonly, dental decay of teeth with reserve crowns and roots within the maxillary sinuses is associated with sinus empyema.

A thorough understanding of the biological behaviour of pulp, its response to physical and chemical trauma and the production of secondary dentin, is key to the diagnosis of dental decay and effective case management.

## REFERENCES

1. Guerini V (1909) *A History of Dentistry*. Lea and Febiger, Philadelphia, pp. 12–48.
2. Hofmeyer CFB (1960) Comparative dental pathology (with particular reference to caries and paradontal disease in the horse and dog). *Journal of the South African Veterinary Medical Association*, 29, 471–480.
3. Homma K, Yamakarvi M, Yamouchi S and Hosoya S (1962) Statistical study on the occurrence of dental caries in domestic animals. The Horse. *Japanese, Journal of Veterinary Research*, 10, 31–36.
4. Baker GJ (1974) Some aspects of equine dental decay. *Equine Veterinary Journal*, 6, 127–130.
5. Baker GJ (1979) *A study of dental disease in the horse*. PhD Thesis, University of Glasgow, pp. 66–87.
6. Wafa NSW (1989) *A study of dental disease in the horse*. MVM Thesis, University College of Dublin, pp. 62–72.
7. Easely KJ (1991) Recognition and management of the diseased tooth. *37th American Association of Equine Practitioners Convention Proceedings*, 120–139.
8. Mueller POE (1991) Equine dental disorders: cause, diagnosis and treatment. *Compendium on Continuing Education for the Practicing Veterinarian*, 13, 1451–1461.
9. Dixon PM (1997) Dental extractions in horses: indications and pre-operative evaluation. *Compendium on Continuing Education for the Practicing Veterinarian*, 19, 366–375.
10. Dixon PM (1997) Dental extraction and endodontic techniques in horses. *Compendium on Continuing Education for the Practicing Veterinarian*, 19, 628–638.
11. Miller WD (1889) *Die Mikroorganismen des mundhole*. Liepzig, pp. 163–182.
12. Shafer WG, Hine MK and Levy BM (1963) *A textbook of oral pathology*, (2nd edn). WB Saunders, Philadelphia, pp. 308–377.
13. Bunting RW (1928) Studies of the relation of *Bacillus acidophilus* to dental caries. *Journal of Dental Research*, 8, 222–229.
14. Keyes PH (1960) The infectious and transmissible nature of experimental dental caries. *Archives of Oral Biology*, 1, 304–409.
15. Fitzgerald RJ, Jordan HV and Stanley HR (1960) Experimental caries and gingival pathologic changes in the gnotobiotic rat. *Journal of Dental Research*, 39, 923–930.
16. Stephan RM (1940) Changes in H-ion concentrations on tooth substance and carious lesions. *Journal of Dental Research*, 27, 576–582.
17. Jenkins GN (1961) A critique of the proteolysis-chelation theory of caries. *British Dental Journal*, 111, 311–319.
18. Frank FR (1964) *Veterinary Surgery* (7th edn). Burgen Publishing, Minneapolis, pp. 69–74.
19. Swanstrom OG and Wallford HA (1977) *Prosthetic filling of a cement defect in premolar tooth necrosis in a horse*. Veterinary Medicine/Small Animal Clinicians, 1475–1477.
20. Seltzer S and Bender IB (1990) The dental pulp biologic considerations in dental procedures (3rd edn). Ishiyaken EuroAmerica, St Louis, 1–38.
21. Kirkland KD, Baker GJ, Marretta SM, Eurell JAC and Losonsky JM (1996) Effect of aging on the endodontic system, reserve crown and roots of equine mandibular cheek teeth. *American Journal of Veterinary Research*, 57, 31–38.
22. Stanley HR *et al.* (1983) The detection and prevalence of reactive and physiologic sclerotic dentin, reparative dentin and dead tracts beneath various types of dental lesions according to tooth surface and age. *Journal of Oral Pathology*, 12, 257.
23. Kim S and Trowbridge P (1998) Pulpal reaction to caries and dental procedures. In: *Pathways of the Pulp* (7th edn), eds S Cohen and RC Burns, Mosby, St Louis, Chapter 15, 532–551.
24. Gutmann JL and Harrison JW (1991) *Surgical Endodontics*. Blackwell Scientific Publishers, Boston. pp. 316–383.
25. Goldman M, Pearson A and Darzenta N (1974) Reliability of radiographic interpretations. *Oral Surgery*, 34, 287.
26. Goldman M, Pearson A and Darzenta N (1972) Endodontic success – who's reading the radiograph. *Oral Surgery*, 32, 432.

# 8

# ORAL AND DENTAL TUMORS

Derek C Knottenbelt, BVM&S, DVM&S, MRCVS, Division of Equine Studies, Department of Veterinary Clinical Studies, University of Liverpool, Leahurst, Merseyside L64 7TE

## INTRODUCTION

Tumors of the teeth and oral cavity are relatively uncommon in the horse. Most reports are of single cases rather than series involving several or more. Surveys of equine neoplasia have shown that most of the oral tumors are very rare.[1-6] However, when they do occur they are often important and can be life threatening.[7] Furthermore, as most are not noticed in the early stages even by the most astute owners many are in an advanced state when first presented. This makes the general diagnosis of neoplasia relatively straightforward.[8] However, the gross appearance of many of the masses is remarkably similar and the definitive diagnosis is heavily reliant on histological examination.[9] Confirmation of the exact nature of the tumor may be seriously compromised by concurrent long-standing infections or granulation tissue proliferation. The classification of oral or dental masses is also complicated by the existence of some tumor-like conditions that have many of the clinical features of a neoplasm. Indeed some masses have histological features which support a diagnosis of neoplasia but are, in fact, not cancerous.[10,11,12] For example fibrous metaplasia of the nasal region and hard palate have been described[13,14] and benign neoplastic growths are seen occasionally in association with abnormal germinal tissue of tooth roots.[15] There are also several developmental cystic conditions (such as sinus cysts and conchal cysts) which are sometimes classified as neoplastic but this may not

be entirely justifiable on histological grounds. It is uncertain how these masses develop and their classification is also uncertain. They are however, relatively common compared to true oral or dental neoplasia. Some non-neoplastic conditions such as granulation tissue and hamartomata can present the clinical impression of neoplasia. The variable classification of this type of reaction also makes for difficult initial assessment of the tumors and biopsy is often the only way of establishing the true nature of the mass. Even then however, there are often difficulties as some tumors fall into the undifferentiated or unclassifiable myxoma and spindle cell tumor group[16] which have ill-defined histological characteristics and variable clinical features.

Although there have been some advances in therapeutic options the low incidence of these conditions makes it almost impossible to define the best approach to a specific type of tumor and effective comparative efficacy studies for the various modalities are at best difficult. Treatment options may also be affected by the delayed detection of tumors. Many have a benign character but their size may make it impossible to treat by any currently available means. Clinicians frequently have to make compromises from the ideal treatment options.

In common with other neoplasia, oral and dental tumors can be classified according to their origins[17] (dental, bone, soft tissue) and their behavior (benign/malignant, invasive,

85

proliferative or ulcerative). The prognosis for a particular case is often the primary objective of the clinician. Owners of horses with neoplastic disease are generally more concerned with the prognosis than with the disease itself but some will expect treatment to be successful in every case. As all the conditions are rare it is difficult to provide any realistic and objective assessment of prognosis with or without treatment. While in some cases the course of the condition is relatively predictable the outlook in the large majority is entirely unpredictable.

Oral neoplasia can involve the tissues of:

- teeth (odontogenic tumors)
- bone (osteogenic tumors)
- soft tissues (Fig. 8.1).

## TUMORS OF DENTAL TISSUE ORIGIN (ODONTOGENIC TUMORS)

Tumors in this category are all rare although it has been suggested that they are more common in horses than in other species.[18] Odontogenic tumors are classified according to the inductive effect of one dental tissue on the others.[19] These tumors are almost always benign but are often

locally invasive and aggressive in character. As a general rule dental tumors are best treated by wide surgical removal (to ensure complete ablation of tumor and abnormal tissue) at an early stage in their development when such surgery has a chance of success. In most cases however, the masses are not recognized sufficiently early and so recurrences are common in spite of attempts at wide surgical excision.[20] Most bone and dental tumors are benign in nature but can have serious secondary effects such as nasal obstruction, dental deformity resulting in dysmastication and weight loss, and facial deformity. A summary of the features of odontogenic tumors is shown in Table 8.1.

## AMELOBLASTOMA AND AMELOBLASTIC ODONTOMA

Also known as syn. adamantinoma, odonto-ameloblastoma and enameloblastoma.

### Definition

These tumors are derived from odontogenic epithelial remnants of the tooth germ cells with

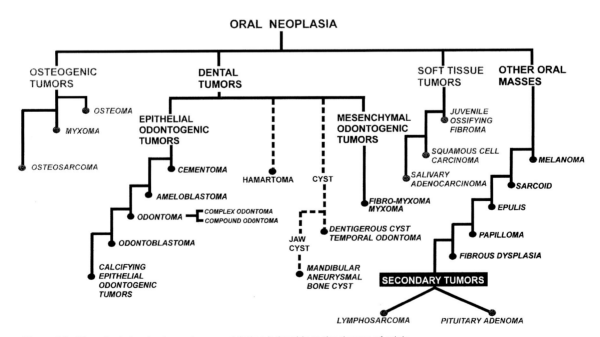

**Figure 8.1.** Flow chart showing tumor types and their relationship to the tissues of origin.

**Table 8.1.** Summary of features of odontogenic tumors based on published characteristics[3,5,34]

| Tumor type | Age group affected | Malignancy | Best treatment option | Prognosis |
|---|---|---|---|---|
| Ameloblastoma | >10 years | benign/locally invasive | surgical excision/ hemimandibulectomy +/− radiation | fair–good |
| Ameloblastic odontoma | < 3 years | benign/locally invasive | surgical excision/ hemimandibulectomy +/− radiation | fair–good |
| Cementoma | Onset uncertain | benign | surgical removal | good |
| Complex odontoma | < 5 years | benign malformation | surgical removal | fair (if removal feasible) |
| Compound odontoma | < 5 years | benign malformation | surgical removal | fair (if removal feasible) |
| Cysts/hamartoma | Various | benign | surgical removal | fair (if removal feasible) |

a fibrous stroma. True ameloblastoma tumors have no inductive changes in the connective tissue and so have no dentin and enamel. The ameloblastic odontoma has a marked simultaneous development of mineralized dental tissues in the tumor including enamel, dentin and epithelium.[19] For clinical purposes the tumors can be grouped together.

## Occurrence

They are more common in the mandibular region of older horses[21–26] but can involve the maxilla and the medullary cavity of the mandible. They have also been found occasionally in the maxillary region.[27] Several cases have also been reported in young foals.[28,29] The reports suggest that ameloblastoma occurs more frequently in the mandible of older horses while ameloblastic odontoma is more often found in the maxilla of younger animals.[30]

## Pathogenesis and histopathological features

These can be recognized histologically by having a mixed proliferative tumor-like appearance with dentin, enamel, pulp tissue and epithelial characteristics. Some have an expanding and destructive nature.

## Clinical features

They may be overtly tooth-like or very mixed, uncoordinated masses of tissue with no obvious tooth tissues. They often develop a cystic central region and cause solid or bony swellings and abnormalities in the associated dental arcade (Fig. 8.2). Occasionally they can present with a discharging sinus onto the side of the face.

## Differential diagnosis

Juvenile ossifying fibroma and other bone tumors of the jaw such as squamous cell carcinoma and myxoma and myxofibroma should also be considered (although the latter tend to be destructive rather than proliferative). Osteosarcoma is singularly rare in the horse. Infections of the tooth roots and adjacent bone can be similar but are associated with extensive necrosis and typical radiographic features often complicated by metaplastic calcification of the maxilla with obvious facial swelling. Jaw fractures and other dental abnormalities including malerupting and supernumerary cheek teeth should also be considered.

## Diagnostic confirmation

Biopsy and radiographic findings are typical but can be similar to other tumor masses. The two

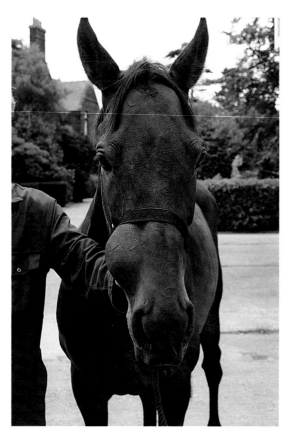

**Figure 8.2.** Facial swelling caused by an ameloblastoma. The tissue contained no obvious dental tissue remnants. This differentiates it from an ameloblastic odontoma.

types can be differentiated radiographically by the presence or absence of enamel and cementum. Ameloblastomas are usually rubbery in consistency and have a roughly spherical or multilocular shape and a cystic radiographic appearance. The ameloblastic odontoma is radiolucent or partially mineralized with specks of enamel tissue mixed throughout. Even when there is extensive ulceration there should be little confusion between this and the carcinomas and sarcomas which have a much more destructive nature.

## Treatment

Surgical removal can be effective if treatment is initiated early and wide excision can be performed. Radiation is probably the best option and has been used successfully.[31]

## Prognosis

The expansive nature of the tumors and the late recognition (particularly in foals and young horses) make the outlook poor.[29] Many horses are destroyed as soon as the tumor is diagnosed although the rate of expansion may be slow and some useful life may be left.

## CEMENTOMA

### Definition

An unusual dysplastic or reactive change typically occurring in the periapical region of the developing tooth and deriving from mesenchymal tissue with no epithelial components.

### Occurrence

Singularly rare. There are few reports of the tumors in the literature but the author has encountered one such tumor that affected the structure of an incisor tooth. It is possible that some of the features of this condition could be found in abnormal or supernumerary cheek teeth.

### Pathogenesis and histopathological features

These present as a complex confluent mass of cementum and fibrocellular stroma in variable proportions situated at the base or on the crown of a tooth. The cementum may be partially or more fully mineralized. Cementifying fibroma is probably a form of this as well as fibroma in which areas of dense mineralized cement are mixed with variable volumes of fibrous tissue. Pathologists can recognize at least four and probably six types of cementoma.

### Clinical features

The location of these tumors (at the base of the tooth) makes their recognition and diagnosis unlikely or impossible at an early stage. Only when there is overt swelling can the possibility be explored. Radiographically they have a distinctive very dense appearance and the tissue contains sheets of cementum-like material.

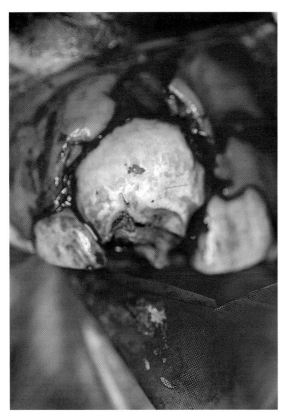

**Figure 8.3.** Cementoma of the crown of an incisor tooth in a three-year-old Hanovarian mare.

Secondary alveolar changes may however, make them harder to recognize. Alterations in the crown structure are unusual but will make the condition easily recognizable (Fig. 8.3).

### Treatment

Removal of the tooth in its entirety is feasible but may be hindered by the ball-like aggregation of tissue at the root of the tooth.

### Prognosis

The masses are benign and removal is curative.

## COMPLEX AND COMPOUND ODONTOMA
### Definition

An irregular tumor-like mass of dental tissues in well-differentiated form. There is a marked inductive effect on mesenchymal tissue in both forms. There is some justification for considering some of these lesions to be hamartomas of dental tissue rather than tumors. Complex odontoma contains all the elements of a normal tooth but the structure is chaotic. Compound odontoma is similar except that the tissue is organized into a recognizable tooth-like structure (although it may be grossly distorted).

### Occurrence

Both young and older horses may be affected.

### Pathogenesis and histopathological features

These are a subtype of the tumors classed as odontoma which contain both dental and epithelial components but complex odontoma lacks the formation of true tooth-like structures which are present in compound odontoma. The mixtures of dental tissues which are characteristic are often better differentiated in young animals. Many of these have effects limited to their space-occupying nature. Cement matrix deposition within the mass may be a unique feature of the tumor in horses.[32]

### Clinical features

Firm painless swellings over the root regions of the maxillary cheek teeth or the premaxilla.[33] Swelling may not be obvious if the more caudal four cheek teeth are involved as the expansion would be contained in the maxillary sinuses (Fig. 8.4).

### Differential diagnosis

Dental disease with new bone formation and lysis. Sinus cysts may in fact be related to these in some cases.

### *Diagnostic confirmation*

The radiographic appearance is characteristic – multiple small lobulated masses within a well-defined cyst-like structure at the root of a maxillary tooth is typical.

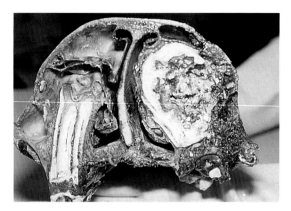

**Figure 8.4.** A complex odontoma in the maxillary sinus.

## Treatment

Surgical removal may be feasible and if so it is curative. Surgical removal and cryosurgery combined can be used but some masses require more than one treatment.[33]

## Prognosis

Full surgical removal should resolve the problem but repeated surgeries may be needed. There are insufficient reports to establish a definitive prognosis but the few that exist do suggest that the outlook is reasonable or even good.

Complex and compound odontoma is reported rarely in horses and is characterized by the presence of a variety of dental tissues, all of which are essentially well formed or normal histologically. The tissues are arranged in a chaotic or random fashion and complete teeth are not formed. This is probably best regarded as a dental malformation rather than a tumor.

## INCIDENTAL TUMOR-LIKE MASSES

Dentigerous cysts are best regarded as benign teratoma and are dealt with elsewhere (see p. 99). They are also known as heterotopic polyodontia. Although they are almost certainly of congenital origin, many are only diagnosed at a later age (often up to 8 years of age,[34] probably because of the relatively insignificant clinical presentation. The masses comprise a variable complex of

tissues but the most have obvious enamel components that make radiographic diagnosis relatively simple. Some cases have a more obvious tooth like nature often with a pseudo alveolus firmly attached to the calvarium. A few however, have no enamel at all (and then comprise a cystic lining alone) or the enamel is not radiographically obvious. Invariably the cystic structure associated with the dental mass has a secretory epithelial lining. This is responsible for the characteristic glairy, mucoid discharge that is almost invariably identified to issue from a small draining sinus tract usually on the leading margin of the pinna about one third of the way up from the base of the ear. It is possibly to probe the sinus and gauge the extent of tooth like tissues. The true extent of the structure can be usefully confirmed by the use of contrast radiography.

Although the condition may be of minor cosmetic significance benign neglect is seldom suggested. In a few cases infection can be significant and so a more aggressive surgical option is usually employed. Surgical resection is probably the only therapeutic option likely to succeed. Where this is performed carefully so as to ensure complete removal of all abnormal tissues the prognosis for cosmetic and functional normality is excellent. Although the surgery may look relatively straightforward however, the dental structures that have to be removed are often closely attached to the calvarium. Aggressive chiselling is sometimes required and can be potentially dangerous. It is probably unwise to attempt this surgery without general anaesthesia. Failure to remove the entire structure or application of inappropriate cyst cautery or flushing will inevitably lead to recurrence and possibly to unwanted secondary consequences such as ear deviations, infection and continued discharge.

There is no reported tendency for these masses to become neoplastic as has been reported in man.[35]

Congenital sinus cysts may be related to dental tissue because in some cases dental tissues can be identified histologically in the contents or bony 'capsule'. There is some debate about the apparently acquired sinus cysts which occur in adult horses (usually around 7 to 10 years of age). These are sometimes very similar in appearance to the congenital form but are commonly linked to progressive ethmoid hematoma in spite of a firm bony cyst lining and some calcification of the structure.

# TUMORS OF BONE ORIGIN (OSTEOGENIC TUMORS)

Primary bone tumors, including osteosarcoma, osteoblastoma, chondrosarcoma and fibrosarcoma, have been described. They are all very rare in horses but there have been several reports of these in the regions of the jaws and the mandible in particular.[20] The histological characteristics of bone derived tumors has been described[36–38] and the classification of the group of tumors is based on these features.

## OSTEOSARCOMA AND OSSEOUS CARCINOMA

### Definition

A malignant mesenchymal tumor in which the tumor cells produce a modified or distinctive bone matrix in haphazard arrangement.

### Occurrence

These are very rare tumors. Over 80 per cent of reported osteosarcomas involve the head[39] and the majority are reported in the mandible.[20,30,40,41] There is a report of a case of osteosarcoma in the mandible of a 6-month-old quarter horse colt which suggests that age is probably not a significant factor,[39] although typically younger horses appear to be more prone to oral or dental neoplasia than older ones.

### Pathogenesis and histopathological features

At least 12 distinctive types can, theoretically be recognized but this is probably irrelevant with the low reported numbers and poor prognosis which they all carry. Several types are recognized in species where the incidence is higher but it is so rare in horses that it is probably unwise to extrapolate from these. The tumor tissue is however, usually not densely cellular with formation of fibrillar stroma, bone or osteoid tissue. The cells have a high mitotic index and an atypical irregular morphology. Trauma is implicated in some cases although this is often impossible to confirm.

### Clinical features

Painful, hot progressive swelling of the mandible with a characteristic 'sun-burst' appearance of bone lysis and irregular deposition of trabecular bone[20] (see also Chapter 11, pp. 137–168).

### Differential diagnosis

Infection resulting in osteitis or osteomyelitis can be very destructive. Various cystic structures such as ameloblastoma, ossifying fibroma and fibrous dysplasia can be similar but usually have characteristic and definite differences even on radiography.

### Diagnostic confirmation

The radiographic appearance is highly suggestive but biopsy provides the only definitive diagnosis.

### Treatment

Radiation offers the only hope of success but the tumors are likely to be highly malignant and so treatment is usually not contemplated. However, some progress relatively slowly and are therefore at least tolerable for limited periods. Euthanasia is the only realistic option.

### Prognosis

There is insufficient data to suggest a true prognosis. However, the highly aggressive nature and rapid course as well as the likely malignancy suggest a hopeless prognosis.

## OSTEOMA

Other osteogenic oral and facial tumors include osteoma, a benign, solitary tumor of bone enclosing marrow and fat which many pathologists regard as a developmental abnormality or hamartoma, i.e. an abnormal accumulation of a normal tissue type in a normal or abnormal location. They are reported in all ages of horse with most being in the head region, in the mandible in particular.[42] The tumors are slow growing and protrude from the surface of the bones of the jaw or face. They are singularly benign but they may reach sufficient size to cause some difficulty.

## TUMORS OF SOFT-TISSUE ORIGIN

The clinical features of common equine oral, soft-tissue tumors are shown in Table 8.2.

### EQUINE JUVENILE OSSIFYING FIBROMA
#### Definition

A poorly defined group of proliferative fibro-osseous, tumor-like, solitary masses which typically develop in the rostral regions of the mandible of young horses.

#### Occurrence

Most are encountered in very young horses. They may not however be observed until the animal is handled at 12 to 14 months of age by which time there may be significant distortion and ulceration of the buccal mucosa.[38]

### Pathogenesis and histopathological features

They may develop from the periodontal membrane and represent alterations in the growth characteristics of the membrane cells or of the developing tooth. The masses are reported to arise from a sessile base on the surface of the bone and expand to replace and displace the normal tissue with a dense fibrous or fibro-osseous tissue. There is a characteristically abrupt transition from fibroblastic stroma to osteoblasts, which form spicules of bone-like tissue. The dense gritty nature of the mass sometimes makes biopsy difficult.

### Clinical features

Lesions may rarely develop in the maxilla and in very rare cases can be bilateral. They often reach considerable size and are initially at least covered by a normal smooth oral mucosa. Later some ulceration is common (Fig. 8.5). Gross distortions

**Table 8.2.** Clinical features of the more common equine oral soft-tissue tumors

| Tumor type | Age group affected | Malignancy | Best treatment option | Prognosis |
|---|---|---|---|---|
| Equine juvenile ossifying fibroma | 2 months–2 years | low | surgical excision | fair to good |
| Myxomatous tumor | n/k* | probably high | n/k | poor to hopeless |
| Squamous cell carcinoma | 5–14 years | low but can be very destructive | radiation cisplatin | guarded |
| Sarcoid | all | negligible but malevolent form can be very aggressive | radiation cisplatin surgery (nodular type only) | very guarded |
| Melanoma | > 7 (gray horses) | low | benign neglect cisplatin cimetidine (by mouth) | fair but a few are malignant |
| Oral papilloma | < 2–3 years | negligible | leave alone surgical excision | good but some persist |
| Epulis | > 10 years | nil | dental hygiene and descaling | good |
| Salivary adenocarcinoma | > 10 years | high | radiation possible | hopeless |

* n/k = not known or insufficient reports to make a judgment.

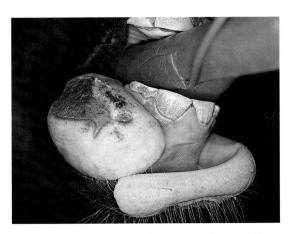

**Figure 8.5.** Juvenile ossifying fibroma in a 14-month-old thoroughbred gelding. Note the generally smooth outline of the firm swelling. The superficial ulceration only developed late in the condition.

of the lip and the associated teeth are likely. The expanding tumor causes loosening of the teeth and consequent dysphagia. Although the tumor should be obvious they are often only identified late probably because there is usually little call to examine the mouth of very young horses.

### Diagnostic confirmation

Radiographically the dense tissue is obvious with only a few showing the calcification more commonly encountered in other species. The more ulcerated and secondarily infected tumors may resemble myxoma or myxofibrosarcoma tumors or the ulcerated epitheliogenic sarcomas.

### Treatment

Surgical excision is curative provided that sufficient attention is paid to the true extent of abnormal tissue. Extensive surgical debulking followed by Cobalt-[60] teletherapy radiation has been successful.[20] Radiation using Cobalt-[60] teletherapy alone in a standing sedated horse has also been used successfully.[43]

Hemimandibulectomy is also an effective option.[9,44] Limited disabilities and acceptable cosmetic effects have been reported.[9] Cases subjected to this surgery recovered well and were able to lead active normal lives. However if extensive excision is required it may leave an unacceptable cosmetic and functional deficit.

### Prognosis

Regrowth of tumor is common because of the difficulty of identifying the margins of the abnormal tissue. All tissue removed should therefore be submitted for histological examination.

## SQUAMOUS CELL CARCINOMA

### Definition

Malignant neoplasm derived from stratified squamous epithelium but which may also occur in sites where glandular or columnar epithelium is present.

### Occurrence

Squamous cell carcinoma, despite being the most common oral neoplasm is still rare. Although mucocutaneous junctions are commonly involved and there is an apparent correlation with non-pigmented skin and high levels of ultraviolet light, many of the most severe and aggressive tumors occur within the mouth.[45] There is often a suggestion that the primary tumor develops in the paranasal sinuses or nasal cavity and the destructive tissue then extends into the hard palate.[46]

### Pathogenesis and histopathological features

The tumors possibly arise in chronically irritated hyperplastic alveolar epithelium in cases of chronic periodontitis. Tumors which develop in the oral mucosa can extend into the nasal cavity[46] and those developing in nasal mucosa can extend into the mouth. In either case the tumor has a dramatic effect on the integrity of the alveolar ligaments. Loss of teeth is common (Figs 8.6a and b). The role of ultraviolet light in the pathogenesis of facial and lip carcinoma is uncertain but the Clydesdale breed and horses with non-pigmented skin on the face and lips are more often affected than other breeds and colors. Histologically the tumors present distinctive characteristics with irregular cords of

DENTAL DISEASE AND PATHOLOGY

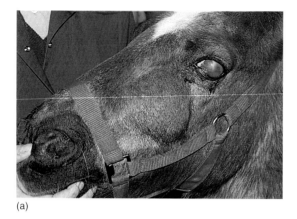

(a)

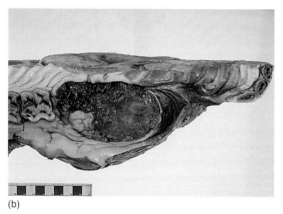

(b)

**Figure 8.6a and b.** Facial distortion due to naso-palatine squamous cell carcinoma in a 12-year-old pony gelding. Note the extensive tissue destruction and the loss of the maxillary teeth (from Prof. D Kelly, with permission).

downward-invading highly mitotic keratinocytes. The deposition of variable amounts of keratin in the deeper layers produces the 'keratin pearls'. The more differentiated cells produce more keratin and so, possibly, this signifies a less dangerous tumor type than those in which almost no obvious keratinocyte structure can be recognized. Tumors originating in the nasal cavity are reported to have a less keratinized nature while those in the oral cavity are usually highly keratinized. Careful histological examination should therefore be able to identify the original site of development.[47]

## Clinical features

The tumors are characteristically slow growing. They can be proliferative but are usually very

destructive and highly infiltrative into local tissues of the mouth including the buccal mucosa, hard palate (Fig. 8.6b) and the lips (Fig. 8.7). Metastases to local lymph nodes are reported and in theory at least may disseminate to the lungs and elsewhere but this is very rare in oral forms of squamous cell carcinoma.[48] Oral tumors may extend to the hard palate (and thence to the nasal cavity),[46] the tongue[49,50] or oral mucosa. It is also quite common for oral squamous cell carcinoma tumors to invade the nasal cavity and the paranasal sinuses (often to the point of gross distortion or obstruction to airflow).[51] Some extend to the pharynx and can physically affect its function (Fig. 8.8). In the former case there is altered airflow (or even complete obstruction of the ipsilateral nostril). In the latter case the patient may be presented with dysphagia of progressive, insidious onset. In both cases weight loss and poor general health are common. More extensive spread may involve the orbit and the cranial cavity with appropriate secondary organ involvement. It is also quite common for nasal squamous cell carcinoma to invade the hard palate and then it might create an oronasal fistula. In all cases there may be extensive soft tissue disruption and consequent loosening and shedding of the teeth (see Fig. 8.6b).

The location of the tumors often means that cases are detected late in their course when a large invasive mass may be present projecting from the gum or hard palate as a grayish, ulcer-

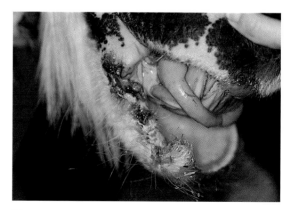

**Figure 8.7.** Ulcerative (destructive) squamous cell carcinoma of the lip of an aged pony gelding.

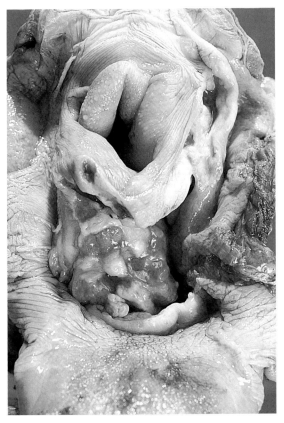

**Figure 8.8.** Squamous cell carcinoma of the pharynx which was identified some 3 months after a lesion had been detected in the hard palate. It is possible that this developed independently or that it was an extension of the earlier lesion.

ated and bleeding mass. Where the tumor surrounds a tooth this may become dislodged and in almost all cases there is a fetid, necrotic odor in the mouth.

## Differential diagnosis

The differential diagnosis includes other proliferative and invasive lesions of the lips such as hemangiosarcoma, myxomatous carcinoma, basal cell carcinoma and equine sarcoid.

## Diagnostic confirmation

Biopsy is characteristic. Fine-needle aspirates can be used but may be misleading. Radiographic examinations can be used to identify masses in the sinuses and the extent of bone destruction.

## Treatment

While surgical excision of oral squamous cell carcinoma lesions has been reported to be successful[52] this on its own can be very difficult. There is a very high rate of recurrence following such attempts. Small discrete tumors may however be amenable to surgical removal and extensive excision involving hemimandibulectomy such as has been described for other tumors of the mandible[44] will also possibly resolve the condition, but may leave an unacceptable cosmetic or functional deficit.

Squamous cell carcinoma appears in the author's experience to be relatively sensitive to gamma radiation and this offers the best prognosis with a reasonably high success rate. Teletherapy is logical and can be finely controlled but repeated fractionated doses need to be used and the horse therefore needs repeated general anesthesia. The number of centers where this can be performed is small and the procedure is very expensive. The much simpler iridium-[192] brachytherapy using linear platinum-sheathed wires has been used by the author to good effect. There are serious logistic complications however and limits to size and location of the tumors which can be treated.

Some cases will respond to intralesional cisplatin* (either in water-soluble form with frequently repeated injections) or as an emulsion of the solution containing 1 mg/ml with an equal volume of sesame or almond oil. The use in oral neoplasia has apparently not been reported in the literature.

The response to immunomodulation using mycobacterial protein materials such as Bacillus Calmette Geurin (BCG) is disappointing in horses in the author's experience.

Treatment of labial squamous cell carcinoma with 5 per cent fluorouracil cream applied topically has been shown to resolve some cases and improve others[53] but cures may be difficult to effect using this alone. It is however a very useful adjunct to other forms of treatment and is

---

*cis-diamminedicloroplatinum or cis-DDP, cis-Platinum.

particularly applicable to small, ulcerated buccal and lip lesions.

## Prognosis

The tumors are usually locally invasive but slow to metastasize and so while the clinical prognosis is inevitably poor many cases can survive even with quite extensive involvement. Secondary complications such as facial or oral distortion, dysphagia, loosening of teeth and nasal obstruction will inevitably suggest a poor prognosis. However, oral squamous cell carcinoma is not reported to be malignant and tends not to metastasize beyond the local lymph node. However, it is probably unwise to assume that this will be the case in all affected patients.

## MYXOMATOUS TUMORS OF THE JAW

### Definition

These are very rare tumors deriving from embryonal connective tissue. Pathologically the tumors are easily recognized by their characteristic stellate cells surrounded by an abundant collagen and proteoglycan matrix without evidence of cartilage formation.

### Occurrence

Older or mature horses are probably more often affected but there are so few reported cases that even this aspect cannot be established with certainty. The maxilla is the commonest site.[30]

### Pathogenesis and histopathological features

The tumors have a gelatinous soft appearance, are highly infiltrative and have a high tendency to metastasize. Histologically there are characteristic stellate cells with abundant soft, amorphous extracellular matrix.

### Clinical features

In horses these may occur particularly in the maxillary region (and possibly the mandibular region) and are characteristically destructive (Fig. 8.9). The combined destruction and proliferation of tumor tissue (consisting mostly of a loose gelatinous material with strands of collagen produced by the characteristically stellate cells of the tumor) creates obvious distortion of the maxilla with secondary nasal and sinus occlusion.

Invasive odontogenic epithelial sarcoma is a highly aggressive, ulcerative and destructive tumor (Fig. 8.10) which develops from the dental epithelium. These can be classified in this group of tumors but really fall into the odontogenic group of neoplastic conditions.

## Diagnostic confirmation

Biopsy is essential to differentiate it from squamous cell carcinoma. Severely ulcerated juvenile ossifying fibroma can resemble these but are usually slow growing and expansive rather than

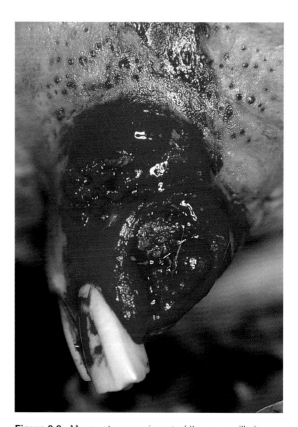

**Figure 8.9.** Myxomatous carcinoma of the premaxilla in a 14-year-old hunter gelding. Note the extensive destruction that is very similar to squamous cell carcinoma. The diagnosis can be confirmed relatively easily by biopsy.

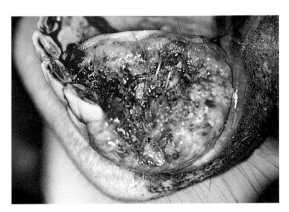

**Figure 8.10.** Invasive odontogenic epithelial sarcoma in the mandible of a 9-year-old thoroughbred mare. Note the extensive destruction and ulceration with proliferation that caused lip distortion.

destructive. Radiographically there is an aggressive lytic appearance with a diffuse mixture of bone and soft tissues often in a partially loculated form. The cardinal radiographic signs of the more malignant forms however are the combined destruction of normal bone and bizarre irregular new bone formation in random arrangement.

## Treatment

Treatment options are very limited – the margins of the tumor and the locality make surgical excision virtually impossible. There are no definitive reports of metastatic spread of these tumors but this may reflect the short local course, which inevitably results in euthanasia before secondary tumors develop elsewhere.

## Prognosis

These tumors are very unpredictable in behavior and so while some are slow and rather more benign others are highly aggressive and so carry a poor or hopeless prognosis.

Other neoplastic and neoplastic-like tumors of the mouth, face and jaws are described in the following section.

## MELANOMA

A tumour of melanocytes occurring in the skin and in other organs (including the mouth). Most melanomas are encountered in grey horses – indeed almost every grey horse over 5–8 years of age will have some melanoma involvement in some site. Other colours may rarely be affected also. The lips and gums may become sites for melanoma development but they are infrequent (Fig. 8.11). There is a strong tendency for melanoma to develop in the parotid salivary glands and the parotid lymph nodes. The development in these sites is usually obvious on inspection. In spite of some tumours having an aggressive appearance and high growth rate the large majority are very benign in character. It is not easy to characterise the degree of malignancy in many of these tumours. Oral lesions are usually very benign but can reach considerable size. Tumours on the lips and gums are often only noted when they reach considerable size. Their rate of growth is usually low and they have no other systemic effects (others may

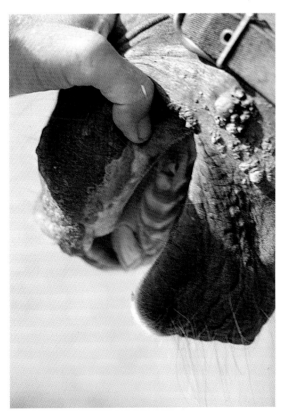

**Figure 8.11.** Malignant sarcoid with extensive involvement of the cheeks and surface erosion into the mouth. This form of sarcoid can be very extensive.

however be developing simultaneously in many other organs). Equine sarcoid and mast cell tumours should be considered in the differential diagnosis (mast cell tumours are commoner in young male horses). The diagnosis of melanoma is easy to confirm from clinical features and fine-needle biopsy or Trucut column biopsy.

Surgical excision is feasible and usually effective but many are left alone without any significant problem. Prolonged daily oral administration of cimetidine at doses of up to 7.5 mg/kg bodyweight has been suggested as being effective but the results are not convincing in many cases.[54,55] Treatment of single or few oral tumours on their own probably does not warrant this approach. The prognosis is usually very fair as the majority have no metastatic tendency but occasional tumours are very aggressive (melanosarcoma) with extensive metastatic spread and serious secondary effects.

## SARCOID

The equine sarcoid is a common fibroblastic tumor of the skin and can involve the mouth.[56,57] There are usually two forms that affect the mouth itself (as opposed to the skin of the lips and cheeks). The nodular form remains subcutaneous and is most often located at the angle (commissure) of the mouth. The malignant form[50,57] also occurs in the tissues of the cheeks in particular and can ulcerate into the mouth (Fig. 8.11). Treatment of buccal forms of the disease is notoriously difficult with radiation, cryosurgery, hyperthermia, laser excision and intralesional cisplatin carrying some chance of success.

## ORAL PAPILLOMA

Viral papilloma is a relatively common occurrence on the skin of the mouth and lips and in some cases they can extend into the oral cavity. A host-specific equine papilloma virus causes them and most often affect young horses in their first year or two at grass. Less usually they affect older horses.

Typically they appear as multiple, discreet or coalescing wart like masses with a grey-pink coloration. They seldom ulcerate except when they are traumatised. The diagnosis is usually simply based on epidemiology and clinical appearance but they can closely resemble the equine sarcoid.

Most cases will resolve spontaneously over some months but individual lesions may be persistent, often for many years. Oral papillomas may be very persistent and should then be subjected to surgical removal or cryonecrosis. Therapeutic measures have included autogenous vaccines prepared from wart tissues and various topical chemicals such as podophyllin. Individual lesions that prove troublesome can be subjected to surgical excision or cryosurgery. The anecdotal efficacy of many less well-defined methods of treatment probably relies upon the high rate of spontaneous resolution.

## EPULIS

These tumor-like gingival masses develop from the fibrous tissue of the gingiva. In horses they are much less common than in some other species such as the dog and cat and seldom reach significant proportions (Fig. 8.12). They can easily be overlooked but are benign and can safely be removed surgically. In many cases they arise from chronic local irritation due to persistent infection or the presence of dental tartar. Removal of the causative factors usually results in complete resolution. There are no reports that they are precursors to more malig-

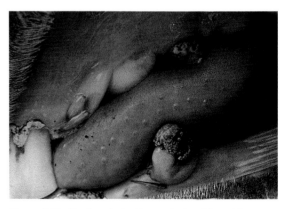

**Figure 8.12.** Benign gingival hyperplasia arising at the gingival margin of the canine tooth (tush). Histological examination confirmed its benign nature but 6 years later a squamous cell carcinoma developed at the site.

nant genuine tumors such as squamous cell carcinoma but the author has experience of a single case which developed a carcinoma some years after a benign epulis was removed from the base of the canine tooth. It is probably unwise to draw any causative inference from this case however. Also, there is a poor histological characterization of the epulis probably because they are easily recognized and usually easily and effectively treated so that few are subject to diagnostic biopsy. Many cases will spontaneously resolve if any dental tartar or damaged dental or soft tissue structures are removed.

## ORAL HEMANGIOSARCOMA

This is a malignant neoplasm of vascular endothelial cells that can arise in any part of the body. They are reported to metastasize early and so tumors in any locality may be primary or secondary. There are a few reports of this tumor in the mouth.[58,59] Aged horses are more likely to develop them and they may be secondary to tumors elsewhere.

## SALIVARY ADENOCARCINOMA

These tumors are very rarely reported but their recognition is important because they are often highly malignant possibly up to 33% will develop pulmonary secondary tumors.[3,60]

## NEOPLASTIC-LIKE DISORDERS OF THE JAWS AND TEETH
### MANDIBULAR ANEURYSMAL BONE CYST

Although bone cysts are relatively common in long bones and in particular in their epiphyseal regions, mandibular cysts are very rare. They probably arise from circulatory disturbances within the bone structure[61] or traumatic alteration of the blood supply to a small area of bone.[62] While such structures might be expected in young horses[12] they may also occur in older horses probably as a result of trauma.[10]

The likely clinical presentation is a sterile, firm, expanding swelling on the ventral man-

dible which can be explained by progressive destruction of cortical bone with thin plates of new bone being laid down under the periosteum. Aspiration may reveal a yellow or reddish-orange fluid in small volumes. The radiographic appearance illustrates the complex, loculated cyst-like structure of bone fragments, cartilage and soft tissue with usually a fine rim of thin bone around the periphery. The structure closely resembles the complex of paranasal sinus cysts that may also arise congenitally or develop at later ages. The rate of expansion may be sufficient to cause disruption and bleeding into the surrounding tissues and may easily suggest a neoplastic lesion. Histologically the lesion resembles a conglomeration of bone fragments, granular debris and fibrovascular tissue with areas of organizing and free blood clot.[12] There is no evidence to suggest that these lesions are of truly neoplastic origin but diagnosis based on radiographic examination alone is probably unwise. While there are no reports of concurrent neoplasia in the horse complexes of tumors and cysts are reported in other species.

## DENTIGEROUS CYSTS (TEMPORAL ODONTOMA)

Temporal odontoma is a rare curiosity in the horse in which dental tissue (which may be instantly recognizable as such) is located at sites away from the jaws (Fig. 8.13). The commonest site is in the temporal region where a discharging sinus tract with glairy, milky discharge can be identified issuing from a discrete opening on the leading edge of the ipsilateral pinna. Sometimes the structure has no obvious dental tissue and comprises a smooth cystic lining lying below the ear. The relationship of dental tissues to sinus cysts (particularly those in young foals) is questionable but many of the lesions have dental structures within them. All these cystic structures are best regarded as simple developmental abnormalities rather than neoplastic lesions.

## FIBROUS DYSPLASIA

Fibrous dysplasia of the bones of the skull has been reported.[13,14,63,64] These are smoothly

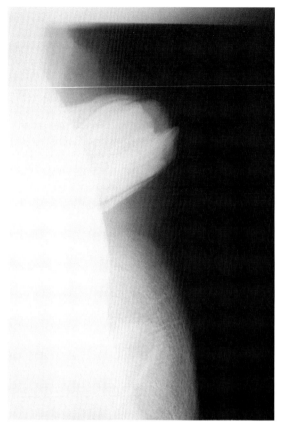

**Figure 8.13.** Temporal odontoma with an obvious tooth-like structure firmly attached to the cranium. There was a discharging sinus tract in the typical site on the leading edge of the pinna.

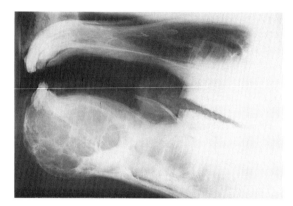

**Figure 8.14.** Fibrous dysplasia of the mandible of a yearling thoroughbred colt.

## SECONDARY TUMORS AFFECTING THE MOUTH AND JAWS

Secondary tumors include those arising by metastatic spread from remote organs and those invading the oral cavity from neighboring areas such as the nasal cavity and paranasal sinuses.

Tumors remote from the mouth and oral structures may have a serious influence on the mouth either through metastatic spread (such as in hemangiosarcoma and lymphosarcoma) or through systemic effects from their functional capacity (e.g. pituitary adenoma-related Cushing's disease).

### LYMPHOSARCOMA

Multicentric (generalized) and cutaneous histiocytic lymphosarcoma may have oral manifestations. Usually the clinical appearance is of ill-defined nodular lesions of variable size embedded in and below the mucosal surface which probably reflect the involvement of the normally diffuse lymphoid tissue in the mouth and pharynx. The gingival mucosa seems to be the area most often affected (Fig. 8.15). A similar nodular appearance is often present in the pharynx where they may have some effect on swallowing and in the sublingual tonsillar tissue. The lesions seldom ulcerate or become infected. Simultaneous submandibular lymphadenopathy and other secondary effects such as

contoured bone deformities arising from an idiopathic loss of bone structure with extensive new formation of a fibro-osseous matrix (Fig. 8.14). The lesion is probably not really a true neoplasm and its major effects in the jaw and face region are due to the expansive space-occupying nature of the slowly expanding mass. The changes are easily recognized histologically[40] but may be confused with neoplastic lesions both radiographically and clinically. Suspicious masses should be subjected to the full range of diagnostic tests including radiography, scintigraphy, biopsy and, where feasible, computed tomography.

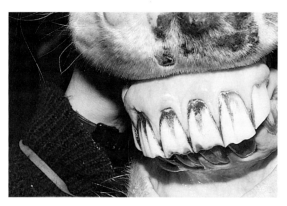

**Figure 8.15.** Cutaneous histiocytic lymphosarcoma with involvement of the gingival tissues. Ill-defined swellings of the gingiva were due to aggregations of abnormal lymphocytes.

anemia, lethargy and weight loss might signify serious systemic involvement. A relationship between the cutaneous histiocytic lympho-sarcoma and granulosa cell tumors in mares has been suggested. All mares with confirmed cutaneous lymphosarcoma should be carefully examined for the presence of an ovarian tumor.

## PITUITARY ADENOMA

Tumors of the par intermedia of the pituitary gland are responsible for secondary oral dis-eases such as extensive non-healing ulcers and dental and alveolar infections. The tumors are the preserve of the older horse (the large major-ity are over 14 to 17 years). Extensive dental and alveolar disease (including periodontal disease and periapical sepsis) develop commonly. This, with advancing, age-related natural degener-ation and the short residual crown of older horses predisposes the affected animals to secondary sinusitis and there may be tertiary consequences from this.

Paraneoplastic changes in the mouth arising as a result of neoplastic disease in other tissues (usually myeloproliferative neoplasia) have also been described[65] and it is important to remem-ber that the mouth may be one of the early sites where clinical evidence of neoplastic disease may be manifest. The lesions seen in the mouth may not be readily attributable to neoplastic disease either at a local or remote site.

## ACKNOWLEDGMENTS

I am grateful to my colleague, Professor Donald Kelly, for the loan of Figure 8.6.

## REFERENCES

1. Jackson C (1936) The incidence and pathology of tumours of domestic animals in South Africa: a study of the Onderstepoorte collection of neoplasms with special reference to their histopathology. *Onderstepoorte Journal of Veterinary Science and Animal Industries*, 6, 1–460.
2. Baker JR and Leyland A (1975) Histological survey of tumours of the horse with particular reference to those of the skin. *Veterinary Record*, 96, 419–422.
3. Head KW (1976) International classification of tumours of domestic animals. XI Tumours of the upper alimentary tract. *Bulletin of the World Health Organisation*, 53, 145–146.
4. Hagdoost IS and Zakarian B (1985) Neoplasms of equidae. Iran *Equine Veterinary Journal*, 17, 237–239.
5. Pirie RS and Tremaine WH (1997) Neoplasia of the mouth and surrounding structures. In: *Current Therapy in Equine Medicine*, ed. NE Robinson, WB Saunders, Philadelphia, pp. 153–155.
6. Sundberg JP, Burnstein T, Page EH, Kirkham WW and Robinson FR (1977) Neoplasms of equidae. *Journal of the American Veterinary Medical Association*, 170, 150–152.
7. Smith P (1996) *Large Animal Internal Medicine*. CV Mosby, Philadelphia, p. 696.
8. Baker GJ (1985) Oral examination and diagnosis: management of oral diseases. In: *Veterinary Dentistry*, ed. CE Harvey, WB Saunders, Philadelphia, p. 217.
9. Richardson DW, Evans LH and Tulleners EP (1991) Rostral mandibulectomy in 5 horses. *Journal of the American Veterinary Medical Association*, 199, 1179–1182.
10. Purdy CM (1985) Mandibular aneurysmal bone cyst in a horse. *Equine Practice*, 7, 22–24.
11. Verstraete FJM and Ligthelm AJ (1988) Excessive granulation tissue of periodontal origin in a horse. *Equine Veterinary Journal*, 20, 380–382.
12. Lamb CR and Schelling SH (1989) Congenital aneurysmal bone cyst in the mandible of a foal. *Equine Veterinary Journal*, 21, 130–132.
13. Gibbs C (1974) The equine skull; its radiographic investigation. *Journal of the American Veterinary Radiological Society*, 15, 70–78.
14. Wyn-Jones G (1985) Interpreting radiographs 6: radiology of the equine head (part 2). *Equine Veterinary Journal*, 17, 417–425.
15. McIlwraith CW (1984) Equine digestive system. In: *The Practice of Large Animal Surgery*, ed. PB Jennings, WB Saunders, Philadelphia, p. 579.

16. Moulton JE (1990) *Tumours in Domestic Animals* (3rd edn). University of California Press, Berkeley, pp. 167–168.

17. Head KW (1990) Tumours of the alimentary tract. In: *Tumours in Domestic Animals* (3rd edn), ed. JE Moulton, University of California Press, Berkeley, pp. 347–374.

18. Cotchin E (1977) A general survey of tumours of the horse. *Equine Veterinary Journal*, 9, 16–21.

19. Gorlin RJ, Meskin LH and Brodey R (1963) Odontogenic tumours in man and animals; pathological classification and clinical behaviour – a review. *Annals of the New York Academy of Science*, 108, 722–771.

20. Turrel JM (1995) Oncology. In: *The Horse: Diseases and Clinical Management*, eds CN Kobluk, TR Ames and RJ Geor, WB Saunders, Philadelphia, pp. 1128–1130.

21. Wahl P (1936) Adamantinoma polycysticum ossificans am Unterkiefer eines Pferdes. *Deutche Tierartztliche Waschrift*, 46, 113–117.

22. Peter CP, Myers VS and Ramsey FK (1968) Ameloblastomic odontoma in a pony. *American Journal of Veterinary Research*, 29, 1495.

23. Vaughan JT and Bartels JE (1968) Equine mandibular adamantinoma. *Journal of the American Veterinary Medical Association*, 153, 454–457.

24. Hanselka DW, Roberts RE and Thompson RB (1974) Adamantinoma of the equine mandible. *Veterinary Medicine for the Small Animal Clinician*, 69, 157–160.

25. Jones SL (1991) Ameloblastoma in mandible of horse (clinical quiz). *Journal of the American Veterinary Medical Association*, 199, 630–631.

26. Summers PM, Wells KE and Adkins KF (1977) Ossifying ameloblastoma in a horse. *Australian Veterinary Journal*, 55, 498–500.

27. Nobel TA and Neuman F (1962) Two adamantinomas – in a mule and in a cow. *Rufuah Veterinarian*, 19, 220–221.

28. Lingard DR and Crawford TB (1970) Congenital ameloblastoma in a foal. *American Journal of Veterinary Research*, 31, 801.

29. Roberts MC, Groenendyk S and Kelly WR (1978) Ameloblastomic odontoma in a foal. *Equine Veterinary Journal*, 10, 91–93.

30. Pirie RS and Dixon PM (1993) Mandibular tumors in the horse: a review of the literature and seven case reports. *Equine Veterinary Education*, 5, 287–294.

31. French DA, Fretz PB and Davis GD (1984) Mandibular adamantinoma in a horse; radical surgical treatment. *Veterinary Surgery*, 13, 165–171.

32. Dubielzig RR, Beck KA, Levine S and Wilson JW (1986) Complex odontoma in a stallion. *Veterinary Pathology*, 23, 633–635.

33. Dillehay DL and Schoeb TR (1986) Complex odontoma in a horse. *Veterinary Pathology*, 23, 341–342.

34. Fessler JF (1988) Heterotopic polyodontia in horses: Nine cases (1969–1986). *Journal of the American Veterinary Medical Association*, 192, 535–538.

35. Main DM (1985) Epithelial jaw cysts: 10 years of WHO classification. *Journal of Oral Pathology*, 14, 1–7.

36. Pindborg JJ, Kramer IRH and Torlini H (1971) *Histological typing of odontogenic tumours, jaw cysts and allied lesions*. World Health Organisation, Geneva, pp. 144–145.

37. Schajowicz F, Ackerman LV, Sissons HA, Sobin LH and Torlini H (1972) *Histological Typing of Bone Tumours*. World Health Organisation, Geneva, pp. 9–45.

38. Morse CC, Saik JE and Richardson DW (1988) Equine juvenile mandibular ossifying fibroma. *Veterinary Pathology*, 25, 415–421.

39. Livesey MA and Wilkie IW (1986) Focal and multifocal osteosarcoma in two foals. *Equine Veterinary Journal*, 18, 410–412.

40. Thorp F and Graham R (1934) A large osteosarcoma of the mandible. *Journal of the American Veterinary Medical Association*, 84, 118–119.

41. Jacobson SA (1969) Parosteal osteoma (juxtacortical osteogenic sarcoma) in animals. *American Journal of Pathology*, 58, 85a.

42. Pool RR (1990) Tumours of bone and cartilage. In: *Tumours in domestic animals* (3rd edn), ed. J Moulton, University of California Press, Berkeley, p. 157.

43. Robbins SC, Arighi M and Ottewell G (1996) The use of megavoltage radiation to treat juvenile mandibular ossifying fibroma in a horse. *Canadian Veterinary Journal*, 37, 683–684.

44. Kawcak CE, Stashak TS and Norrdin RW (1996) Treatment of ossifying fibroma in a horse by hemimaxilectomy. *Equine Practice*, 18, 22–25.

45. Strafuss AC (1976) Squamous cell carcinoma in horses. *Journal of the American Veterinary Medical Association*, 168, 61–62.

46. Howie F, Munroe G, Thompson H and Murphy D (1992) Palatine squamous cell carcinoma involving the maxillary sinus in two horses. *Equine Veterinary Education*, 4, 3–7.

47. Noack P (1956) Die Geschwulste der oberen Amtmungswege bei den Haussaugetieren (parts I, II). *Wiss Z. Humboldt-Univ*, 6; 293–314, 373–391.

48. Jubb KVF, Kennedy PC and Palmer N (1992) *Pathology of Domestic Animals* (4th edn). Academic Press, New York, p. 27.

49. Henson WR (1936) Carcinoma of the tongue in a horse. *Journal of the American Veterinary Medical Association*, 94, 124.

50. Knottenbelt DC and Pascoe RR (1994) *Color Atlas of Diseases and Disorders of the Horse*. Wolfe, London, p. 303.

51. Leyland A and Baker JR (1975) Lesions of the nasal cavity and paranasal sinuses of the horse causing dyspnoea. *British Veterinary Journal*, 131, 339–346.

52. Orsini JA, Nunamaker DM, Jones CJ and Acland HM (1991) Excision of oral squamous cell carcinoma in a horse. *Veterinary Surgery*, 20, 264–266.

53. Paterson S (1997) Treatment of superficial ulcerative squamous cell carcinoma in three horses with topical 5-fluorouracil. *Veterinary Record*, 141, 626–628.

54. Goetz TE, Ogilvie GK, Keegan KG and Johnson PJ (1990) Cimetidine for the treatment of melanoma in three horses. *Journal of the American Veterinary Medical Association*, 196, 449–452.

55. Goetz TE and Long MT (1993) Treatment of melanoma in horses. *Compendium of Continuing Education*, 15, 608–610.

56. Pulley LT and Stannard AA (1990) Tumours of the skin and soft tissues. In: *Tumours in domestic animals* (3rd edn), ed. JE Moulton University of California Press, Berkeley, pp. 23–87.

57. Knottenbelt DC, Edwards SER and Daniel EA (1995) The diagnosis and treatment of the equine sarcoid. *In Practice*, 17, 123–129.

58. Fry FL, Knight HD and Brown S (1983) Hemangiosarcoma in a horse. *Journal of the American Veterinary Medical Association*, 182, 287–289.

59. Sweigard KD and Hattell AL (1993) Oral haemangiosarcoma in a horse. *Equine Practice*, 15, 12–13.

60. Stackhouse LL, Moore JJ and Hylton WE (1978) Salivary gland adenocarcinoma in a mare. *Journal of the American Veterinary Medical Association*, 172, 271–273.

61. Biesecker JL, Marcove RC, Huvos AG and Mike V (1970) Aneurysmal bone cysts; a clinicopathological study of 66 cases. *Cancer*, 26, 616–625.

62. Dabezies EJ, D'Ambrosia RD, Chuinard RG and Ferguson AB (1982) Aneurysmal bone cyst after fracture. *Journal of Bone and Joint Surgery*, 64, 617–621.

63. Jacobson SA (1971) *The Comparative Pathology of the Tumours of Bone*. Charles C Thomas, Springfield IL, pp. 355–362.

64. Livesey MA, Keane DP and Sarmiento J (1984) Epistaxis in a Standardbred weanling caused by fibrous dysplasia. *Equine Veterinary Journal*, 16, 144–146.

65. Williams MA, Dowling PM, Angarano DW *et al.* (1995) Paraneoplastic bullous stomatitis in a horse. *Journal of the American Veterinary Medical Association*, 207, 331–334.

# SECTION 3

# DIAGNOSIS OF DENTAL DISORDERS

# 9

# DENTAL AND ORAL EXAMINATION

K Jack Easley, DVM, MS, Equine Veterinary Practice, Shelbyville KY 40066

## INTRODUCTION

Oral and dental disease are a common occurrence in horses as evidenced by the results of incidence studies of dental disease carried out on abbatoir specimens.[1,2,3] Signs of dental disease are often not apparent to the owner until the disease is well advanced. Casual oral or dental examination as part of a complete physical examination is not sufficient to detect most oral or dental problems. This has been demonstrated by the reported high incidence and the comparatively low clinical diagnosis of dental disease.[4,5] Clinical signs of dental disease are often not specific and may be reflected in other body systems. An example of this is horses showing signs of lameness that are alleviated when dental problems are corrected.[6]

Most equine practitioners consider oral examination as simply parting the lips, casually looking at the incisors and placing a finger in the cheek to feel for points on the first few upper cheek teeth. Only a small percentage of equine dental disease will be detected through this type of examination. A complete oral examination includes observing and feeling both oral hard and soft tissues for pathology, anatomy and genetics. The hard tissues consist of teeth and osseous structures. The soft tissues consist of the lips, cheeks, tongue, palate, gingiva and oral mucosa.

The basis of modern clinical therapy is diagnosis. This presupposes that disease can be accurately identified and then efficiently eliminated by the application of appropriate therapy. It would seem, therefore, that information obtained in making a diagnosis is the foundation for successful treatment. Discipline must be exercised in collecting material for a meaningful diagnosis.

Although a comprehensive history and physical examination of every patient seen while performing routine dental work would be a valuable service to clients, this is not practical in most cases. However, one must establish the presence or history of medical problems that may have an impact on safe delivery of dental care. The minimal dental examination process must be thorough enough to detect abnormalities in their early stages of development so that corrective action can be taken to prevent the progression of the pathological process to the point where correction is difficult if not impossible. The extent of the examination will increase depending upon the information obtained in the history and the findings from the minimal examination. The examination process must be performed in a routine fashion to ensure efficiency and quality of the examination. Variations and/or abnormalities detected at the time of the initial examination must be documented. If no notation is made in the record it can be assumed that there was no abnormality at the time of examination. When routine becomes habit, the results are thorough and the time to complete examination is reduced. A standard dental record form can be an invaluable aid in helping develop good examination habits (Fig. 9.13).

A typical examination starts with a brief history while screening the animal from a distance. The screening process should give the veterinarian a general idea of the type of horse, his thriftiness, general use and overall physical condition. The animal's feed and water source should be observed as well as the amount and type of feed being consumed. Attention should be directed to the horse's manure to gain an idea of how well feed is being processed and digested. The head is surveyed for shape, symmetry and obvious abnormalities. The head should be palpated for irregularities or tender areas especially along the upper dental arcade. Then lips are parted, the incisors inspected and age estimated. The oral mucous membranes, intermandibular space and tongue are evaluated. The range of motion of the jaw is viewed and its grinding sound and vibration are evaluated. The oral cavity is then inspected visually and palpated from the labial edges of the incisor teeth, caudal to the buccal recesses distal to the last molar. Subtle details of the examination process are extremely important. This chapter will attempt to detail the complete dental examination. Special examination considerations and procedures will be outlined for horses of various ages and occupations.

## WEANLING EXAMINATION (BIRTH TO 18 MONTHS)

Foals should be examined soon after birth and again at weaning for any congenital defects in head symmetry or masticatory function and evaluated for proper eruption sequence and alignment of the incisors. If facial asymmetry or severe malocclusion are detected at an early age, a genetic consultation and possible surgical or orthodontic correction can be discussed with the owner. The premolars should be examined every 6 months for sharp enamel points, abnormal wear and improper number and position.

## YOUNG PERFORMANCE HORSE EXAMINATION (18 TO 52 MONTHS)

Young athletic horses are asked to respond to bitting when the mouth is most active. During this 3 year period, all 24 of the deciduous teeth are shed and 36 to 44 permanent teeth erupt. Eruption cysts in the gums over erupting permanent teeth, gingivitis, periodontal disease and loose caps or cap slivers can cause oral pain and associated eating and training problems. Asymmetrical shedding of deciduous teeth can unbalance the occlusal table leading to abnormal mastication and tooth wear. Cheek or tongue pain and ulcerations from sharp enamel points on the premolars, molars and wolf teeth, can cause trouble with mastication and severe difficulty for the trainer and/or rider trying to cue the horse from the bit. Unequal eruption of permanent incisors leads to abnormal wear and a smiling or frowning incisor table. This may prohibit normal lateral jaw excursion. Retained or displaced incisor caps or supernumerary incisors can also lead to malocclusion or oral pain.

Wolf teeth can cause bitting problems or interfere with rounding the rostral edges of the premolars for the bit. Horses which have not had previous dental work may have wolf teeth present. Blind, unerupted, displaced or lower wolf teeth should be identified.

The canine teeth should erupt in most male horses between 4.5 and 5 years of age. Some canines may not penetrate the loose oral mucosa that tents up over the crown. This often leads to painful eruption cysts.

All young athletic horses should have a biannual oral examination. Horses that are shedding caps may need attention more often. Keep in mind that when PM 2 caps are shed, the permanent teeth will be in wear and sharp within 3 to 6 months.

## ADULT PERFORMANCE HORSE EXAMINATION (4 TO 10 YEARS)

The adult horse should have a full set of permanent dentition by 5 years of age. Most of these horses have already been exposed to training and bitting. The long-crowned hypsodont teeth continue to erupt into the oral cavity. Discrepancy in occlusal contact will begin to show in the young adult and become progressively worse as the horse ages. In the male horse by middle age, canine teeth are fully erupted and the sharp crowns can be formidable weapons.

It is important to evaluate critically the incisor and molar tables for occlusal contact and balance. Most problems are easy to correct and manage if they are attended to during this stage of life. This group of horses should have annual oral examinations.

The caudal cheek teeth must be thoroughly evaluated by palpation to detect hooks or ramps, sharp buccal or lingual enamel points and arcade balance. The mandible should be moved from side to side with the mouth closed to evaluate lateral jaw excursion and balance. During this part of the examination the incisors should be evaluated for symmetry, balance, length and contact.

## MATURE HORSE EXAMINATION (10 TO 18 YEARS)

Abnormalities of wear are a significant problem in mature horses. Slight malocclusions and uneven wear patterns place abnormal stresses on teeth in the dental arcades. This predisposes the dental table to abnormal crown wear, crown fracture and periodontal disease. Annual dental examinations are the rule, but some horses with dental and facial abnormalities may benefit from more frequent attention. At this age, the reserve crowns begin to show excessive wear and the older upper molars 1 and 2 may begin to suffer from infundibular decay or attrition that can lead to a 'wave' mouth forming on the central portion of the molar arcade. Ramps, hooks and beaks can be quite prominent and may require extensive correction to return the horse to its normal dental form.

Terms that may be encountered in describing abnormalities of wear can cause confusion. Some common terms are ramp, hook, beak and curved arcade. A ramp is an area where the dental arcade gently slopes and the exposed crown is taller at one end of the tooth than the other end. A hook is an abrupt elevation at the rostral or caudal edge of the molar arcade that involves the occlusal surface of the tooth. Quite often a hook will appear as a ramp from the

buccal aspect, but a cupped-out, steep elongation seen on the palatial side of the tooth identifies the formation of a hook as opposed to a ramp. A beak is an enamel point that forms on the rostral or caudal edge of the arcade. Curved arcade describes the occlusal surface where it gently slopes to follow the curve of the jaw and the exposed crown length is the same in the front and the rear of the tooth.

Incisor abnormalities are more prominent in the middle-aged horse than in younger horses. Small discrepancies in occlusion or tooth alignment begin to manifest themselves as abnormalities of wear or as severe tooth angulation deformities. The incisor arcades may take on a grinning, stepped, irregular, tilted or frowning conformation. Horses that have had abnormal masticatory patterns may not wear the incisors evenly on both sides of the arcade leading to a tilted or diagonal bite. Hook formation on the rostral upper and caudal lower edges of the molar arcades cause the arcade to shift caudally and can bring the incisors out of full occlusion. When this occurs the central upper incisors no longer contact the central lower incisors and they become elongated. From the standpoint of correcting oral balance, this is important. When the molar hooks are removed, the lower jaw can shift forward into a more normal position and the elongated incisors will meet in full occlusion. This can bring the molar tables out of occlusal contact and lead to problems with mastication. Correction would entail shortening and balancing the elongated incisor table.

By middle age, canine teeth become formidable weapons in stallions and geldings. Some mares may have small or rudimentary canines. Large, sharp canines can injure the horse's tongue or a groom's hands. Prominent canines can also reduce the space for the tongue and some horses suffer from excess tongue pressure when bitted.

## GERIATRIC HORSE EXAMINATION (18 YEARS AND OLDER)

Most old horses suffer from some form of dental disease. There is an accumulating effect throughout life of occlusal or wear abnormalities. The abnormal wear patterns previously discussed often become more pronounced. Abnormal stresses on teeth with less reserve crown, which results from altered wear and mastication, cause teeth to shift from their normal occlusal position. Tartar accumulation around lower canines is quite common and leads to gingivitis and periodontal disease. Aged horses suffer from a high incidence of periodontal disease.[7]

The importance of a general physical examination should be emphasized before dental procedures are considered. Even though severe dental disease is present, it may not be the main contributing factor to weight loss or poor condition. Many older horses suffer from organ failure such as kidney or liver disease, anemia and low grade sepsis. Neoplasia are also more commonly encountered in the older horse. The heart, liver, kidneys and other body systems should be carefully evaluated before an old horse is sedated or extensive dental procedures, such as extractions, are performed.

Care should be taken when working on an old horse's dentition not to damage, further loosen or accidentally extract teeth. Although, if an old horse's teeth can be digitally extracted with minimal force, then they need to be taken out. Owners should be educated about normal dental attrition and recognize the importance of oral health in keeping the horse productive into old age. All horses wear their teeth to the root if they live long enough. The teeth will become smooth on the occlusal surface because the crown contains enamel and the root does not. These smooth-mouthed horses will develop severe abnormalities of wear in a relatively short time requiring frequent oral examinations and dental maintenance in order to keep the mouth healthy. Since the teeth have lost their sharp enamel edges, mastication and digestion of forage becomes more difficult and less efficient. Therefore, most old horses need to have their diet adjusted by reducing the amount of rough forage that can predispose to esophageal choke or colic from intestinal impaction. The nutritional needs of older horses must be met and can be supplied by processed geriatric diets manufactured today.

## DENTAL EXAMINATION EQUIPMENT

Equipment utilized to examine properly the equine masticatory system is minimal, but certain items are necessary to perform a complete oral examination.

### HALTER AND LEAD

An adjustable halter with a noseband large enough to get the horse's mouth opened wide and not place pressure on the muzzle is suggested. A short lead shank (1–2 meters) with a loop in the end allows the horse to be controlled while the veterinarian works with both hands.[8]

### METAL FRAME DENTAL HALTER

This piece of equipment can be used to restrain the head of a horse in a comfortable position to work in the mouth (Fig. 9.1). This halter can withstand pressure placed on the lead rope without the noseband collapsing around the cheeks. The lead can be pulled down or secured like a martingale to hold the head down. The cheek ring can be placed on the top and a rope suspended from the ceiling to elevate the head of a sedated horse. A 1.38 cm diameter, 1 meter long cotton rope with a quick-release snap works well for either application.

### MOUTH SPECULUM

A mouth speculum is essential for complete evaluation of the equine oral cavity. The two general categories of specula are the gag or wedge type and the full mouth speculum.

There are a number of designs of gag specula. The basic principle is to place a wedge in the mouth between the upper and lower molar arcades to block the mouth open. There are advantages and disadvantages to this type of restraint. The greatest advantage is that the spool or wedge is small and inside the mouth, the device is both lightweight and user safe. It also does not interfere with the incisor teeth which can be worked on with the speculum in place. One disadvantage is that the device does not allow for good observation or room for

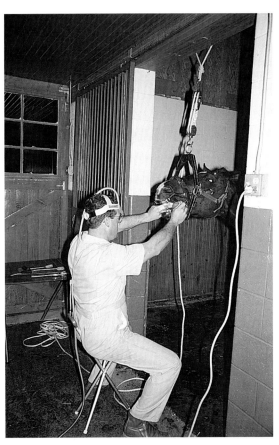

**Figure 9.1.** A sedated horse being examined with its head suspended in a metal frame dental halter. A full mouth speculum is in place. A head light is used to give good illumination to the oral cavity.

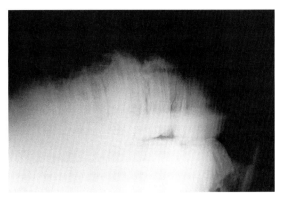

**Figure 9.2.** Radiograph of a fractured upper premolar 3 on a 3-year-old colt. Three weeks prior to presentation, this horse's teeth had been floated by a non-veterinarian. A round spool type mouth gag had been used to hold the mouth during the procedure. It is speculated that the horse fractured this newly erupted tooth while chewing on the gag.

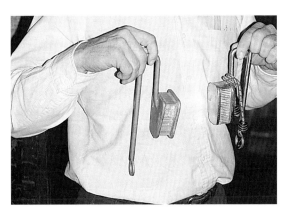

**Figure 9.3.** Wedge type mouth gags are less apt to damage teeth because the masticatory forces are disturbed over several tooth crowns.

digital examination of the oral cavity. Another disadvantage is that a horse chewing on the spool can damage its molar teeth (Fig. 9.2). This occurs particularly in the young horse with erupting permanent teeth or the old horse with short, fragile reserve crowns. These devices can also slip off the molar arcades into the palate and cause damage to the gingiva. Palate lacerations and injury to the palatine artery are also possible.

The types of mouth gags available today vary in size, shape and method of retention. Several of the more common ones are: Schoupe mouth gag, Jeffery gag, and Messer wedge, Bayer mouth wedge, Jupiter Spool, and Meiers dental wedge (Fig. 9.3).

The full mouth speculum restrains the mouth in the open position by applying pressure on the incisor arcades. These types of specula are, as a rule, larger, heavier and more cumbersome than gags. There is also more of a need for chemical restraint when using a full mouth speculum. Since there is the ability to adjust the amount of opening of the speculum, care must be exercised when using these devices to assure that the horse's mouth is not forced beyond a comfortable limit. The speculum should not be left in the open position for an extended period of time – not to exceed 30 minutes – without allowing the horse to relax. Whenever the mouth is opened wide, the buccal mucosa is pulled in against the edges of the upper cheek teeth. Therefore, it is extremely important to remove sharp buccal enamel points from the upper teeth before forcing the mouth open. The greatest advantage of the full mouth speculum is the increased ability for visual and digital inspection of the deep recesses of the oral cavity and greater access to perform dental procedures with good access to the inner oral cavity.

The types of full mouth specula available vary in size and shape. I prefer the McPherson or Hausman type full mouth speculum with adjustable leather straps (Fig. 9.4). Other full mouth specula are: Arnold's mouth gag, Butler's mouth gag, Guenther mouth speculum, Vernell's mouth gag, McAllen mouth speculum, McClelen mouth speculum, Stubbs screw speculum and Meister speculum. Flat gum plates are available with the Hausman type speculum that can be used on cattle (Fig. 9.5). This gum plate can be placed palatally to the upper incisor table to allow oral examination of a horse with a parrot mouth.

## MISCELLANEOUS EXAMINATION EQUIPMENT

Other equipment necessary for oral examinations includes a good light source – a hand held light or head lamp is essential. A flexible cable fiberoptic light can be used to illuminate the deep recesses of the oral cavity and buccal spaces. Various types of cheek retractors can

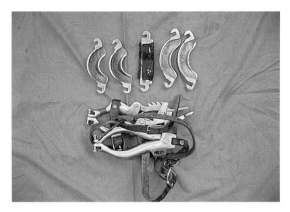

**Figure 9.5.** A stainless steel Hausman type full mouth speculum with large and small incisor plates and a gum plate. The straight gum plate rests on the palate and is handy for examining horses with severe incisor overjet or cattle that lack upper incisors.

allow better visualization in the buccal spaces. A long-handled mechanic's mirror or fiberoptic scope is useful in visualizing the interproximal spaces. A laparoscope with a 45 to 75 degree angled lens can be an invaluable aid in examining between the caudal cheek teeth.

Dental picks and probes are available in various lengths and blade shapes. The complete oral examination can be greatly aided by the use of long dental picks. These devices are especially useful in the examination of older horses, and provide tremendous help in evaluating pockets between and around teeth that cannot be reached with a digit (Fig. 9.6).

A bucket to hold diluted disinfectant (chlorhexidine) solution to rinse the horse's mouth, clean hands and clean equipment are essential when evaluating the oral cavity. A 400 cc dose syringe with a blunt tip is useful to rinse the mouth before oral examination and during dental procedures. Hand care and protection are important factors when working in the mouth. Sharp enamel edges encountered on the teeth and abrasive instruments can cause injuries. Moisture and the bacteriological nature of partially chewed food, always present in the horse's oral cavity, add to the already less than desirable conditions. Moisturizing hand lotion will help lubricate and seal the hands from moisture and dirt. Gloves can be used to protect the hands from abrasions and debris. Soap and

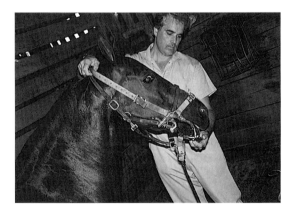

**Figure 9.4.** A McPherson type full mouth speculum being placed on a horse.

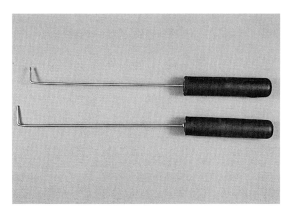

**Figure 9.6.** A set of thin dental picks used to probe and clean out periodontal pockets between cheek teeth.

a nail brush are necessary to clean up properly after performing dentistry (see also Chapter 12).

## DENTAL SIGNALMENT

Data on the horse's owner and trainer/manager/agent/groom should include their name, address and means of contact. This is especially important for the person granting permission to work on the horse and the person responsible for payment for services. The horse's insurance status and type of policy (mortality, loss of use, major medical and surgical) should be recorded. The stable name and address and the horse's location on the premises (barn number, paddock, stall number, etc.) can be helpful for rechecks and follow-up. The horse should be identified on the record by name and described by breed, color, sex, age, type of work and any special identifying markings, scars, brands or tattoos.

## DENTAL HISTORY

The dental history should concentrate on oral, dental or gastrointestinal related areas. Special consideration must be given to other body systems that could be related to masticatory function or the safety of the animal or veterinarian. A history of cardiac abnormalities, respiratory disease, renal problems, hepatic disease or neurological symptoms could affect the way the animal is approached and restrained for examination and therapy. The animal's breed-

ing history and pregnancy status could have an effect on dental care scheduling. Additionally, the horse's show or race schedule may have an impact on when work is performed and whether drugs used to sedate or treat the horse would be considered prohibited substances. The owner should be questioned about the horse's condition and type of exercise, temperament, stable vices, eating and drinking habits, fecal consistency and physical abnormalities. Specific questions asked could begin with these examples. Has the horse gained or lost weight over the past year? Have the horse's temperament or stable habits changed? Does the horse train well and what type of bridle and bit does he wear? Have any changes been noticed in the horse's head carriage or demeanor when bitted? Does the horse make any noises or wear a tongue tie when exercised? Have eating or drinking patterns changed? Such changes might include taking longer than normal to eat, head shaking, tilting when eating, dribbling or quidding feed. Horses with sharp enamel points may pack hay in the buccal space pushing the cheeks away from the upper teeth before eating grain. Inquire about water sources and drinking habits. Find out if excessive salivation, oral odor, or nasal or lacrimal discharge has been noticed. Has the animal experienced any gastrointestinal problems such as choke, colic or changes in fecal consistency?

The horse's vaccination and deworming status should be determined. This is a good time to discuss these important preventative health topics. Tetanus toxoid may need to be given if corrective dental procedures such as wolf tooth extraction or abrasion from a sharp float rasp break the oral mucosal barriers. The owner should be questioned about the animal's history of infectious disease as well as the presence of infectious or contagious disease on the farm. This information may affect the degree of sanitation used between patients on the premises and the degree of disinfection or sterilization of equipment and personal items between farms.

If the equine patient is being seen for a particular dental complaint, a complete history of the problem should be ascertained and documented. A complete history is important as it has been statistically proven that horses presented with a dental complaint are 5.8 times as likely to have one or more selected dental abnormalities.[4] However, do not let a complaint of a dental problem distract or deter from taking a complete dental history and performing a thorough dental and physical examination. A systematic approach to history taking may quickly identify a primary problem that could be related to the animal's age, use, a previous accident, illness or a behavioral problem.

## PATIENT OBSERVATION

Observation of the animal in its normal surroundings can provide information about stable management, eating habits and vices. The area where the dental examination is performed must allow for safe restraint. The area should be free of obstacles that could injure the horse, an attendant or the veterinarian. A high-ceiling area

shaded from bright sunlight with solid walls and a soft non-slip floor is ideal. Access to warm water and electricity may be a consideration.

The horse should be observed and his temperament assessed. Hair, coat and body condition should be evaluated by observation and palpation. Record the body condition score.[9] Condition scores range from 1 to 9, with 1 describing an extremely emaciated animal and 9 being an obese one (Table 9.1). The optimal condition score is between 5 and 6 on the scale (Fig. 9.7). Objective data such as photographs and weight measured with a scale or tape can be recorded. This data can be a valuable tool in management of dental health and patient nutrition. The animal's posture and stance should be observed and abnormalities brought to the attention of the groom and noted in the record. Abnormalities such as swellings, injuries and hoof problems may go unnoticed by the owner or attendant until after you have performed dental procedures.

**Table 9.1.** Description of the Condition Score System

| Score | Description |
|---|---|
| 1 | *Poor:* Emaciated. Prominent spinous processes, ribs, tailhead and hooks and pins. Noticeable bone structure on withers, shoulders and neck. No fatty tissues can be palpated. |
| 2 | *Very Thin:* Emaciated. Slight fat covering over base of spinous processes. Transverse processes of lumbar vertebrae feel rounded. Prominent spinous processes, ribs, tailhead and hooks and pins. Withers, shoulders and neck structures faintly discernible. |
| 3 | *Thin:* Fat built up about halfway on spinous processes, transverse processes can not be felt. Slight fat cover over ribs. Spinous processes and ribs easily discernible. Tailhead prominent, but individual vertebrae can not be visually identified. Hook bones appear rounded, but easily discernible. Pin bones not distinguishable. Withers, shoulders and neck accentuated. |
| 4 | *Moderately Thin:* Negative crease along back. Faint outline of ribs discernible. Tailhead prominence depends on conformation, fat can be felt around it. Hook bones not discernible. Withers, shoulders and neck not obviously thin. |
| 5 | *Moderate:* Back is level. Ribs can not be visually distinguished but can be easily felt. Fat around tailhead beginning to feel spongy. Withers appear rounded over spinous processes. Shoulders and neck blend smoothly into body. |
| 6 | *Moderate to Fleshy:* May have slight crease down back. Fat over ribs feels spongy. Fat around tailhead feels soft. Fat beginning to be deposited along the sides of the withers, behind the shoulders and along the sides of the neck. |
| 7 | *Fleshy:* May have crease down back. Individual ribs can be felt, but noticeable filling between ribs with fat. Fat around tailhead is soft. Fat deposits along withers, behind shoulders and along the neck. |
| 8 | *Fat:* Crease down back. Difficult to palpate ribs. Fat around tailhead very soft. Area along withers filled with fat. Area behind shoulder filled in flush. Noticeable thickening of neck. Fat deposited along inner buttocks. |
| 9 | *Extremely Fat:* Obvious crease down back. Patchy fat appearing over ribs. Bulging fat around tailhead, along withers, behind shoulders and along neck. Fat along inner buttocks may rub together. Flank filled in flush. |

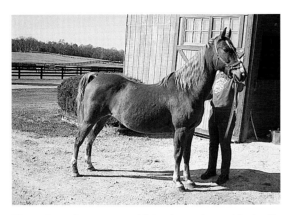

**Figure 9.7a.** A pregnant saddlebred mare in good flesh with a nice fall hair coat and a body condition score of 6.

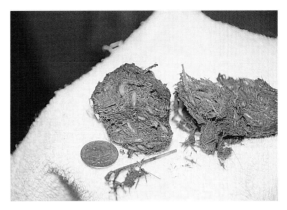

**Figure 9.8.** Abnormal equine manure. Notice the whole grain and large forage stems, these are signs of poor masticatory function. The coin is for size reference (2.5 cm diameter).

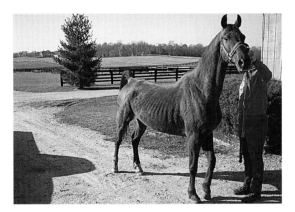

**Figure 9.7b.** A thin saddlebred mare with a rough hair coat and a body condition score of 3.

The stable floor should be surveyed for grain dropped from the horse's mouth or partially chewed boluses of hay that appear much like a cow's cud. This would indicate quidding. Feces should be examined for volume and consistency as this can reflect how well the horse is masticating its feed (Fig. 9.8). Normal manure should be semi-moist and fecal balls should be formed. Feces with long forage stems or whole grain indicate poor mastication. Long stems in poorly masticated feed can predispose the horse to esophageal choke or intestinal impaction colic.

The horse's body and head type should be assessed and recorded. Head conformation can be reflected in the conformation of the dental arcades. Horses with short dished faces typical of the Arabian breed may have a more curved arcade with the last two lower molars ramped up in the curve of the mandible (Curvature of Spee). Breeds that typically have long straight heads (thoroughbred and some warmblood breeds) are predisposed to malocclusion of the molar arcades leading to rostral and caudal hook formation. Miniature horses and ponies are more prone to dental crowding and misplaced or malerupted dentition.

## EXTRAORAL PHYSICAL EXAMINATION

During the basic physical examination (temperature, pulse, respiratory rate, auscultation of heart, lungs and abdomen) the clinician can assess the horse's temperament. The examination should be carried out with patience using techniques of good horsemanship that will gain the confidence of the horse and owner.

The head should be evaluated for symmetry, balance and gross abnormalities which may give clues to dental problems. Standing at the horse's side, assess the head shape and conformation. Look for bumps or protuberances. Young horses between the ages of 2.5 and 4 years of age will have symmetrical, non-painful bony enlargements on the mandible and/or over the maxillary region. These enlargements are the result of normal tooth crown and root development of erupting permanent teeth and the shedding of deciduous caps. If these enlargements are hot, swollen, asymmetrical or associated with a draining tract, tooth pathology should be suspected.

The eyes should be clear and free from lacrimal discharge. The facial contour should be even and any swellings or protuberances noted. Standing directly in front of the horse, evaluate the head for symmetry. The ears, eyes, facial crests and nasal bones should be the same on both sides of the head. Observe and palpate the temporalis and masseter muscles and temporomandibular joints.

Open the mouth slightly and percuss the frontal and maxillary sinuses. Palpate the parotid salivary glands and intermandibular lymph nodes. Manual examination should course the ventral aspect of both sides of the mandible for enlargements noting the vessels and parotid salivary duct at the rostral edge of the masseter muscle. Place open hands under the noseband of a loose halter and exert pressure on the cheeks at the level of the upper dental arcade (Fig. 9.9). Palpation from the level of the medial canthus of the eye, progressing rostrally over the masseter muscle to the level of the nasal notch allows detection of abnormal wear patterns on the upper dental arcades. If the horse resists this maneuver by tossing its head, it is most likely the result of pain from sharp enamel points piercing against the buccal mucosa. If sharp points are present, they should be floated off prior to employment of a full mouth speculum into the oral cavity. Otherwise, as the

mouth is opened, the cheeks are pushed tightly against the sharp enamel points and the horse will object to opening its mouth. Thus, a normally painless examination procedure will cause excruciating pain for the patient and/or subsequently the examiner.

Observe the nasal passages and palpate the false nostrils. Asymmetry of air flow, odor or discharge from the nostrils should be noted. Observe and palpate the lips for bit injuries, noticing especially any scars or ulcers in the commissures. The lips of gray horses are a common area to find melanomas. The upper lip should be rolled up and the underside examined for a tattoo (Table 9.2). The labial mucosa should be salmon-pink in color and glisten with saliva. Ulcers or erosions should be documented and their cause determined. Keep in mind the possibility of vesicular stomatitis which is a reportable zoonotic disease. If any abnormalities are detected from the history or examination, con-

**Table 9.2.** A note on lip tattoos

Most horses that race in the USA are permanently identified with a freeze brand on the neck or a tattoo on the upper lip. Each breed registry has a different alpha-numeric system for identifying horses by their upper lip tattoo.

The Jockey Club of North America uses an alpha-numeric system that consists of a letter of the alphabet followed by numbers. The letter corresponds to the year the horse was foaled with 1997 starting a new 26 letter series. Therefore, 1996 would be Z and 1998 would be B. Horses imported into the USA are identified with an asterisk (*) at the beginning instead of a letter.

The American Quarter Horse Association uses a more random alpha-numeric system of five numbers in older horses and more recently, four numbers followed by a letter.

The American Paint Horse Association uses a numbering system that consists of five digits. The first digit corresponds to the last digit of the horse's year of birth. These first digits would be repeated every ten years.

Since 1982 the United States Trotting Horse Association has been using a system starting with A followed by three or four numbers. That would make foals born in 1998 have an upper lip tattoo that would start with the letter T followed by three or four digits. Horses born prior to 1982 were tattooed with three digits followed by a letter.

Arabian and Appaloosa horses that race in the United States require lip tattoos for identification. Their six-digit registration number is tattooed on their upper lip.

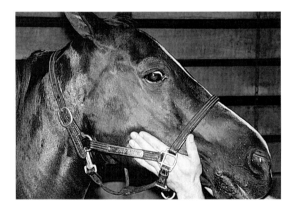

**Figure 9.9.** The palm of the hand is placed under the loose noseband of the halter and pressure placed against the cheeks. Sharp enamel points as well as uneven upper dental arcades can be detected.

sider observing the horse eating. This is best done before the mouth is washed for the oral examination and before sedation is administered.

When evaluating the horse's eating patterns, make a distinction between the horse having trouble with prehension and mastication and the horse that is unable to swallow. Prehension requires neuromuscular coordination and an intact jaw and incisor arcade. Mastication is usually altered by tooth problems or abnormalities in the bones, muscles or temporomandibular joints. Lesions to the tongue or basal ganglion problems can adversely affect prehension and mastication. Swallowing is a more complex process and neurological, muscular or mechanical abnormalities in the pharynx or esophagus should be considered over a dental problem. Rabies is a fatal zoonotic disease that, in its early stages in the horse, mimics other types of eating abnormalities. Equine practitioners and any assistants working in horses' mouths should be vaccinated for rabies and have an antibody titer check periodically in those parts of the world where rabies is endemic.

Standing in front of the horse, part the lips and examine the incisor arcade. Evaluate the incisor teeth for number, shape and symmetry. The incisors should be checked for anatomical characteristics used in assessing the horse's dental age. Compare the estimated age to the horse's real age as a discrepancy between these two could indicate abnormal incisor development or wear.[10] Important to keep in mind is the variation between horses of the same and different breeds in their dental characteristics and real age.[11–14] Observe the incisors while the jaw is moved through a full range of motion. This is best done by standing to one side of the horse and holding the head stationary with a hand on the bridge of the horse's nose. The other hand is used to grasp the mandible and while pressing the mouth shut, moving the jaw from side to side.

During this maneuver, the jaw moves laterally from pivot points at the temporomandibular joints. As the jaw is moved from one side to the other you can determine the range of lateral motion before tooth contact is made with a sloped portion of the molar table. Remember,

the more rostral portion of the arcade will contact first. This will work more caudal as the jaw moves farther to each side. Horses that have had the table surface from the rostral cheek teeth reduced in height will have to move further to one side before the sloped upper and lower molar tables grind over one another and the incisors gradually separate.

Two distances are noted during this maneuver. First, the lateral distance before the sloped molar tables make the upper and lower incisor arcades begin to separate. The second distance noted is the total lateral distance the mandible travels. By observing the incisors, and listening to and feeling the molar arcades grind on one another, one can gain information about the slope of the molar tables and symmetry of the occlusal contact of the upper and lower arcades.[15] Normal lateral excursion will possess a relatively even, subtle to moderate vibration and sound. Deviations from this can be an indication of abnormal dental contact due to long or tall teeth, hooks, etc. (see Chapter 13). It must be kept in mind that this maneuver does not mimic the chewing motion of the horse as outlined in Chapter 2. Remember, if the horse resists this part of the dental examination, sedation may be indicated to help the horse relax and allow a more thorough physical examination. Detomidine (10–40 mcg/kg i.v.) or xylazine (0.05–1 mg/kg i.v.) alone or in combination with butorphanol (0.025–0.1 mg/kg i.v.) will give satisfactory sedation even in particularly fractious horses. With sedation, a complete dental examination can be carried out safely and thoroughly.[16]

## ORAL EXAMINATION

The mouth is the window into the body. The oral mucous membrane is a thin sheet of tissue that permits the veterinarian to view changes in vessels and connective tissue beneath the oral mucosa. Lift the lips and observe the glistening mucosa covered by a thin layer of saliva. There are relatively few sensory nerve endings in the gingiva which makes it a safe area to depress for observing vascularity and capillary refill time.

The oral examination begins with the interdental space and adjacent structures. This area often reveals the performance horse's bitting history. The lip commissures, bars of the lower jaw, tongue and palate are evaluated. In male horses over 4 years of age canine teeth can be observed. The lower canines lie rostral to the upper canines making for a longer lower diastema. The uppers erupt in the suture between the incisive and maxillary bones and usually break through the mucosa 2 to 8 months after the lowers. Young adult stallions and geldings between the ages of 4 and 6 years of age may have canine teeth in various stages of eruption. It bears repeating that long sharp canine teeth can be a danger to the examiner and care should be exercised to avoid injury when manually examining the mouth. These teeth can be shortened and blunted to aid in examination. About 25 per cent of all mares have between one and four rudimentary canine teeth.[17] Dental plaque or tartar accumulation around the canines leading to gingivitis will often be seen in older horses. Eruption cysts or tenting of the mucosa with ulceration over these teeth can cause oral pain and bitting problems.

The upper and lower interdental space should be observed and palpated. Firmly run a thumb over the mucosa, feeling for protuberances above or below the gum line and observe the horse's response to pressure. The lower bars should be checked for sharpness, bony irregularities, mucosal ulcers or thickenings. The presence of lower first premolars can be detected in horses and should be palpated for, just rostral to the lower first cheek teeth. The upper edge of the diastema is palpated for bony abnormalities and upper first premolars. These caniniform teeth are referred to as 'wolf teeth' and erupt between 6 and 18 months of age. If present, they can be found along the edge of the maxillary and palatine bones from the palatial side of the upper PM 2 to the 2 to 3 cm rostral. These teeth usually erupt through the oral mucosa but can migrate under the mucosa and remain there as bumps. The unerupted wolf teeth, referred to as 'blind wolf teeth', can cause oral discomfort and training problems in bitted horses. Wolf teeth come in a vast array of shapes and sizes with the visible crown shape having no relation to the size or shape of the root.

The tongue should be checked for function and any anatomical abnormalities noted. Tongues are frequently injured from harsh bits or neglected tongue ties. Calluses or ulcerations are the result of chronic trauma from sharp teeth. Observe and palpate the hard palate. Lampas, or thickening of the palatial mucosa just behind the upper incisors, is common in young horses that are erupting permanent dentition. The hand can be introduced into the interdental space and a thumb pressed on the hard palate to make the horse open its mouth.

The non-speculum intra-oral inspection and palpation is carried out next. Each clinician should develop their own technique for oral palpation and inspection as a prelude to rinsing the mouth and insertion of the full mouth speculum. The horse should be encouraged to open its mouth either by pushing a finger from the outside of the cheeks between the dental arcades or by hooking a thumb into the commissures of the lips. Great care should be exercised whenever a finger is placed in the mouth to avoid serious injury.

In the two-handed method, the right side of the dental arcade is palpated by approaching the horse from the left side. The left labial commissure is parted with the right hand and the tongue is grasped and pulled through the left interdental space. Care should be taken that the tongue is not traumatized by canine teeth of males or geldings. The cheek teeth of the right maxilla can then be examined by manipulating the right side of the lips with the left hand and by inserting the left hand into the horse's mouth. This process is then reversed to permit a similar inspection of the left arcades. A flashlight, head light or snake light greatly facilitates this examination. The examination must not be conducted in a leisurely fashion because it may annoy the horse to have its tongue grasped for long periods.

For experienced operators, the one-handed technique is recommended. The horse is approached from the front and the right side and the mouth is palpated by inserting the right hand into the right interdental space with the palm facing laterally. The hand should be slightly flexed and the back of the hand is then used to force the tongue between the left cheek teeth arcades. This keeps the horse from completely closing the mouth and enables the examiner's fingers to run quickly along the arcades palpating both the upper and lower arcades for hooks, spaces, overgrowth and irregularities. The procedure is then repeated on the other side of the mouth using the left hand to examine the left dental arcades. As previously stated, when using the two-handed technique it is best to carry out this procedure as quickly as possible.[6] The hand is examined when removed from the mouth, taking note of unchewed feed materials and/or odor. This method is certainly not suitable for attempting to demonstrate specific lesions to owners. At this point the mouth should be rinsed taking notice of the volume, consistency and smell of material flushed from the mouth.

The distance from the commissures of the lips to the rostral edge of the first cheek teeth should be noted as this varies among horses. This distance will affect the ease with which one works on the rostral teeth and may affect the comfortable position of the bit in a working horse.

The easiest and safest way to thoroughly evaluate the oral cavity is by using a full mouth speculum. To place the speculum in the mouth, the examiner stands to the left side of the horse. With the left hand holding the mouthpiece and the right hand holding the poll strap, the mouthpiece is introduced between the incisors in the same manner as a bit. The left thumb and forefinger are used to open the mouth and guide the mouthpiece into place between the incisors while the right hand applies steady tension to the halter strap from behind the horse's poll. When the speculum is properly positioned, the left hand is maneuvered to the halter's buckle to adjust the strap length until the speculum strap is snug. The mouthpiece is adjusted from the front to square it with the incisors. A final check is made to ensure that the teeth and incisor plates are free of tongue, lips and examiner's digits so they are not pinched when opening the speculum. It is important to adjust the noseband and chin strap to allow a stable yet comfortable fit on the horse. Horses with sharp buccal points on the upper dental arcade may resist the full mouth speculum and floating the upper arcades may be beneficial before this part of the examination is attempted. The jaws of the speculum are opened one notch at a time alternating each side until the jaws are opened two to three notches. If the mouth resists being opened with the speculum in place, the temporomandibular joints and bony structures of the jaw should be carefully evaluated before excessive force is placed on the jaw. At this point the oral cavity is ready for visualization and palpation (Fig. 9.10).

To visualize the oral cavity, good illumination is critical. A battery-operated halogen light or transilluminator with a 7 to 15 cm extension will work. A head light provides good illumination while allowing both hands to be free for instrumentation inside the mouth. A blade retractor fitted with an illuminator will aid in the evaluation of the buccal recesses. A basket retractor designed by Stubbs will keep the tongue and buccal mucosa pulled away from the teeth for good visual access to the last few cheek teeth (Fig. 9.11) (RC Stubbs, personal communication, 1997). A flexible fiberoptic scope or rigid laparoscope or intraoral camara has proved useful in obtaining a close up and detailed view of the caudal recesses of the mouth. The oral soft tissues should be observed with special attention paid to the palate, tongue and buccal mucosa. The teeth should be evaluated for conformation, position and number.

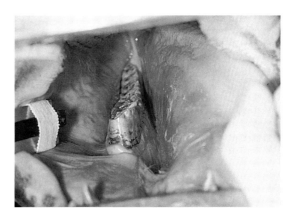

**Figure 9.10.** The oral cavity of a restrained horse can be visualized with a full mouth speculum, cheek retractor and a good light source.

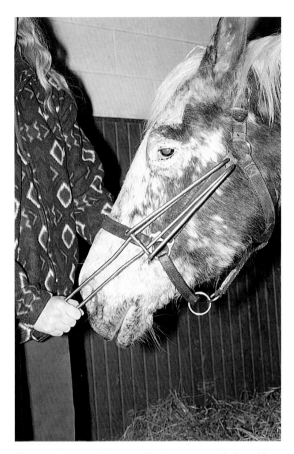

**Figure 9.11.** A stainless steel basket retractor designed by Stubbs will keep the cheek and tongue out of the field of vision while performing an oral examination.

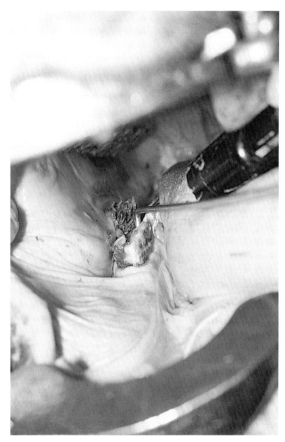

**Figure 9.12.** A dental pick being used to remove feed from a gingival pocket adjacent to fractured 407.

Common premolar findings would include hooks, ramps, erupting teeth or loose caps or cap slivers. In the center of the molar table, one may observe long teeth, wave mouth, cupped out or decayed infundibula, missing teeth or split or misplaced crowns. The caudal dental arcades should be inspected and noted buccal ulcers, sharp enamel points or hooks, supernumerary or missing teeth or ramped dental arcades. The mesial and distal dental margins should be inspected for abnormal tooth contact or feed packed into gingival pockets. A 3.5 mm diameter dental pick with a 31 cm long shaft can be used to probe the four corners of the cheek teeth to detect and clean out periodontal pockets (Fig. 9.12). A calibrated pick can be used to measure gingival pocket depth which will range from 0.5 mm to 12 mm for normal teeth. It

has been shown that gingival pocket depth measures at the corner of the teeth significantly increased with periodontal disease.[18] Defects have been found on the occlusal surfaces of a large number of periapically infected teeth.[3] These defects can be detected by carefully probing the occlusal surfaces of suspect teeth.

The oral cavity should be palpated feeling the buccal, occlusal and lingual surface of all four arcades. The gingival margins of the cheek teeth should be uniform with no feed packed between them. The crown height should be the same on the mesial and distal aspect of each tooth. The crown height should be longer on the buccal aspect of the uppers and the lingual aspect of the lowers. This reflects the normal 10 to 15 degree slope of the molar arcade. Any deviation or asymmetry in molar table height or angle should be noted. Each exposed tooth crown should be grasped between the thumb and forefinger and checked for stability noting any movement. The occlusal surfaces of the arcades should be palpated noting any defects or asymmetry in the occlusal crown surface. Keep in mind that any defect in one arcade will usually be reflected in a wear abnormality or defect in the opposite occlusal arcade.

## ANCILLARY DIAGNOSTIC TESTS

If the initial dental examination findings reveal signs of dental disease, other diagnostic techniques can be employed to make a more definitive diagnosis. A more thorough oral examination can be carried out on a sedated restrained or anesthetized horse. Endoscopic examination of the nasal passages, larynx and oral cavity is often indicated. Skull radiographs, both plain and contrast film studies, give added information about dental, osseous and sinus structures. Sinus centesis or sinuscopy singularly or combined with culture, cytology and/or histopathology can help differentiate primary sinus conditions from sinusitis secondary to dental disease or oral contamination. Other imaging modalities such as ultrasonography, computerized tomography, nuclear scintigraphy or fluoroscopy may reveal a more accurate picture of some dental pathologies.

Radiographic examination of the equine skull can add valuable information to physical examination, oral examination and endoscopic findings. Details of skull radiology are outlined in Chapter 11. Most equine practitioners have access to portable radiographic equipment making this a routine part of the complete work-up of any case with suspected dental pathology. Standing skull films with the mouth open, can give the veterinarian a more complete assessment of the occlusal pattern of the dental arcade.

Radiology is indicated before major dental corrections can be safely carried out in many cases. Other imaging modalities such as ultrasonography, digital radiology, computerized tomography and gamma scintigraphy are also available to many practitioners. These diagnostic tools can aid in making an accurate diagnosis.

Cases of dental disease that involve the upper last four cheek teeth may be associated with sinus disease. The most common presenting sign for sinus disorders is a unilateral nasal discharge. Percussion of the maxillary and frontal sinuses with the mouth open may help in the detection of masses or fluid that fill the sinuses.

Endoscopy of the nasal passages can confirm whether or not the discharge is coming from the nasomaxillary opening. The nasomaxillary area cannot be directly observed with endoscopy, but drainage limited in the caudal aspect of the middle nasal meatus suggests sinus drainage. Malerupted teeth have been seen to narrow the nasal passages which can make passing the scope difficult if not impossible on the affected side.

Standing radiography of the head is a practical, routine procedure to aid in the diagnosis of sinus involvement or disease. Fluid accumulation in the sinuses or dense masses confirm the presence of sinus disease. Sinus centesis or trephination and biopsy can be carried out in the standing horse under local anesthesia. Cytologic evaluation of fluid collected from the sinus can help in the differential diagnosis of sinus infection, tumor or cyst. Bacteriologic culture of the aspirate can be helpful in differentiating primary sinus disease from a pure culture of one bacterial species as opposed to a mixed growth of bacteria from diseased tooth roots. Bacterial sensitivity testing can indicate the correct antimicrobial agent to use for therapy. Care must be taken in evaluating microbiological results because of the presence of secondary organisms superimposed over primary infections or neoplastic conditions.

A good description of the examination of the paranasal sinuses using an arthroscope has been described by Ruggles, Ross and Freeman.[19] This examination can be performed utilizing local anesthesia in the standing sedated horse or under general anesthesia. The reference describes portals for examining the frontal, caudal, and rostral maxillary sinuses. Examination of the dorsal conchal and spheno-palatine sinuses is performed using the frontal sinus and caudal maxillary sinus portals. Sinuscopy has been valuable in diagnosing and treating some sinus disorders without the need for exploratory flap sinusotomy.[20] Lavage can be accomplished through the arthroscope cannula and suction can be used to remove ancillary debris and fluid. Endoscopic examination has proven useful in the diagnosis of sinusitis, neoplasia, cyst formation, tooth root abscesses and primary hemorrhage.

## ORAL AND DENTAL CHARTING

Charting is the process of recording the state of health or disease of the teeth and the oral cavity.[21] To properly chart the mouth, the dental formula and anatomical locations in the mouth must be standardized to make documentation consistent. Use of standard abbreviations for dental terms to describe anatomical boundaries, pathology and diagnostics and therapeutic procedures have made communication possible between colleagues in both the veterinary and human dental professions.

The American Veterinary Dental College Nomenclature and Classification Committee has endorsed the use of the Triadan tooth numbering system. Numbering is based on a fully phenotypic dentition made up of 44 teeth. This three digit system uses the first digit to designate the quadrant and arch location and whether the dentition is deciduous (primary) or permanent (adult). The quadrant implies the right or left side of the individual. The arch denotes maxillary or mandibular. The numbering sequence is upper right, upper left, lower left and lower right. The permanent (adult) dentition utilizes numbers 1 to 4, and the deciduous (primary) dentition uses numbers 5 to 8. In each quadrant, the first or central incisor is always 01, with incisors numbered 01 to 03, the canines, whether present or not, take up the 04 position in the formula. The premolars are numbered 05 to 08 and the molars are numbered 09 to 11.[22,23]

To fully understand equine tooth development and anatomy and to properly document abnormalities for dental record keeping, certain oral topographical terms have been defined. For a unique identification of each surface of a tooth, the following descriptions are used:

| | |
|---|---|
| apical | – toward the apex or root |
| buccal | – toward the cheeks |
| coronal | – toward the tooth crown |
| distal | – posterior or caudal (interproximal surface farthest from mandibular symphysis) |
| labial | – toward the lips |
| lingual | – toward the tongue in the lower arcade |
| marginal | – border or edge near the gingival margin |
| mesial | – anterior or rostral (interproximal surface nearest to mandibular symphysis) |
| occlusal | – occlusing or masticating surface |
| palatal | – toward the palate in the upper arcade |
| proximal or interproximal | – between the teeth. |

Computerized dental charting and record keeping is being used in human and veterinary dentistry. Standard abbreviations and record forms are essential to make this transition into equine practice. Some common dental abbreviations are listed below.

SP – sharp enamel points
BI (L, A or U) – buccal injury (laceration, abrasion, ulcer)
LI (L, A or U) – lingual injury (laceration, abrasion, ulcer)
CH – crown hook
BK – beak
RP – ramp
Sp – step
Wa – wave
ETR – excessive transverse ridges
Cup – cup in central portion of crown
TC – tall crown
PD – periodontal pocket
Fx – fracture
CAL – calculus
DT/R – deciduous root sliver or fragment
CA – cavity
SN – supernumerary
O – missing tooth

WC – worn crown
ROT – rotated
X – extraction.

Other shorthand systems have been used to grade dental lesions.

### Grades of Periodontal Disease[3]

+ Local gingivitis with hyperemia and edema
++ Erosion of the gingival margin
+++ Periodontitis with gum retraction
++++ Gross periodontal pocketing and destruction of alveolar bone.

### Grading the Severity of Dental Caries[3]

Grade 1 Caries of the infundibular cementum
Grade 2 Caries of infundibular cementum and surrounding enamel
Grade 3 Caries of infundibular cementum, enamel and dentin
Grade 4 Splitting of the tooth as a result of caries
Grade 5 Loss of tooth due to caries.

This system is utilized on the sample dental charts provided. A dental chart can be used to record the examination, assessment and pathology. A second diagram can be used to denote the specific treatment and post treatment result or a single diagram can be used as a combined report form (Fig. 9.13).

## DENTAL RECORDS AND TREATMENT PLANNING

The horse's signalment, use and management should be recorded. Pertinent history should be noted with special emphasis on digestive system or performance problems. The horse's general body condition should be recorded and a numbered body score assigned. The results of the masticatory system examination should be recorded and problems listed in order of significance. A plan for treatment of each problem should be outlined based upon the results of history, clinical findings and oral examination before proceeding with any dental work. This problem-orientated approach is important because the owner and/or trainer should be informed of any abnormalities, given a plan for treatment and an estimate of the cost before any correction procedure is carried out. An owner consent statement is often included in record forms and can minimize problems should a legal claim be filed against the veterinarian or a bill come in dispute for collection.

## CONCLUSION

The basis for a complete equine dental examination is the development of a routine treatment plan that is used on each patient. By utilizing proper restraint techniques and equipment, a thorough examination can be performed with minimal stress to the horse and risk of injury to the veterinarian. Finally, a complete written record of the dental examination, findings, treatment plan and follow-up recommendations is essential for the long-term management of equine oral health.

### REFERENCES

1. Kirland K (1994) *A survey of equine dental disease and associated oral pathology.* Abstract, *Proceedings of the 3rd World Veterinary Dental Congress*, Philadelphia, 103.
2. Baker GJ (1997) Some aspects of equine dental disease. *Equine Veterinary Journal*, 2, 105.
3. Baker GJ (1979) A study of Equine Dental Disease. PhD Thesis. University of Glasgow, pp. 78–82.
4. Uhlinger C (1987) Survey of selected dental abnormalities in 233 horses. *Proceedings of the 33rd Annual Meeting of the American Association of Equine Practitioners*, December, 33, 577–583.
5. Orsini P (1989) *Handout notes from Orsini's Presentation at the Eastern States Veterinary Conference*, Orlando, FL.
6. Baker GJ (1998) Dental physical examination. *Veterinary Clinics of North America Equine Practice*, August, 1998, 247–257.
7. Dixon PM (1997) Equine cheek teeth disease: Is periodontal disease still a problem? *World Equine Dental Congress*, April 2, Birmingham, 6–12.
8. Fischer DJ and Easley J (1993) Equine dentistry: proper restraint. *Large Animal Veterinarian*, 48, 14–22.
9. Henneke DR (1985) A condition score system for horses. *Equine Practice*, 7, 13–15.
10. Galvayne S (1886) *Horse Dentition: Showing How to tell exactly the age of a horse up to thirty years.* Thomas Murray and Son, Glasgow, p. 16.

DIAGNOSIS OF DENTAL DISORDERS

EQUINE DENTAL EVALUATION AND MAINTENANCE FORM

(SPACE ABOVE LEFT BLANK FOR ADDRESS OF DVM)
MEMBER  AMERICAN ASSOCIATION OF EQUINE PRACTITIONERS

DATE _____    STABLES _____
OWNER _____    TRAINER _____
ADDRESS _____    _____

_____    _____

PHONE- _____    PHONE _____

HORSE _____ BREED _____ COLOR _____ AGE _____ SEX _____
PROBLEMS _____

| SOFT TISSUE | WOLF TEETH | INCISORS | | CANINES | | MOLARS |
|---|---|---|---|---|---|---|
| NORMAL | PRESENT | NORMAL | OVERBITE | NORMAL | NORMAL | FLOAT |
| LIPS | ABSENT | TILTED | UNDERBITE | UNERUPTED U L | HOOKS F R | CUT-FLOAT |
| TONGUE | UNERUPTED | SMILE | BROKEN TEETH | CUT | HIGH TEETH | CUT-FLOAT |
| PALATE | REMOVE | FROWN | | BUFF | WAVE | CUT-LEVEL |
| GUMS | ROOT FRAGMENT | STEP | | REMOVE TARTAR | STEPPED | CUT-LEVEL |
| BARS | | CAPS | | EXTRACT | SHEAR | CUT-LEVEL |
| CHEEKS | | ALIGN | | | RAMP | CUT-LEVEL |
| | | TOO LONG U L | | | RIMS | FLOAT |
| | | SHORTEN | | | SEPARATION | BROKEN TEETH |
| | | FLOAT | | | CUPPED OUT | |
| | | DREMEL | | | CAPS REMOVED | |
| | | | | | TABLE ANGLES L___ R___ | |

FEE _____         FEE _____         FEE _____         FEE _____

SEDATION: DETOMIDINE _____ BUTORPHANOL _____ XYLAZINE _____ ACEPROMAZINE _____

FEE _____         FEE _____         FEE _____         FEE _____

OCCLUSION RIGHT _____ _____
LEFT _____

| 111 | 110 | 109 | 108 | 107 | 106 | 105 | 104 | 103 102 101 201 102 103 | 104 | 105 | 206 | 207 | 208 | 209 210 211 |

gum line

gum line

| 411 | 410 | 409 | 408 | 407 | 406 | 405 | 404 | 403 402 401 301 302 303 | 304 | 305 | 306 | 307 | 308 | 309 310 311 |

A = ABSENT   CH = CHIPPED   C = CUT   R = REDUCE   E = EXTRACT

TRIP FEE _____ COMMENTS _____

**Figure 9.13a and b.** Equine dental evaluation and maintenance form.

| DATE | OWNER | | FARM NAME/PHONE | | | WORK PHONE | |
|---|---|---|---|---|---|---|---|
| ADDRESS | | CITY | | STATE | ZIP CODE | HOME PHONE | |
| HORSE REG. NAME | | STABLE NAME | COLOR | | BREED | SEX | YR. FOALED |

Hair Coat:     EX     VG     G     P
Condition Score: _____
Lateral Jaw Excursion:     N     AB
History: _____
_____

D. Age _____ Reg. Age _____
Feces:     Fine     Med     Coarse
Palpation Response:     +     −
Soft Tissue _____

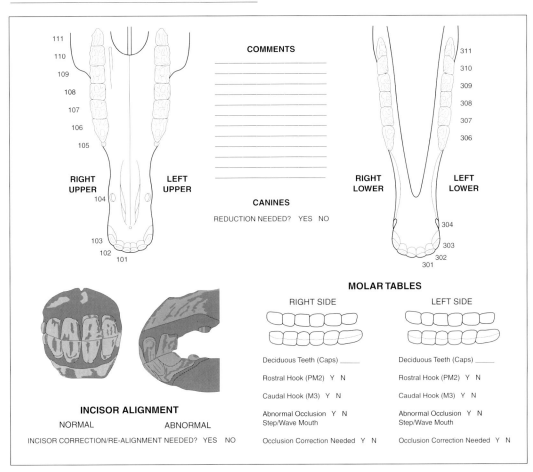

**COMMENTS**

**CANINES**

REDUCTION NEEDED?   YES   NO

RIGHT UPPER    LEFT UPPER

RIGHT LOWER    LEFT LOWER

**INCISOR ALIGNMENT**

NORMAL          ABNORMAL

INCISOR CORRECTION/RE-ALIGNMENT NEEDED?   YES   NO

**MOLAR TABLES**

RIGHT SIDE                    LEFT SIDE

| Deciduous Teeth (Caps) _____ | Deciduous Teeth (Caps) _____ |
|---|---|
| Rostral Hook (PM2)   Y   N | Rostral Hook (PM2)   Y   N |
| Caudal Hook (M3)   Y   N | Caudal Hook (M3)   Y   N |
| Abnormal Occlusion   Y   N Step/Wave Mouth | Abnormal Occlusion   Y   N Step/Wave Mouth |
| Occlusion Correction Needed   Y   N | Occlusion Correction Needed   Y   N |

CHARGES
Farm Call
Professional Exam
Sedation/Tranquilization
Anaesthesia
Xeroradiography
Anti-inflammatory
Antibiotics
Medication/Treatment Other
_____
Problem _____
_____
_____
_____
_____

Initial Est          Actual Amt Chrg

**RE-EXAM NEEDED**

+++++++
DATE

**TOTAL AMOUNT DUE**

+++++++

All services are strictly cash and must be paid at the time of service.

**Figure 9.13b**

11. Walmsley JP (1993) Dental aging in horses between five and seven years of age. *Equine Veterinary Education*, 5, 295.

12. Richardson JD, Lane JG and Waldron KR (1994) Is dentition an accurate indication of age in the horse? *Veterinary Record*, 135(2), 31–34.

13. Richardson JD, Cripps PJ and Lane JG (1995) An evaluation of the accuracy of aging horses by their dentition. *Veterinary Record*, 137(5), 117–121.

14. Muylle S, Simoens P and Lauwers H (1996) Aging horses by an examination of their incisor teeth: an (im)possible task. *Veterinary Record*, 138(13), 295.

15. Rucker BA (1996) Incisor procedures for field use. *Proceedings of the 41st Annual Convention of the American Association of Equine Practitioners*, 22.

16. Baker GJ and Kirkland KD (1995) Sedation for dental prophylaxis in the horse: a comparison between detomadine and xylazine. *Proceedings of the 42nd Annual Convention of the American Association of Equine Practitioners*, 40.

17. Miles AEW and Grigeon C (1990) *Colyer's Variations and Disease of the Teeth of Animals*, (revised edn). Cambridge University Press, Cambridge, p. 121.

18. Stock S (1997) Periodontal parameters in the normal and pathological equine tooth. *Proceedings of the World Equine Dental Congress*, Birmingham, April 2, 1997, pp. 92–95.

19. Ruggles AJ, Ross MW and Freeman DE (1991) Endoscopic examination of normal paranasal sinuses in horses. *Veterinary Surgery*, 20, 418–423.

20. Ruggles AJ, Ross MW and Freeman DE (1993) Endoscopic examination and treatment of paranasal sinuses in 16 horses. *Veterinary Surgery*, 22, 508–514.

21. Wiggs RB and Lobprise HB (1997) *Veterinary Dentistry Principles and Practice*, Lippincott-Raven Publishers, Philadelphia, New York, p. 96.

22. Floyd MR (1991) The modified Triadan system: nomenclature for veterinary dentistry. *Journal of Veterinary Dentistry*, **8**, No. 4, 18.

23. Foster DL (1993) Nomenclature for equine dental anatomy based on the modified Triadan system. *Proceedings from the Annual Meeting of the International Association of Equine Dental Technicians*, Detroit, p. 35.

# THE SYSTEMIC EFFECTS OF DENTAL DISEASE

Derek C Knottenbelt, BVM&S, DVM&S, MRCVS, Division of Equine Studies, Department of Veterinary Clinical Studies, University of Liverpool, Leahurst, Merseyside L64 7TE

## INTRODUCTION

The ability to prehend and chew food is of paramount importance to the horse. Although the digestive process is heavily reliant upon bacterial digestion and fermentation in the large colon and cecum, chewing appears to be a major prerequisite for this process.

Animals which fail to chew effectively for whatever reason (physical malfunction, pain or neuromuscular abnormality) exhibit a variety of clinical signs ranging from weight loss to diarrhea and colic resulting from impaction of the large colon and, to a lesser extent perhaps, the stomach and small intestine. The clinical detection of dental disease may, at times, be difficult because of the subtlety of signs. These may include reluctance to start eating, slow or intermittent eating and dropping of food from the mouth. Sometimes these are only detectable by careful direct observation of the eating process involving several different foods. This can be time consuming but it can be unwise to accept the owner's reports of 'normal eating'.

Some of the most important secondary effects of dental disease relate to the close relationship between the cheek teeth in particular and the nasal cavity and paranasal sinuses. Sepsis of the cheek teeth commonly results in either nasal or paranasal sinus sepsis, or respiratory obstruction, or both of these. It is easy to forget the role of the teeth in apparent nasal disease.

The secondary systemic effects of dental disease or abnormality include some clinically important behavioral and metabolic effects. While the former are possibly more difficult to define they can themselves nevertheless lead to metabolic consequences. There are few reports of the critical evaluation of the role of dental disease in the horse. This is somewhat disappointing in view of the enormous advances in dental medicine in other species.[1,2]

## BEHAVIORAL CONSEQUENCES OF DENTAL DISEASE

Behavioral problems are commonly attributed, perhaps unjustifiably in many cases, to dental problems that ostensibly cause pain or discomfort. Behavioral abnormalities have been attributed to:

- the presence of wolf teeth (vestigial PM 1),
- eruption of both incisor and molar permanent teeth, dental capping is a term usually applied to the erupting permanent cheek teeth
- sharp enamel edges on the buccal margin of the upper cheek teeth and the lingual edge of the lower cheek teeth[2]
- painful dental or oral disorders.

The consequences of these can be fairly dramatic but in many cases the problem fails to resolve after treatment, implying that the problem was not due to dental disease or abnormality.

## HEADSHAKING AND FACIAL PAIN

Some cases of headshaking, tossing of the head and poor responsiveness when ridden have been attributed to dental disease. Headshaking behavior is often ascribed to the presence of the wolf teeth (vestigial PM 1) in particular, and to their position and size. There is considerable debate about whether this is entirely justified.[4] Horses showing headshaking symptoms specifically related to the wolf teeth resolve quickly once the teeth are removed. While it is certainly true that removal of the teeth can resolve the problem in these few cases, many are removed without any noticeable benefit.

Normal molar and incisor eruption has also been identified as a possible cause of transient behavioral problems with ridden work. Where this is genuinely so, resolution of the behavioral patterns follows correction of the underlying dental pathology whether spontaneously or through clinical intervention.

Dental disease has also been suggested as a cause of facial pain and this may lead to behavioral responses that are usually classified as a form of headshaking. The putative relationship between facial pain and headshaking has occupied clinicians for many years but has not stimulated much research interest. It is entirely possible that facial pain or irritation can be caused by dental disease. This may be mediated via indirect or secondary effects on the mental or infraorbital nerves. Most such cases are associated with gross pathology of the alveolus and the surrounding alveolar bone of either the maxilla or mandible. Maxillary sinus disease arising secondarily to dental disease (pp. 134–135) or to oronasal neoplasia (Chapter 8) may also have a profound effect on the infraorbital nerve (Fig. 10.1). The pathogenesis of this is uncertain but direct inflammation or physical distortion may be involved.

The diagnosis of dental-related headshaking or bit resentment may be relatively easy in cases with obvious dental disease but is often very difficult in animals with no overt evidence of this. Gamma scintigraphy can be used to identify dental disease at a subclinical level but again it is hard to be certain of the relationship between the two problems.

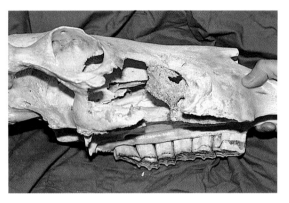

**Figure 10.1.** This horse developed a severe headshaking behavior. Hyperesthesia and persistent rubbing of the right nostril and face caused chronic dermatitis and hyperkeratosis. Facial pain was ascribed to secondary sinus involvement from extensive periodontal disease. The caudal three maxillary teeth had been lost and much of the maxillary and lacrimal bones had been destroyed. The infraorbital canal was also virtually destroyed and the exposed infraorbital nerve ran through the inflamed and infected tissues.

## BITTING PROBLEMS

Horses with resentment to the bit may have oral problems such as the case of mandibular inter-dental-space microfractures in polo ponies but many are not resolved by alteration in the bit type, even to the point of using a bitless bridle. Fractures of the wolf teeth (caused either by trauma from the bit or from careless attempts at extraction) can cause significant harness resentment but there are many other possible causes of this behavior and dental or oral diseases are not usually involved. In the event that such a diagnosis is made the wolf teeth can be extracted or a different harness method can be used.

## BIT GNATHISM

Pain or discomfort associated with dental disease can cause salivation (ptyalism). Some horses will persistently mouth at the bit – often to the extent of dramatic frothing at the mouth. In some cases this has been attributed to dental problems, again involving the wolf teeth or erupting incisors. It is possible that 'dental pain' is involved and in these cases it can be possible to identify the cause and resolve the problem. However, most are behavioral in origin and it is seldom possible to relate the dental abnormalities with the clinical problem.

## RELUCTANCE TO EAT

Anorexia or pica can often be directly attributed to painful dental, oral or jaw disease. There are, of course, many other causes including gastric ulceration and esophageal disease. Dental conditions such as premolar capping (transient non-shedding of the temporary residual crown), tooth or alveolar infection, impaction of molar teeth and displacement of cheek teeth can cause significant pain and therefore a reluctance to eat. However, even horses with severe dental or oral disease may not show overt evidence of pain although secondary effects of dysmastication (masticatory disability) are encountered with some frequency. Conversely some horses with even minor oro-dental disease (such as buccal ulceration from sharp enamel edges) may show obvious discomfort or even overt pain and consequent reluctance to eat normally. A history of quidding of hay but ability to eat grass and other foods without difficulty is commonly reported in horses with sharp enamel edges or periodontitis.[2] Weight loss as a result of reluctance to eat is subtle rather than dramatic in most cases.

## LAMPAS

Edema of the hard palate mucosa was historically regarded as a distinct pathological condition deriving from dental 'disease'. It was regarded as clinically significant when the hard palate mucosa was below the level of the occlusal surface of the upper incisor teeth (Fig. 10.2). The condition is now known to be a normal local circulatory consequence of incisor (or sometimes cheek tooth) eruption. No treatment is warranted and there is certainly no justification for the barbaric firing of the palate with a red-hot iron, which is still practiced in some areas of the world. Problems with inappetance and chewing are commonly found during the eruption of teeth but it seems likely that this is due to the dental problem itself and not the lampas. In any case there would rarely be any long-term consequences from it.

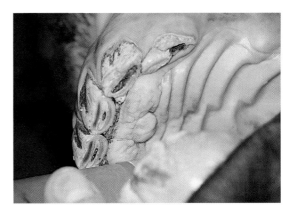

**Figure 10.2.** Edema of the hard palate (lampas) due to the physiological effects of incisor eruption. Note the level of the hard palate is below the occlusal margin of the upper incisor teeth.

## DYSPREHENSION

Difficulty with prehension of food is remarkably rare in the horse in spite of some severe abnormalities of the congruity of the upper and lower jaws or severe dental disease. Prehension also relies heavily on the normal function of the major cranial nerves and upon the musculoskeletal components of the jaws and face. By far the commonest cause of dysprehension is pain in the musculoskeletal structures of the jaws or hyoid apparatus. The metabolic consequences of dysprehension are related to the failure to ingest food, i.e. weight loss, poor nutritional status or dysmastication (impaired or abnormal mastication) (see pp. 129–130).

## DEGENERATIVE JOINT DISEASE OF THE TEMPOROMANDIBULAR JOINT

Pain or physical limitations originating in the temporomandibular joint (or in the hyoid apparatus) may prevent a horse from opening its mouth effectively to prehend food (Fig. 10.3). Usually these changes are insidious in onset and it is often difficult to establish the origin of the problem.

In some cases temporomandibular joint disease arises as a secondary consequence of primary dental disease – long-term (even minor) alterations in jaw movement being the primary

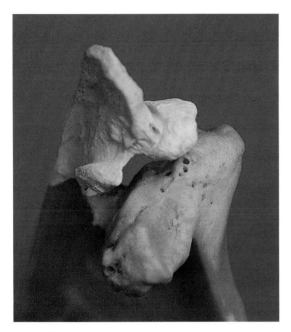

**Figure 10.3.** Degenerative joint disease of the temporomandibular joint, which caused severe progressive pain with dysprehension and dysmastication, with progressive overgrowth of the cheek teeth resulting in a severe shear mouth. No lateral movement of the mandible was possible due to a 2 cm overgrowth of the buccal aspect of the maxillary cheek teeth. Severe, chronic weight loss was the reported primary sign.

cause. A diagnosis is difficult to make without recourse to intra-articular analgesia, radiography and/or gamma scintigraphy. It is also very difficult to establish whether the dental deformity is the cause of the joint degeneration or its result. Horses with grossly abnormal jaw movement as a result of physical or pain-related restriction of movement will inevitably develop dental deformities which reflect the deficiency of occlusal attrition. Secondary joint disease may arise from long-standing abnormal function and this may serve to create further limitations on movement.

A vicious cycle of disability, progressive deterioration in chewing ability and alteration in joint function culminates in an irresolvable dental deformity known as 'Shear Mouth'. The major problem with these disorders is that they are often only recognized when significant clinical consequences such as weight loss are beyond the stage at which any treatment can be instituted. Treatment is palliative at best, usually relying on the provision of a tolerable diet.

## DYSMASTICATION

Dysmastication is an inability to masticate food effectively. Affected horses usually show obvious difficulty with mastication which often manifests as quidding or loss of partly masticated, saliva-sodden food from the mouth (Fig. 10.4). In some cases the condition can be so severe that little food is actually swallowed in spite of a ravenous appetite (Fig. 10.5). In others the signs are more subtle and slow eating or food pouching in the cheeks may be all that is noticed. Food pouching

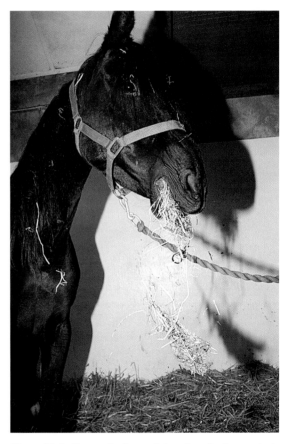

**Figure 10.4.** Dysmastication and dropping of saliva-soaked wads of hay (quidding) as a result of chronic dental infection in a 3-year-old Arabian colt which presented for weight loss over the previous 6 months. A very limited amount of hay was actually swallowed. Soft food and grass were eaten almost normally.

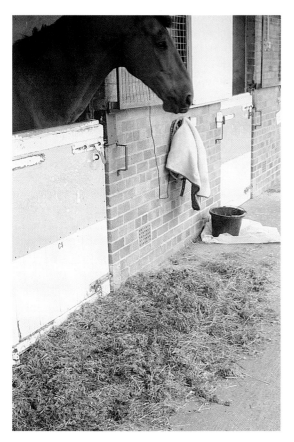

**Figure 10.5.** Severe quidding in a 6-year-old thoroughbred gelding as a result of chronic dysmastication caused by multiple dental abnormalities (including gross dyscongruity of the occlusal surfaces (shear mouth) and temporomandibular degenerative joint disease – see Fig. 10.3). This pile of semi-chewed food was accumulated overnight. The horse had a ravenous appetite but was quite unable to chew any fibrous food. Severe weight loss was reported.

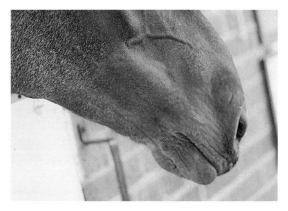

**Figure 10.6.** Food pouching in the cheek is suggestive of dental abnormality but can be a result of neuromuscular disorders affecting the cheeks, face or mouth.

in the cheeks is a common sign of and consequence of dysmastication (Fig. 10.6) which can be attributed in some cases to dental disease. However, it is also a potential sign of neuromuscular disorders of the face, mouth, jaws and tongue.[3]

The presence of dysmastication can be obvious in some cases but can also be very difficult to confirm unless extra time is taken to observe the horse during feeding periods. Some foods will be easier to manage and so again it may be subtle changes that are present.

The cheek teeth are held in place extremely firmly by strong alveolar tissues, but a few meta-

bolic conditions result in either a weakness in this, for example nutritional secondary hyperparathyroidism (bran disease or big-head) alveolar infection (periodontal disease) or neoplastic disease. An inability to exert normal downward and lateral masticatory pressures causes loss of grinding efficiency and consequent loss of digestive efficiency. Such horses will often eat very slowly and some loss of saliva-soaked food (quidding) can usually be seen (although in many cases this is not always obvious).

Dysmastication has several distinct systemic and metabolic consequences which are well recognized by most clinicians but which are poorly reported in the literature. These include:

- oral ulceration
- weight loss
- obstruction and impaction of the esophagus, stomach, jejunum, ileum, cecum, large colon or small colon
- diarrhea.

## ORAL ULCERATION

Oral ulceration is a common cause of anorexia and although it is often a result of dental disease there are other important causes. The full extent of the ulceration may not be obvious during a casual inspection of the mouth (even with the help of a torch or head lamp). The value of oral endoscopy cannot be overemphasized – careful examination of the mouth in this way can be one of the most valuable diagnostic tools in the investigation of dental or oral disease (see Fig. 10.7). Horses with significant oral ulceration (including those where the lesions are located at sites which are consistent with dental disease) should be investigated for other possible primary causes. Horses with non-healing oral ulcers that fail to respond to appropriate dental care often have other underlying pathology including Cushing's disease or advanced renal failure. Other causes of oral ulceration include:

- chemical and caustic burns (including Blister-beetle toxicity and mercuric blister contact)
- drug toxicity (particularly with non-steroidal anti-inflammatory drugs and oral organophosphate anthelmintics)
- plant irritations
- systemic auto-immune vesico-bullous disorders (including pemphigus vulgaris and bullous pemphigoid)[5]
- some infectious diseases (including viral stomatitis, the larval stages of *Habronema musca* and *Gastrophilus* spp. infestation can also cause and sustain oral ulceration).

Usually a careful clinical examination and a full historical investigation will help to establish the likely primary disorder. Where this resolves, the underlying oral ulceration should clear quickly – the mouth has a remarkable ability to heal quickly and without any residual scarring. The most common oro-dental disorder in the horse is buccal (and to a lesser extent lingual) ulceration and laceration (Fig. 10.7) caused by sharp enamel overgrowths (the enamel points) on the lateral edges of the maxillary (and more rarely the lingual edges of the mandibular) cheek teeth.[6] This is probably the most common cause of dysmastication and quidding and these ulcers heal rapidly once the underlying problem has been resolved. Testing saliva for occult blood is sometimes helpful as means of detecting oral ulceration (a urine dipstick applied to the oral mucosa is often sufficient).

While dental disease such as enamel overgrowth and maleruption is a common cause of oral ulceration there are many other causes. Infectious causes include viral stomatitis and migrating larvae of *Gastrophilus* spp. Non-infectious causes include direct trauma, caustic burns, auto-immune disease, renal failure and internal neoplasia. A flow chart for the differential diagnosis of oral ulceration is shown in Figure 10.8.

## WEIGHT LOSS

Digestive efficiency depends heavily on effective mastication. Normal mandibular movement results in the characteristic, self-sharpening, highly efficient wear patterns of the cheek teeth.[7] There is little doubt about the relationship between dental disease, dysmastication and weight loss but there are few documented reports of the extent of the effect. Even in cases where the dental disorder is relatively innocuous in appearance the inability to chew effectively has significant and serious metabolic consequences. Failure to disrupt fibrous food results in impaired simple digestion of soluble nutrients and an inefficient fermentative digestive process in the large colon and cecum. Fecal consistency often reflects this with a high fibrous content with prominent long fibers. This can arise from a number of dental disorders including:

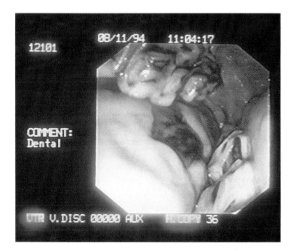

**Figure 10.7.** Oral (buccal) ulceration resulting from overgrown enamel edges on the caudal cheek teeth. The horse ate slowly and saliva tested positive for blood using a urine dipstick. The lesions were not very obvious when viewed in the conscious horse but endoscopy was usefully employed to establish the nature of the problem.

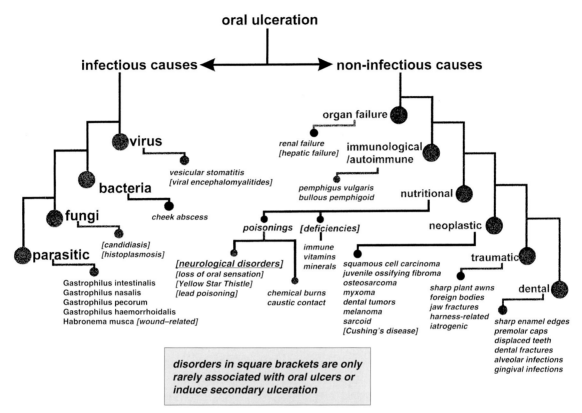

**Figure 10.8.** Oral ulceration: a flow chart to facilitate the investigation and diagnosis of oral ulcers.

1 failure of normal lateral movement (arising primarily from dental abnormality or secondarily from temporomandibular joint disease)

2 loss of occlusal efficiency arising from dental pain or deformity which prevents normal occlusion, and also from musculoskeletal pain or weakness

3 inefficient grinding surface on the occlusal surface of the cheek teeth ('smooth mouth') however caused (chronic ingestion of sharp sand, over enthusiastic floating or rasping of the teeth, old age and hypoplasia of the enamel ridges have been identified as possible causes)

4 absence of cheek teeth

5 severe or progressive physical deformity of the dental arcades.

Shedding of teeth as a result of alveolar, dental or connective tissue disease can also have a pro-found influence on masticatory efficiency. The shedding of the molar teeth in old age (see Chapter 4) reflects the ultimate loss of dental efficiency although this is not really a dental disease. This has historically been regarded as one of the primary causes of geriatric or natural death in the horse – the teeth being a common organ of failure in old age.[8] Horses with poor tooth structure, disease or a faster rate of natural attrition (arising from inherent dental weak-nesses or from dietary factors) might then be expected to have shorter lives than those with good, normal dental function. However, appro-priate adjustments to the diet can prolong life significantly and maintain body condition. Weight loss in a very old horse can often be directly attributed to natural attrition of the cheek teeth and this aspect should always be considered.

A further natural change which develops in older cheek teeth is the loss of the enamel ridges responsible for grinding efficiency. Thus the simple presence or absence of the cheek teeth may not be the only cause of reduced dental efficiency. It is therefore necessary to examine thoroughly the mouth and the teeth, as well as the process of eating, in all horses that suffer from acute, sub-acute or chronic weight loss.

## ALIMENTARY TRACT OBSTRUCTION AND IMPACTION

### Choke

Failure to chew effectively can result in esophageal obstruction with the typical signs of choke such as salivation, nasal regurgitation of food, water and saliva, often accompanied by some distress. Metabolic consequences of choke include inhalation pneumonia, water and food deprivation and in some severe cases esophageal damage resulting in ulceration and stricture. This consequence of dental disease is unusual and other causes of choke should be explored first.

### Colic (impaction)

There is a widespread recognition (but few documented reports) of the relationship of dental disease to non-strangulating obstructive colic. However, in some cases the two are also unjustifiably linked. Failure to chew food certainly results in the ingestion of a high proportion of long-fiber material. Significant impaction develops in the stomach, ileum, cecum and large colon – particularly at the pelvic flexure and more rarely in the jejunum and small colon.[9] It is easy to overlook the possible etiological role of dental disease in colic cases.

Gastrointestinal obstructions characteristically cause low-grade, persistent or recurrent colic. Individual episodes can be more severe, largely depending on the degree and site of the obstruction and any secondary consequences. The extent to which the consistency of the ingesta is responsible for the impaction is often impossible to establish categorically but it is certainly true that some impactions are made up of long-fiber ingesta tangled into a dense rough aggregation. Some ingested materials are more liable to induce impaction and obstruction anyway and some of these are impossible or difficult to masticate, even in a normal horse (e.g. synthetic nylon fibers, wood shavings or wood turnings). A close examination of fecal consistency in relation to the dietary components may provide useful information. In the event that surgery is necessary to relieve the obstructions the true nature of the obstruction can usually be established. It is important to realize however, that some obstructions, such as ileal and pelvic flexure impaction, occur relatively often in horses with normal dental structure and function.

## DIARRHEA

There are few documented reports on the role of dental disease in diarrhea but occasionally dental disease is implicated. Coarse, badly chewed ingesta may cause excessive water retention, particularly in the large and small colons. The consistency may also have a significant effect on intestinal motility. Where dental disease is the primary cause the consistency of the feces can be very variable ranging from overt diarrhea in which extensive long-fiber strands can be found in profuse diarrheic feces to 'softer than normal' feces (which also have a high long-fiber content). The feces may be intermittently normal with variable episodes of obvious diarrhea. A few cases will show a mixture of normal fecal balls with plentiful watery fluid particularly at the beginning and end of defecation. There are few reports of these effects in the literature but most practicing veterinarians will recognize the symptoms. When investigating a clinical case of diarrhea it is easy to ignore the possibility of dental disease (Fig. 10.9).

## DYSPHAGIA

The term dysphagia is used to describe difficulty with swallowing but it is also often used to cover broader difficulties with eating. True dysphagia is very rarely related to dental disease, being more often caused by physical or neuromuscular problems in and around the pharynx and is therefore not discussed here.

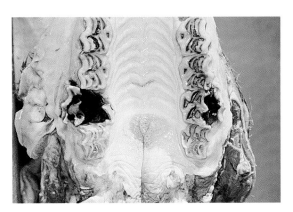

**Figure 10.9.** Diarrhea and severe weight loss were attributed to failure of masticatory efficiency in a 2-year-old pony. The feces contained significant amounts of unchewed long-fiber food. The pony had considerable difficulty chewing but managed to swallow reasonable amounts of hay and concentrate food and was diagnosed with severe decay of both fourth cheek teeth.

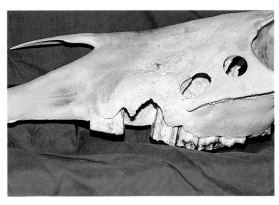

**Figure 10.10.** Metaplastic calcification involving the maxilla around a decayed, infected second maxillary cheek tooth.

## SECONDARY CONSEQUENCES OF DENTAL DISEASE

Some of the secondary consequences of dental disease are discussed here.

## METAPLASTIC CALCIFICATION

Dental infections, and particularly those which affect the cheek teeth, can be very destructive to the bone of the alveolus. Infection is characterized in some cases by simultaneous bone destruction (osteolysis). Metaplastic conchal calcification, where the conchal cartilage becomes progressively calcified as result of dental disease (particularly disease affecting the rostral three maxillary cheek teeth), has been well described.[10] When affecting the first three cheek teeth this change may also cause facial swelling (Fig. 10.10) which is easily identified radiographically. The changes are relatively common and very typical and although, in theory at least, neoplastic bone disease might be mistaken for it, the latter is very rare.

## CONCHAL NECROSIS[11,12,13]

The close relationship of the apices of the maxillary cheek teeth to the paranasal sinuses and the

nasal structures means that destructive dental disease may affect the nasal cavity with or without any outward sign of facial swelling. The first two cheek teeth are most likely to involve the nasal cavity while the more caudal ones will probably show sinus involvement. Periapical infection of the first two maxillary cheek teeth (and occasionally the third) in younger horses will sometimes discharge into the nasal cavity producing a unilateral nasal discharge instead of the more usual facial sinus tract. In older horses with less reserve crown the infection will usually drain around the tooth directly into the mouth.

Discharging sinus tracts associated with dental disease affecting the mandibular teeth and the rostral two maxillary cheek teeth are relatively common. The metabolic consequences are dependent upon the underlying cause of the problem. These can be periapical sepsis, infundibular necrosis, maleruption or supernumerary teeth (with or without gross abnormalities). For the most part however, the secondary consequences are not severe.

## FACIAL DISTORTION AND DEFORMITY

Physical abnormality in the outline of the mandible is a very common finding in young horses as a result of normal dental eruption. The extent of the characteristically firm swellings in the mandible can sometimes be alarming. They are more common in the rostral cheek teeth. As the third cheek tooth is the last to erupt it is possible for it to become impacted by the firmly erupted second and fourth teeth. Where this occurs there is a progressive swelling of the face over the apex of the third tooth (usually level with the end of the facial crest). This is called an eruption cyst. Under normal conditions this cystic structure will resolve spontaneously after occlusal contact is achieved. In some cases however, the teeth are impacted and so the third tooth (in maxillary or less commonly the mandibular arcades) are unable to erupt effectively. This may induce significant secondary osteitis and fistula formation over the site of the tooth.

## EPISTAXIS

Epistaxis can arise from dental disease either directly through erosion and ulceration of the alveolus into the nasal cavity (cheek teeth 1/2) or the paranasal sinuses. Such decay of alveolar bone (whether from dental disease or neoplasia) is usually accompanied by a fetid odor (which is restricted to the ipsilateral nasal cavity). Blood or purulent material may be seen endoscopically within the nasal cavity but only that directly restricted to the drainage angle of the maxillary sinuses can be justifiably identified as of sinus origin. There are of course many other causes of blood and purulent discharges from the nasal cavity.

## SINUSITIS

One of the best-known secondary consequences of maxillary dental disease affecting the more caudal four maxillary cheek teeth is sinusitis.[14,15] The primary dental disease can take a number of forms including maleruption, primary or secondary dental fractures, alveolar infection and periodontal disease or infundibular necrosis.

While in theory any of the four most caudal maxillary teeth can be involved there is a higher incidence of maleruption, fracture, infection and alveolar disease in the third and fourth teeth. This means that rostral maxillary sinusitis is possibly more common than infections of the caudal maxillary sinus.[16] The clinical conse-

quences vary from a mild, purulent nasal discharge (Fig. 10.11) to severe fetid, postural (possibly hemorrhagic discharge) with dysmastication and dysphagia. A diagnosis is reliant upon the combined use of radiography, sinus trephination, endoscopy (with sinuscopy)[17] and scintigraphy. Typically for any chronic septic focus there may be metabolic effects which are not instantly recognizable as being of dental origin. These include weight loss, anemia and poor general health status including loss of athletic performance (see Fig. 10.12).

## RESPIRATORY OBSTRUCTION

Swelling of the tissues around the apices of the rostral two maxillary teeth can cause significant respiratory obstruction. Usually the extent of obstruction is not severe unless the case is advanced and long standing but altered or asymmetrical air flow may be recognizable at an earlier stage. By the time the nasal septum has been distorted sufficiently to cause contralateral obstruction of air flow the animal will almost certainly have shown some other recognizable signs. Nevertheless it is quite common to encounter horses with severe and often life-threatening nasal obstruction as a result of infection or maleruption of the first two cheek teeth. Sinus cysts and oronasal neoplasia are also common causes of respiratory obstruction (see Chapter 8 Figs 8.3, 8.5, 8.9).

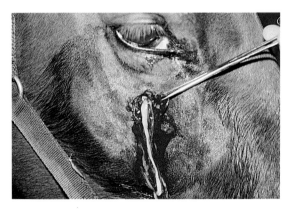

**Figure 10.11.** Maxillary sinusitis that was caused by dental sepsis involving 108.

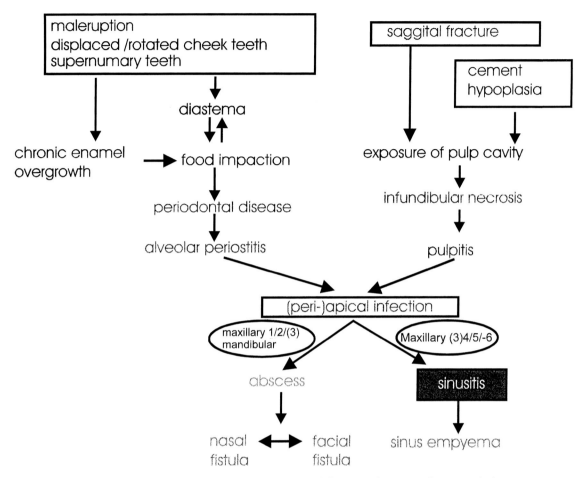

**Figure 10.12.** Algorythm showing the clinical consequences of dental disease on the surrounding anatomical structures.

### REFERENCES

1. Dixon PM (1993) Equine dental disease: a neglected field of study. Editorial in *Equine Veterinary Education*, 5, 285–286.
2. Lane JG (1994) A review of dental disorders of the horse, their treatment and possible fresh approaches to management. *Equine Veterinary Education*, 6, 13–21.
3. Dixon P (1997) Dental Disease. In: *Current Therapy in Equine Medicine*, ed. NE Robinson, WB Saunders, Philadelphia, pp. 149–153.
4. Knottenbelt DC and Pascoe RR (1994) *Color Atlas of Diseases and Disorders of the Horse*. Wolfe, London.
5. Williams MA, Dowling PM, Agarano DW *et al.* (1995) Paraneoplastic bullous stomatitis in a horse. *Journal of the American Veterinary Medical Association* 207, 331–334.
6. Dixon PM (1997) *Examination and Pathology of the Oral Cavity*. Proceedings of the 5th Geneva Congress of Equine Medicine and Surgery, 14–16 December, Geneva, pp. 9–14.
7. Kilic S, Dixon PM and Kempson SA (1997) A light microscope and ultrastructural examination of calcified dental tissues of the horse: 1 The occlusal surface and enamel thickness. *Equine Veterinary Journal*, 29, 190–197.
8. Dixon PM and Copeland AN (1993) The radiological appearance of mandibular cheek teeth in ponies of different ages. *Equine Veterinary Education*, 5, 317–323.
9. Booth AJ, Hansen TO, Mueller POE and Williamson L (1995) Diseases of the large intestine causing colic. In: *The Equine Manual*, ed. AJ Higgins and IM Wright, WB Saunders, London, pp. 483–485.
10. Richardson JD and Lane JG (1993) Metaplastic conchal calcification secondary to chronic dental periapical infection in seven horses. *Equine Veterinary Education*, 5, 303–307.
11. Baker GJ (1982) Dental disorders in the horse. *Compendium of Continuing Education*, 4, 508–514.

12. Baker GJ (1985) Oral examination and diagnosis: management of oral diseases. In: *Veterinary Dentistry*, ed. CE Harvey, WB Saunders, Philadelphia, p. 217.

13. De Moor A and Verschooten F (1982) Empyaema and necrosis of the nasal conchae in the horse. *Deutsche-Diergeneeskundig-Tijdschrift*, 51, 173–191.

14. Baker GJ (1982) Diseases of the teeth and paranasal sinuses. In: *Equine Medicine and Surgery* (3rd edn), American Veterinary Publishers, Santa Barbara, pp. 437–458.

15. Laverty S and Pascoe JR (1997) Sinusitis. In: *Current Therapy in Equine Medicine*, ed. NE Robinson, WB Saunders, Philadelphia, pp. 419–421.

16. Honnas CM and Pascoe JR (1996) Diseases of the paranasal sinuses. In: *Large Animal Internal Medicine* (2nd edn), ed. BP Smith, Mosby, CV New York, pp. 615–618.

17. Chan C and Munroe G (1995) Endoscopic examination of the equine paranasal sinuses. *In Practice*, 17, 419–422.

# DENTAL IMAGING

Christine Gibbs, BVSc, DVR, PhD, MRCVS, University of Bristol

## INTRODUCTION

Imaging is a widely used and constantly evolving diagnostic aid in many spheres of equine clinical practice and is particularly indicated for the investigation of disorders of the head because some of its components are relatively inaccessible to direct visual or manual evaluation. It has been recognized for many years that conventional radiography can make an important contribution to the demonstration of certain dental conditions, particularly those affecting the relatively secluded maxillary and mandibular cheek teeth.[1-15]

Although basic X-ray units of the type available in most veterinary practices generate sufficient radiation to produce images of acceptable quality, radiographic examination is often considered to be too technically demanding for routine use in equine dentistry. This is probably because the anatomical complexity of the area under investigation imposes a need for intricate radiographic techniques and represents a challenge to radiological interpretation. However, the combination of air spaces and mineralized tissue in the equine head produces excellent radiographic contrast which allows demonstration of relatively minor gross pathological changes, provided that suitable projections are selected and accurately executed. Alterations in the number, size, shape and configuration of teeth can be identified, together with associated disruption of skeletal components and abnormal proliferation or loss of bone. Accumulation of fluid or soft tissue material in the paranasal sinuses and nasal airways may also be detected.

The limitations of conventional radiography have prompted consideration of the use of alternative imaging techniques. Computed tomography (CT)[16-18] generates high-quality images in multiple planes, but requires expensive and sophisticated equipment. The main clinical disadvantage of this procedure is the requirement for prolonged general anesthesia. In contrast, nuclear scintigraphy and ultrasound have the virtue of being suitable for use in standing horses. Scintigraphic studies show promise for localization of subtle osseous or vascular changes which may be associated with dental disease[19] (JC Boswell, personal communication, 1997) and facilities for such investigations are becoming more widely available. High resolution ultrasound equipment is now available in many equine practices and examinations can be performed with minimal interference to the patient at a low cost. Although this technique has limitations in anatomical regions in which bone and gas predominate, it may have a place in the evaluation of dental disorders associated with major disruption of alveolar bone and soft tissue swelling.

Despite the increasing popularity of alternative modalities, for the foreseeable future, radiography is likely to remain the imaging procedure most commonly used for the demonstration of dental disease in horses. With knowledge, care and experience, valuable clinical information can be obtained from radiographs in a wide range of disorders. The objective of this chapter is to help the reader acquire the necessary skills for successful radiography and radiological interpretation.

# RADIOGRAPHIC TECHNIQUES

## EQUIPMENT

### X-ray machines

Any type of X-ray unit can be used for equine dental radiography. Generally speaking, exposure requirements are not high, so even low-output portable machines are suitable.

Of greater importance is the system used for mounting or suspension of the X-ray tube, because it is sometimes necessary to carry out dental radiography with the horse standing. A facility must therefore be provided for directing the horizontal X-ray beam at high level. It is also an advantage if the tube head can be moved through a range of angles in order to permit a variety of oblique projections. The most effective arrangement is a telescopic ceiling mount with a range of vertical travel between 75 and 200 cm and a tube connection which allows both vertical and horizontal rotation through an angle of 180°. A horizontal travel facility in two directions is desirable but not essential. Column-mounted X-ray tubes, either fixed or mobile, tend to be less convenient to manipulate and often have limited facilities for tube rotation and angulation. In this case, positioning of the patient becomes more critical and sufficient space must be available around the machine to allow the horse to stand at a variety of angles to the X-ray beam. If no custom-made tube support is available, it is perfectly feasible to obtain satisfactory radiographs by improvising a tube stand from a step ladder or a combination of articles such as tables, stools or boxes available in most stable yards!

It is a great advantage if the light beam diaphragm unit is swivel-mounted, so that it can be adjusted to provide accurate primary beam collimation in any plane. Whenever possible, equine dental radiography should be carried out in conditions of low environmental light intensity. This maximizes visibility of the margins of the light beam making accurate collimation easier.

## Imaging systems

The choice of imaging system (film and screen combination) must always be a compromise between the desirability of fine image detail and the need to keep exposure factors as low as reasonably possible. For most equine dental radiography it is advantageous to use an imaging system with a wide range of exposure latitude and photographic contrast. This is because the structures of the skull have intrinsically high radiographic contrast, particularly in the region of the caudal maxillary arcades, where heavily mineralized dental and osseous tissue lie adjacent to the radiolucent air spaces of the paranasal sinuses and nasal chambers.

Although the high-speed versions of traditional calcium tungstate intensifying screens are generally satisfactory, more recently developed phosphors which are salts of rare-earth metals have the advantage of increased light emission and relatively lower exposure requirements. Rare-earth screens are now available in a wide range of speeds and detail. For most equine dental examinations involving the cheek teeth, medium speed and medium detail screens give acceptable results (e.g. Lanex Regular, Kodak Ltd). If a high-output generator (> 300 mA) is available, the use of slower speed, finer detail imaging systems can be considered. Very fast screens should be avoided, not only because detail and contrast are sacrificed, but also because exposure factors are more critical and may be difficult to select reliably. For the incisors and canines, intra-oral examinations of the cheek teeth and the full dentition of young foals, a fine detail system is desirable (e.g. MinR, Kodak Ltd, which uses a single screen and film emulsion).

## Accessory equipment

**Grids.** It is rarely necessary to use a grid for equine dental radiography. This is because there is little bulky soft tissue in the regions under investigation so that the amount of scattered radiation produced is relatively small. The use of grids in standing animals should be positively discouraged, because of the increased exposure requirement and difficulties associated with alignment for oblique projections. The only examination in which sufficient scatter is produced to justify routine use of a grid is the ventrodorsal view of the caudal arcades, where a great thickness of mandibular bone must be penetrated in addition to the partially superimposed cheek teeth. As this projection is normally obtained with a vertical beam in the recumbent, anesthetized animal, radiation hazards can be well controlled.

**Cassettes.** For external placement and intra-oral positioning for the incisor and canine teeth, any type of rigid film cassette can be used, but lightweight plastic construction is preferred for ease of handling.

To obtain intra-oral radiographs of individual cheek teeth, it is necessary to place the film far back in the oral cavity and the only feasible way of doing this is to employ a flexible film package or cassette. The use of human dental film packs has recently been described in detail,[14] but they have the disadvantages of being small ($5 \times 7.5$ cm approximately) and requiring manual processing. Non-screen film prepacked in larger paper envelopes can also be used and some types are suitable for automatic processing. Unfortunately, their market in the human medical field is declining, so production is likely to be discontinued in the foreseeable future. Plastic envelope cassettes containing either one or two intensifying screens mounted on firm, but slightly flexible card, have recently appeared as a substitute for envelope-wrapped non-screen film. They are suitable for equine intra-oral use, but radiographic sharpness may be marred by less than perfect film–screen contact. The standard rectangular shape ($13 \times 18$ cm) and relatively thick seams on the packets also present some limitations to the anatomical areas which can be included on the radiograph. An alternative is to improvise cassettes of a more suitable shape for the equine oral cavity (i.e. $10 \times 25$ cm approximately) by double wrapping the film and card-mounted intensifying screen or screens, cut down to size, in closely fitting

light-proof bags. The most suitable material is heavy-duty black polythene, the edges of which are closed with light-proof adhesive tape. The inner bag, which remains open at one end, fits the screens and film tightly. The outer bag is very slightly larger and is slipped over the inner bag from the open end. The outer bag is then temporarily sealed with tape which can easily be opened to allow removal of the film for processing. Again, the weakness of this system is poor screen–film contact. Films in flexible cassettes are susceptible to pressure damage (see Fig. 11.5) so care must be taken when removing them from between tightly clenched teeth.

**Cassette holders.** For dental radiography of standing horses it is essential to use some kind of cassette holder whenever possible. The potential need for a variety of oblique projections means that a flexible and readily adjustable system is required. In this respect, the standard vertical suspension linked to the X-ray tube used in many fixed units may not be entirely suitable, particularly if the cassette holder is not capable of a full range of independent movement. A simple method of suspending a cassette in a vertical position which allows free movement is to place it in a fabric bag hanging from a mobile drip stand. Adjustable ties at each side allow varying heights and angles to be used (see Fig. 11.2). The small rigid cassettes used for intra-oral radiography of the incisor dental arcades can conveniently be held at a distance by grasping them with long-handled hoof trimmers or farriers' pincers (see Fig. 11.1).

**Labelling and positioning aids.** Radiographic markers suitable for indicating sides, projections, centering points and anatomical landmarks should be available. Positioning aids such as sandbags and radiolucent foam pads will be needed for radiography of recumbent patients.

## RADIATION PROTECTION

Use of a horizontal or near horizontal X-ray beam at high level increases the risk of radiation exposure to the upper bodies, heads and necks of human attendants. Obviously, generally accepted protection practice must be observed,[20,21a] but special precautions may also need to be taken.

Conscious animals should be restrained by one person only, from a position which enables them to be at least 1 m and preferably 2 m from the nearest margin of the primary beam. All persons present during radiography should wear protective lead aprons and those whose hands are at risk of being closer than 2 m to the primary beam must be provided with protective gloves or sleeves.

Cassettes and holders should be manipulated by members of staff experienced in the techniques being used. For those required to undertake such procedures regularly, consideration should be given to providing extremity dosemeters and thyroid protection. Should an occasion arise when the need to hold a cassette is unavoidable, the largest size available should be used and held at arm's length by the corners of a short side. The X-ray beam must be closely collimated and centered as far as possible from the hands.

## RESTRAINT AND SETTING UP

It may be possible to radiograph quiet, sensible horses in the standing position without the use of pharmacological restraint, but it is essential that they are cooperative enough to keep still for several minutes in a predetermined position while equipment is moved around them. They must also stand voluntarily with the head low enough to accommodate the range of travel of the X-ray tube. It is not acceptable to use manual restraint to retain the head in the required position.

Sedative and tranquilizing drugs are now used routinely for restraint of horses for clinical examinations, including radiography. Care should be taken to avoid overdosing when there is a tendency for the head to be held too low and postural instability may predispose to sudden movement. It is often expedient to perform radiography in conjunction with other investigations requiring sedation. In such cases, it is best that the examination is done before any invasive procedure such as dental rasping or direct sinus endoscopy.

Manual restraint should be confined to prevention of roaming activity by loose control of the head. A simple rope or webbing halter without metal components should be used with a lead rope at least 2 m long.

Two people are needed to set up the tube and film cassette. The radiographer must be clearly aware of the exact projections and centering points required and position the X-ray tube accordingly. An assistant, under the guidance of the radiographer, should then position the cassette. At this stage it is often helpful if the person restraining the horse checks alignment in the third dimension from a position at right angles to the primary beam. Immediately before exposure, all participants must retreat as far as possible from the path of the primary beam.

Under general anesthesia, restraint is perfect, but it is positioning which presents the challenge. To obtain accurate and reproducible oblique radiographs it is preferable, whenever possible, to keep the head in a standard laterally recumbent posture and obtain the desired projections by manipulating the X-ray tube and cassette into the required relative positions (see Fig. 11.3).

For laterally orientated projections, image quality is usually optimal if the animal lies on the affected side, although this entails the inconvenience of turning it before further clinical evaluation or intervention can take place. As it is not usually feasible to re-turn the animal during or immediately after surgery, intra- and postoperative radiographs must be taken in less than ideal circumstances, with the affected side uppermost (see Figs 11.3 and 11.8). In some cases, particularly when ventrodorsal or near ventrodorsal views are required, it may be necessary to withdraw the endotracheal tube.

The design of some operating tables makes it difficult to obtain a full range of movement of the X-ray tube around the patient's head, thus restricting projection options. In such cases, it may be necessary to devise some form of extension platform onto which the head and neck can be drawn to give surrounding unobstructed space.

# PROJECTIONS

## Introduction

In equine dental radiography, the correct choice of projection is critical. While the incisor arcades and canines can be demonstrated with ease, the anatomical conformation and location of the cheek teeth present a major radiographic challenge. Various projections and techniques have been reported in the literature.[7,10,13,14,21b,22–26] The standardized projections described below are in regular use and have stood the test of time. However, it may sometimes be necessary to resort to tube and film positions contrived specifically to show a particular lesion. Such projections are referred to as 'lesion orientated oblique'.

## Incisors and canines

**Standardized projections (Fig. 11.1).** The film cassette is positioned intra-orally. For the upper arcade, the primary beam is directed from the dorsal aspect and centered on the midline of the muzzle between the nostrils at an angle approximately 20° rostral to the perpendicular plane. This angle matches approximately the lie of the incisors in the premaxilla and therefore helps to compensate for image distortion caused by their curved conformation. For the lower arcade, the X-ray beam is directed from the ventral aspect and centered on the prominence of the chin using a similar rostral beam angle.

**Other projections.** Lateral radiographs tend to be relatively unhelpful because of superimposition of right and left sides, but may be indicated in cases where there is gross displacement of teeth or to check fracture displacement and alignment after repair.[27] Lesion orientated oblique projections may occasionally be indicated for demonstration of individual incisors and for the canines, a modification of the standard lateral oblique projection for the cheek teeth can be used (see the next section).

## Maxillary cheek teeth

**Lateral projection (Fig. 11.2).** Although superimposition of the right and left arcades prevents identification and evaluation of individual teeth, true lateral radiographs are of value for demonstrating associated disease processes in the maxillary bones and paranasal sinuses. This projection is easily obtained in the standing

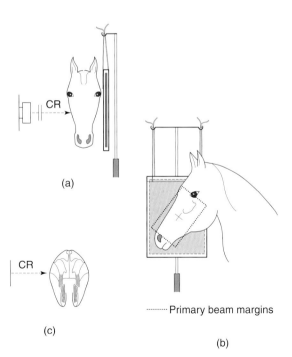

(a)

(c)

·········· Primary beam margins

(b)

**Figure 11.2.** Diagrams showing a system for cassette suspension and X-ray beam to film orientation for lateral radiography of the cheek teeth in standing horses, (a) frontal (DV) view, (b) lateral view and (c) rostrocaudal view represented by a section through the head at the level of PM 4. X = centering point (1– 2 cm rostral to the facial crest at the level of PM 4).

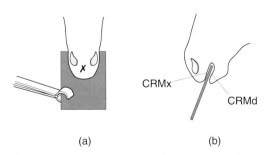

(a)                    (b)

**Figure 11.1.** Diagrams showing relative positions of cassette and X-ray beam for (a) dorsoventral (DV) and (b) ventrodorsal (VD) intra-oral radiographs of the incisors and canines. X = centering point, CRMx = central ray for DV projection; CRMd = central ray for VD projection.

horse. The cassette is positioned vertically on the clinically affected side, parallel with the outer contour of the face and as close as possible to it. The X-ray beam is centered at the level of the facial crest, 1–2 cm rostral to its rostral extremity. To avoid unnecessary distortion, it is essential that the primary beam is exactly perpendicular to the centering point in both rostrocaudal and dorsoventral planes. This means that in standing horses, individual adjustments need to be made to accommodate the angle at which the head is being held. To obtain a lateral projection in a recumbent horse under general anesthesia, the muzzle must be raised on a foam pad or sandbag so that the sagittal plane is parallel with the film. For general evaluation the radiographic field should cover the whole facial area, including the nasal chambers and maxillary and conchofrontal sinuses. To achieve accurate collimation, the light beam diaphragm unit should be rotated so that alignment of the X-ray beam conforms with the angle of the head. If selected sections of the dental arcades are required, centering and collimation can be modified accordingly.

**Dorsolateral–lateral and ventrolateral–lateral oblique projections (Fig. 11.3a).** Oblique projections provide the most convenient method for obtaining radiographs of the right and left arcades of the maxillary cheek teeth separately. Because accurate positioning is critical and awkward to obtain in the standing animal, this technique is best performed with the patient under general anesthesia. The relationship between head and cassette is the same as for the lateral projection, except that the cassette must be offset so that it is correctly aligned with the point at which the X-ray beam emerges from the head. Less distortion of dental images occurs if the arcade being radiographed is closer to the film (dorsolateral–lateral oblique). Image sharpness is also marginally improved. The beam is angled from the dorsal (maxillary) aspect and the film offset ventrally. Acceptable, but incomparable images of the upper arcade can be obtained by angling the X-ray beam the same amount in the opposite direction, ventrally, toward the mandible (ventrolateral–lateral oblique). In the sedated or anesthetised horse a block placed between the

incisors will separate the cheek teeth arcades. For adult horses with average or broad conformation of the head, a suitable beam angle is 30° from the vertical. A slightly larger angle (up to 45°) is required for young and narrow heads in which the dental arcades are closer together.

**Intra-oral oblique projection (standardized) (Fig. 11.3b).** A system for obtaining intra-oral projections of the apices and reserve crowns of individual cheek teeth has recently been described in detail.[14] Envelope wrapped human dental film 5 × 7.5 cm is recommended. The anesthetized patient is positioned in lateral recumbency with the side to be examined uppermost. The film is placed in the oral cavity, closely applied and parallel to the hard palate at the level of the tooth of interest. This location is determined by reference to a lateral radiograph on which the distance from the rostral aspect of the first incisor to the desired centering point is measured. The film is introduced taped to a perspex ruler, so that the required distance can be confirmed. For most teeth, the X-ray beam can be directed at an angle of 60° to the horizontal, but for the longer reserve crowns in 2-year-old horses, increased incident angles of 70°–80° were required. The centering point is at or up to 6 cm dorsal to the facial crest, depending on the length of the tooth being radiographed. The disadvantage of this technique is that if the affected tooth is not identified beforehand, several exposures may be required.

**Ventrodorsal projection.** The true ventrodorsal projection usually provides little information about the teeth themselves, but may be used to evaluate intercurrent disease of the paranasal sinuses, nasal chambers and maxillary bones. When setting up for this projection, meticulous care must be taken to ensure that the head is absolutely straight. Even slight tilting produces sufficient asymmetry to preclude a meaningful comparison of right and left sides. The centering point is on the midline at the rostrocaudal level of the region of interest.

**Ventrodorsal projection (offset mandible) (Fig. 11.3c).** Using this projection, it is possible to demonstrate the buccal surfaces, alveoli and adjacent

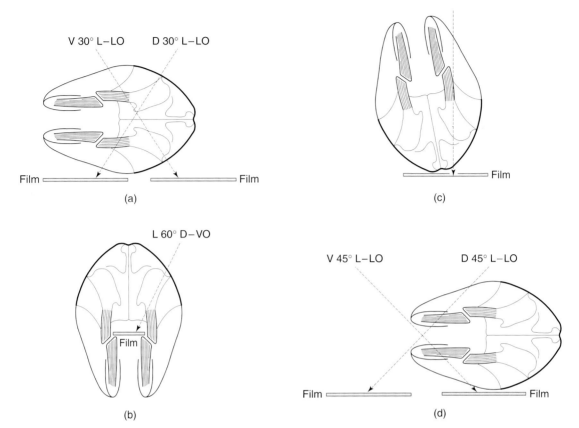

**Figure 11.3.** Diagrams of a section through the head at the level of 108, showing beam direction and cassette position for projections of (a) maxillary arcades [lower; dorso-30°-lateral–ateral oblique (D30°L–LO): upper; ventro-30°-lateral–lateral oblique (V30°L–LO)], (b) intra-oral for individual maxillary teeth [lateral-60°-dorsal–ventral oblique (L60°D–VO)], (c) abaxial margins of the rostral maxillary arcade (VD with offset mandible and slight rotation) and (d) mandibular arcades [lower; ventro-45°-lateral–lateral oblique (V45°L–LO): upper; dorso-45°-lateral–lateral oblique (D45°L–LO)].

maxillary bone of the cheek teeth. From a ventro-dorsal position, the mandible, which is slightly mobile, is displaced to the contralateral side and its position is maintained by applying tension to a snare placed around the mandibular diastema. The X-ray beam is tightly collimated to minimize scattered radiation. For the rostral premolars, it may be necessary to rotate the head slightly away from the affected side. This projection is particularly useful for demonstrating subtle alveolar disease and maxillary osteitis.

**Lesion orientated oblique projections.** Oblique projections customized to demonstrate specific lesions must be set up with care. The indication is usually a clinically identifiable abnormality,

such as swelling or obvious disruption of teeth or bone. It is important to arrange the X-ray beam and film so that the area to be examined is shown to best effect, which is usually obtained by placing the lesion on the 'skyline'.

### Mandibular cheek teeth

**Lateral projection.** True lateral projections of the mandibular cheek teeth are rarely indicated but might provide some useful information in cases where there is major disruption as a result of trauma or neoplasia. The technique is the same as for the maxillary teeth except that the centering point is more ventral, midway between the diastema and angle of the jaw.

**Ventrolateral–lateral and dorsolateral–lateral oblique projections (Fig. 11.3d).** These are the most effective projections for demonstrating the roots and reserve crowns of the mandibular cheek teeth. As for the equivalent projections of the maxillary arcades, the film cassette must be positioned parallel to the head and as close to it as possible. To obtain an image of the arcade nearer the film, which will be the lower if the horse is recumbent, the X-ray beam is directed from the ventral aspect (ventrolateral–lateral oblique). For the farther (upper) arcade, the beam is angled from the dorsal aspect (dorsolateral–lateral oblique). The centering point and primary beam margins are selected according to the tooth or teeth under investigation. As the mandibular arcades are closer together than their maxillary counterparts, the angle of the beam to the vertical needs to be increased. For heads of average conformation and the central portion of the arcade, 45° is suitable. A slightly increased angle of about 50° may be needed for narrower heads and the more rostral teeth (PM 2 and 3). For the more caudal teeth (M 2 and 3), a lower angle (35°–40°) can be used. The increased beam angles mean that the degree to which the cassette must be offset is also increased.

**Intra-oral ventrodorsal projection.** It is possible to obtain ventrodorsal radiographs of the mandibular cheek teeth by using intra-oral films, but the relatively high exposures required to penetrate the dense mandibular bone and superimposed dental crowns tend to produce images of low contrast. Poor screen/film contact may also impair film quality (see Fig. 11.19b).

**Lesion orientated oblique projections.** Customized projections of the mandibular teeth and surrounding structures can be obtained by either external or intra-oral techniques and are most likely to be useful for investigating traumatic disruption or swellings arising at atypical sites.

## EXPOSURE SELECTION

The choice of exposure factors will depend on the output of the X-ray machine and speed of the imaging system in use. To maximize radio-graphic contrast between mineralized tissue and adjacent air spaces, a relatively low tube voltage of the order of 55–60 K V should be used. For low-output machines this may cause problems with the concomitant requirement to increase exposure times, so compromise may be necessary, particularly when radiographing standing horses. Distance is the factor which requires special consideration in equine dental radiography, particularly when setting up for oblique views. To limit the effects of magnification, a tube/film distance of at least 1 m is desirable, but to overcome positioning constraints, it may sometimes be expedient to compromise by using shorter distances, in which case the tube output factors will need appropriate adjustment.

## QUALITY EVALUATION

Before attempting to identify pathological changes, it is important that each radiograph is inspected carefully, the quality of the image assessed, and any shortcomings which might interfere with interpretation noted. A decision must then be made as to whether the defects present are acceptable in the circumstances of the particular case under investigation, or whether it is necessary to obtain repeat or additional radiographs. Some of the factors to be considered are discussed in the next sections.

### Exposure and development

In the maxillofacial region, correct exposure is particularly critical for assessing the relationship between mineralized structures and adjacent air spaces. It is important that the contents of the paranasal sinuses and nasal chambers are not over-exposed (too dark), when subtle changes in their soft tissue content will be obscured. For all projections over-exposure at the periphery of the image is an inherent problem, and this is exacerbated along the ventral border of the rostral mandible in 45° oblique views. It may therefore be necessary to use bright-light transillumination to examine these dark areas. In some cases an additional radiograph may be required using lower exposure factors. Under-development gives rise to poor radiographic contrast and can be recognized by paleness or uneven blackening of the background of the image.

### Centering and field size

A check should be made that the X-ray beam is centered so that the area of interest is represented on the radiograph without unacceptable distortion. It is also essential that all structures about which information is required are included within the beam margins.

### Projection

The relative positions of anatomical landmarks should be checked to ensure that the head, film and X-ray beam were correctly aligned to produce the desired projection.

### Artefacts

A search should be made for artefacts which might confuse interpretation. Extraneous marks may be caused by traces of mud or contamination from lotions, ointments or dressings. Images of rope or webbing restraining devices may be visible (see Fig. 11.7c). Pressure marks on films from flexible intra-oral cassettes appear as light under-exposed linear streaks (see Fig. 11.5).

## RADIOGRAPHIC ANATOMY
### DECIDUOUS TEETH
#### Incisors (Di 1–3)

Temporary incisors are shell-like in appearance and can be distinguished from their permanent counterparts by the absence of elongated roots (see Fig. 11.5).

#### Premolars (Dp 2–4)

Temporary premolars have short, spicular roots. Figure 11.4 shows that they can be distinguished from developing molars by their greater mineral content, relative lack of internal structure and small or radiographically absent alveoli (dental sacs).

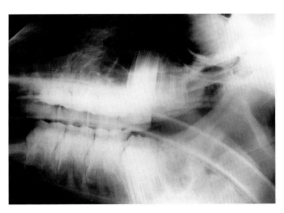

**Figure 11.4.** Lateral radiograph of the facial and mandibular areas of a yearling pony under general anesthesia showing the right and left arcades of cheek teeth partly superimposed. D-1-3s are erupted and in wear; they are short and dense and their spicular root conformation can be seen well in the mandible. The germs of 06, 07 and 08's are not yet visible. 09's are well developed, erupted in the maxilla and partially erupted in the mandible. 10s are in a fairly advanced stage of development and contrast with the appearance of the deciduous premolars by their lesser radiopacity, striated pattern and radiolucent dental sacs delineated by lamina dura.

### PERMANENT TEETH
#### Incisors and canines (I 1–3; C)

On standardized DV and VD intra-oral radiographs, as shown in Figure 11.5, the incisor roots and crowns are closely packed. Curvature of the arcade leads to partial superimposition of the roots of I2 and I3, but inter-dental spaces should be visible between right and left I1 and I1 and 2. Normally, only parts of the periodontal membranes and lamina dura can be seen. On correctly exposed radiographs, the pulp cavities should be clearly defined. In recently erupted teeth, the infundibular spaces can be recognized on the obliquely projected occlusal surfaces and in those which have been longer in wear, traces of cement may be visible as thin elliptical or inverted conical radiodense shadows (see Figs 11.14a and 11.18). In this projection, the images of the canine teeth are superimposed on the roots of I3, so if specific information is required about either structure, customized oblique projections would be required. Although often unerupted, canines are usually present and quite well developed in mares.

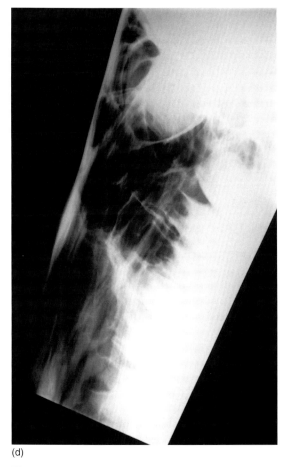

(d)

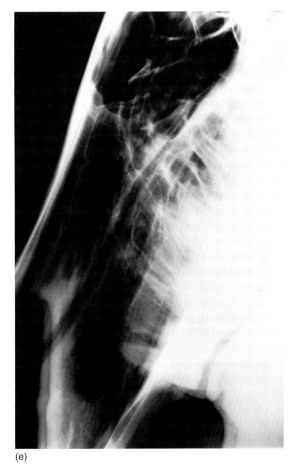

(e)

**Figure 11.7.** *continued.*

There are marked variations in the size and shape of the paranasal sinuses in individual horses. 'Dish-faced' Arabians have relatively small airspaces, while those in 'Roman-nosed' heavy horses are much more capacious. The course of the infra-orbital canal is also conformation-related, so the position of the reserve crowns relative to this structure is not a reliable guide to age or dental wear. The rostral walls of the maxillary sinuses are consistently seen at the level of 108 and 208 and are usually caudal to the rostral radicles. There is often an indistinct condensation of bone in this area, giving rise to an increase in radiopacity which obscures the apices of 108 and 208 and may be difficult to distinguish from pathological proliferation. The position, integrity and course of the bony septa separating the rostral and caudal compartments of the maxillary sinuses are more variable and sometimes differ considerably between right and left sides. They may not be clearly distinguishable from other shelves of bone within the sinuses, but usually traverse them in a dorsal direction, originating from an area between the roots of 109, 209, 110 and 210. The clarity with which the nasal turbinate bones (conchae) can be seen is highly variable. The ventral conchae are well shown in Figure 11.7e.

If present, the wolf teeth 105 and 205 can be seen on lateral radiographs (Figs 11.7c, 11.16a, 11.22a, 11.29). They vary in dimensions from a few millimeters to about 2 cm and are triangular or trapezoid in shape. In a survey of radiographs of 134 horses,[11] the frequency of occurrence of

PMs1 was 30 per cent, but this may not be a true reflection of their incidence because of the common practice of 'therapeutic' removal.

**Standardized oblique radiographs.** Figure 11.8a shows the relationship between individual cheek teeth of the right maxillary arcade on a left dorso-30°-lateral–right lateral oblique radiograph of an 8-year-old horse with normal dental roots and reserve crowns. Relative under-penetration of M 3 and dense blackening of the maxillary sinus area illustrate the problem of obtaining correct exposure of all teeth in the arcade and normal sinus air spaces. (Normal M 3 are shown more clearly in Figs 11.21 and 11.23b). The size distribution of interdental spaces is fairly consistent between horses, but the width of the spaces is variable, (see Fig. 11.23b). Inconsistent

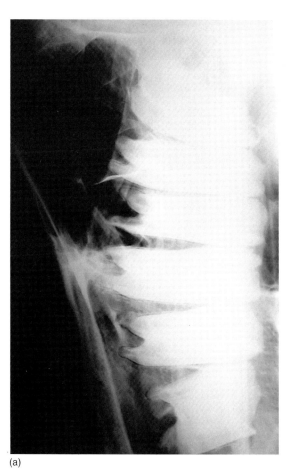

(a)

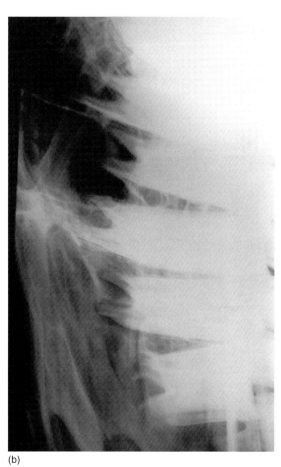

(b)

**Figure 11.8.** Standardized oblique radiographs of the right maxillary arcade of an 8-year-old hunter. (a) Left dorso-30°-lateral–right lateral projection (right side closer to film). M 3 can not be evaluated accurately because of relative under-exposure. The dental apices are variable in shape, but mostly pointed, except rostral 107 and 111. The interdental spaces are relatively large between 106 and 107, 107 and 108, and 108 and 109 and much narrower between 109 and 110, and 110 and 111. Parts of the periodontal membranes and lamina dura can be seen around the root apices and reserve crowns. In no tooth are they complete. The rostral border of the maxillary sinus can be seen through a hazy radiopaque area and arises at the caudal tip of the rostral radicle of 108. A vertically orientated, sharp linear opacity superimposed on the rostral radicle of 110 and the infra-orbital canal may represent part of the septum separating the rostral and caudal compartments of the maxillary sinus. (b) Right ventro-30°-lateral–left lateral projection (right side farther from the film) showing the effects of magnification and distortion. Compared with (a) the dental images are longer and the roots appear more spicular. The distal reserve crowns are superimposed on their contralateral counterparts. Note that in this projection, the periodontal membranes and lamina dura tend to be less clearly delineated. The linear opacity which probably represents the inter-compartmental septum of the maxillary sinus is more clearly demonstrated on this view.

demonstration of the lamina dura and periodontal membranes is a normal feature of this radiographic projection. These structures are visible only where the X-ray beam passes through them tangentially. Thus, their absence or partial absence is not necessarily an indication of alveolar disease. The line of the occlusal surface of the arcade often undulates slightly. The rostral wall of the maxillary sinus should be clearly delineated and its site of origin in relation to the radicles of PM4 can normally be identified. The inter-compartmental septum is less well defined but may be partly represented by a highly radiodense linear shadow extending dorsally from a point adjacent to the root of M2. The images of the infra-orbital canal are widely separated, but the one on the contralateral side may not be visible because of relative over-exposure.

A right ventro-30°-lateral–left lateral oblique radiograph of the same arcade of the same horse is shown in Figure 11.8b, which illustrates the characteristic elongation of the dental images which is a feature of this projection. The occlusal surfaces of the teeth cannot easily be evaluated because of superimposition on the contralateral arcade. Despite magnification, image sharpness usually remains fairly good, although details of root anatomy, periodontal membranes and lamina dura tend to be less clear than in the dorso-30°-lateral–lateral projection.

**Ventrodorsal radiograph (offset mandible).** This projection is illustrated in Figure 11.9 in which the radiographic field is collimated to show the right maxillary cheek teeth. The relationships between the wall of the maxillary sinus and buccal surfaces of the reserve crowns of 108 and the molars are clearly shown, but details of crown structure cannot be appreciated. 106 and 107 and rostral 108 are superimposed on the lateral wall of the maxilla. To reveal the junction between them, slight leftward rotation of the head would be required (see Fig. 11.26).

**Intra-oral radiographs (Fig. 11.10).** A customized projection using intra-oral film is illustrated in Figure 11.10. To demonstrate the lower reserve and exposed crowns of the maxillary arcade, the film was wedged at an angle close to the lingual

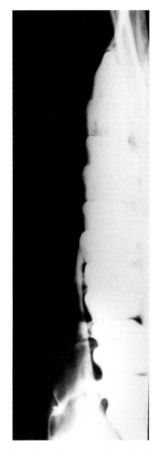

**Figure 11.9.** Ventrodorsal radiograph centered 2 cm rostral to the right facial crest showing the maxillary cheek teeth which have been exposed by displacing the mandible toward the left. The abaxial surfaces of caudal PM4 and M1–3 are clearly shown in contrast with the air-filled maxillary sinuses surrounding them.

surfaces of the teeth and the X-ray beam directed about 20° dorsal to lateral.

## Mandibular cheek teeth

The gross anatomical effects of aging on the mandibular cheek teeth has been illustrated by radiographs of specimen hemimandibles in two recent studies.[28,29] Young roots are tubular in appearance with open apices. They are surrounded by large, rounded radiolucent areas which represent the soft tissue content of the dental sacs. These 'eruption cysts' are most prominent around 307, 407 and 308, 408 and between the ages of 2 and 4 years. The mandi-

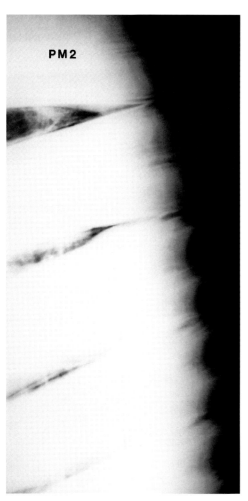

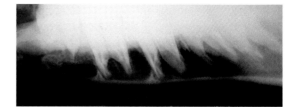

**Figure 11.11.** Left ventro-45°-lateral–right lateral oblique radiograph of the right hemimandible of a 9-year-old horse. The cortex is straight, but variable in thickness, and the teeth lie well above its endosteal border. From 307 back, the roots become more caudally orientated and the slope of the reserve crowns increases. Despite earlier eruption, the apices of 306 remain rounded. The buttresses of cortical bone rostral to the apices of 307 and 308 are normal variants. The normal appearance of a younger mandible is shown in Fig. 11.19b.

**Figure 11.10.** Intra-oral oblique radiograph showing the reserve and exposed crowns of 206–208 and 209, 210 of a 7-year-old hunter. The slight unsharpness of the images of the more caudal teeth is due to poor screen/film contact. Note the sharply pointed margins of the occlusal surfaces and caudally decreasing interdental spaces. The distinctive shape and caudal angulation of 206 is clearly demonstrated. Periodontal membranes and lamina dura can be seen in the interdental spaces through which the X-ray beam has passed tangentially.

bular cortex below them tends to be thin and bulges ventrally. As the teeth mature and migrate orally, the root apices become more pointed, but the pulp canals remain open and the periodontal membranes and lamina dura are often indistinct or incomplete. The radiographic configuration of a 5-year-old hemimandible in the ventro-45°-lateral–lateral oblique projection

is shown in Figure 11.19b. Figure 11.11 shows the same projection in a middle-aged horse. M3 is not included. More-caudal centering, a smaller beam angle and higher exposure factors would be required to demonstrate it to best effect. The degree of pointing of the roots of PM3 and 4 and M1 and 2 reflects the relative ages of the teeth. The distinctive configuration of PM2 is a consistent feature.

## CLINICAL INDICATIONS

Radiography is generally used to confirm or provide additional information about dental problems already suspected or identified by more direct clinical examination.

Cases involving trauma to the facial bones or mandibles severe enough to consider interventional management should be radiographed routinely and checked carefully for dental involvement (see Figs 11.18–11.20).

Gross disorders of the exposed crowns are normally recognized easily by inspection, but radiography may contribute to making a decision about the most suitable management strategy. In contrast, disease of the roots and reserve crowns of the grinding teeth may not be associated with visible dental abnormalities and the presenting signs of nasal discharge, facial swelling, discharging tracts and sometimes pain are non-specific. In such cases, radiography plays a crucial part in diagnostic confirmation and identification of the affected tooth or teeth. It should be remembered that although direct maxillary sinus endoscopy gives visual access to the roots of the caudal cheek teeth, chronic inflammatory changes within the cavity may obscure the clarity with which they can be seen.

Radiography makes an important contribution to a number of interventional procedures. Landmark guides can be established by taking radiographs immediately preoperatively with radiopaque markers placed externally to assist in identification of an individual diseased tooth at surgery (Fig. 11.12a). Intra- or postoperative radiographs are indicated routinely to check for removal of all dental fragments following repulsion of diseased grinders (Fig. 11.12b) and to confirm correct alignment following fracture stabilization or reduction.

Follow-up radiographs may be indicated to check the progress of healing in trauma cases or to investigate complications arising from earlier interventions (see Fig. 11.21).

# RADIOLOGICAL INTERPRETATION
## DEVELOPMENTAL DISORDERS

Abnormalities may occur in the number, size, shape and position of the teeth and often several problems occur in combination. External effects on the exposed crowns can be evaluated visually, but radiography is useful for showing the full effects of any defects by revealing the structure and location of the roots and reserve crowns.

### Malformation

Deformity of the permanent 201 is illustrated in Figure 11.13. It is not possible to determine

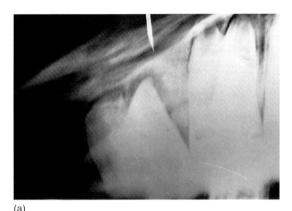

(a)

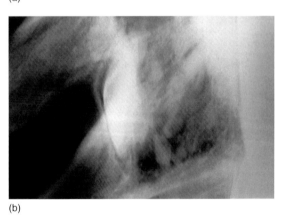

(b)

**Figure 11.12.** Dorso-30°-lateral–lateral oblique radiographs showing (a) a radiopaque external marker (hypodermic needle) used as a guide to the location of a diseased tooth (206) and (b) close-up postoperative study following removal of the tooth showing retained dental fragments, some of which are large.

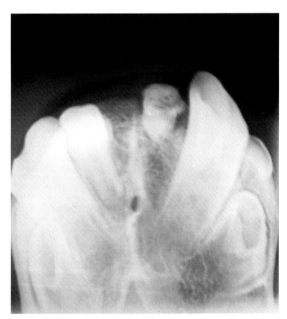

**Figure 11.13.** Malformation. Dorsoventral intra-oral radiograph of the premaxilla of a 3-year-old filly showing a small, distorted 201. The root is surrounded by an uneven radiolucent halo but the crown is erupted. 101 is more normal in shape, but both root and crown are small and eruption is not complete. 102 and 202 are normal in size and erupted. Dis3 are still present and 103 and 303 are well formed but not yet erupted. Centering was not accurate and the asymmetry between right and left is probably due to slight rotation.

whether this is a true congenital anomaly or whether the affected teeth were damaged during development.

## Maleruption

Figure 11.14a shows grossly abnormal eruption of 102 and 202, which is bilaterally symmetrical. The affected and adjacent teeth are relatively normal in size and shape. In Figure 11.14b 106–110 show varying degrees of deformity and maleruption.

## Malocclusion

Any abnormality of eruption of a permanent tooth which interferes with the integrity of the arcade in which it is situated predisposes to abnormal wear of the opposing arcade and a tendency to malocclusion. In the case illustrated in Figure 11.15, absence of an erupted 209 has led to rostral migration of 210 and 211. Although the space is almost obliterated, a

defect in the occlusal surface remains and as a consequence the opposing mandibular 309 was overgrown. The presenting signs of oral discomfort and general malaise were attributed to this problem. Retention of permanent cheek teeth is an unusual but well-described developmental anomaly.[30]

## Anadontia

Complete absence of individual teeth can give rise to dramatic effects of malocclusion. The case illustrated in Figure 11.16 had severe problems with mastication and was in poor body condition. Absence of mandibular 403 had led to complete lack of wear of the opposing maxillary deciduous tooth and severe malocclusion. The condition was bilateral.

## Temporal terratoma (dentigerous cyst)

Development of anomalous dental tissue in the parieto-temporal region of the calvarium is a

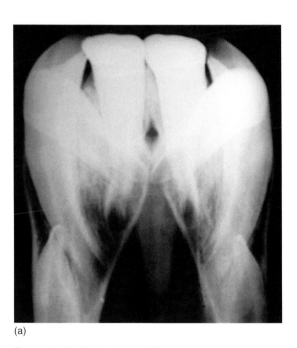
(a)

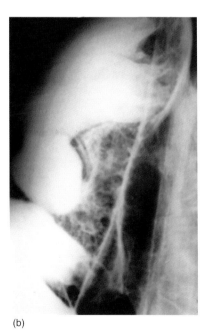
(b)

**Figure 11.14.** Maleruption. (a) Dorsoventral intra-oral radiograph of the premaxilla of a 5-year-old pony gelding showing maleruption of 102–202. The root apices lie medial and rostral to those of I 1 and the alignment of the teeth is at an angle of about 40° abaxial to their normal location. 103 and 203 appear to originate from a normal position, but they are elongated and curved. The large infundibular spaces indicate relatively recent eruption. (b) Intra-oral lesion orientated oblique radiograph of a 5-year-old part-thoroughbred horse showing 106 is abnormally directed caudally, 107 is bent caudally at the middle of the reserve crown and 108 is rotated through 90° from its normal position to be viewed end on. 109 appears to be unaffected.

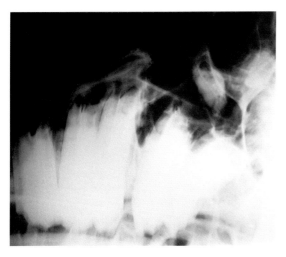

**Figure 11.15.** Retention and malocclusion. Right dorso-30°-lateral–left lateral oblique projection of the left maxillary cheek teeth of a 6-year-old Arabian mare. A small, fusiform mass of mineralized tissue is situated in the position where 209 should be. 206–208, appear normal. 210 and 211 are erupted but have migrated rostrally so that the space normally occupied by 209 is almost closed. There is a marked defect in the occlusal surface at this site. There are two radiopaque mineralized masses in the caudal compartment of the maxillary sinus. The more rostral is homogeneous in texture and probably represents an accumulation of cement. The other, which is partly superimposed on the ethmoturbinate, has a striated pattern suggesting that it is part of a deformed tooth. There is no evidence of any other pathological change in the sinus cavity or maxillary bone.

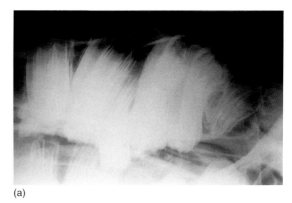

(a)

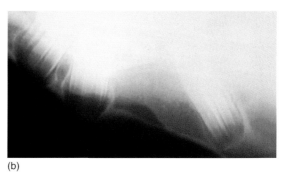

(b)

**Figure 11.16.** Anadontia and malocclusion. (a) Left dorso-30°-lateral–right lateral oblique and (b) left ventral-45°-lateral–right lateral oblique radiographs of the right maxilla and mandible of a 2-year-old thoroughbred horse showing absence of (mandible) 407 and (permanent) 408 (b) and abnormal elongation of maxillary (deciduous) 107 (a). 108 is abnormally angled rostrally and the developing 109 is narrow and also rostrally orientated. 01 and (mandible) 02 are still present and there is a well-developed 105. The molars appear normal; 111 is in the mid-stages of development. 406 and 407 appear relatively normal. 108 is fully developed, but its rostral angulation is exaggerated. 110 and 111 are not included in the radiographic field.

widely recognized cause of discrete, hard swellings and discharging tracts on the heads of young horses. Figure 11.17 shows a well-developed terratoma which was situated just rostral to the base of the right pinna. Radiography contributes to accurate localization and preoperative evaluation of the size and structure of the lesions (see Chapter 8, p. 99).

## TRAUMA

The use of radiography for evaluation of mandibular fractures is illustrated in Figures 11.18 and 11.19. Figure 11.20 shows multiple fractures of the maxillary and nasal bones and molar teeth. The injury was of 11 days duration and clinical signs of severe sinusitis had already developed. The radiographic findings of gross disruption of permanent teeth contributed to the decision to recommend euthanasia rather than attempting salvage surgery. Figure 11.21 is a radiograph taken 3 months after removal of a diseased M 1. The iatrogenic fracture of M 2 probably explained why clinical signs of maxillary sinusitis had persisted.

## DENTAL INFECTION

### Maxillary periapical disease

Infection involving the roots of the caudal cheek teeth (M 1–3) appears high on the list of differential diagnoses of unilateral purulent nasal

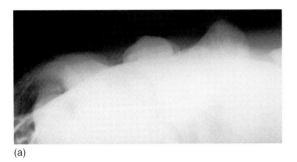

(a)

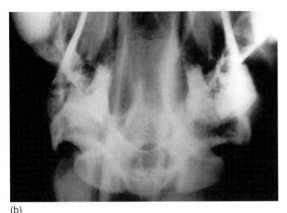

(b)

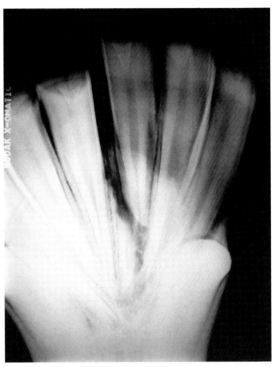

**Figure 11.17.** Temporal teratoma. (a) Lesion orientated oblique and (b) ventrodorsal radiographs of the caudal skull of a yearling thoroughbred colt. On (a) an ovoid, laminated structure can be seen partly superimposed on the parietal bone. On (b) the same structure can be seen immediately abaxial to the left petrous temporal bone. A radiolucent margin and thin outer shell are visible caudally. This appearance is typical of a temporal terratoma.

**Figure 11.18.** Rostral mandibular dental fracture. Ventrodorsal intra-oral radiograph of the rostral mandible of a 7-year-old gelding showing a fracture through the left side. All three left incisors are displaced rostrally. There is an oblique fracture through the root of 301 and the abaxial border of 303 is separated from the alveolar bone. Note the clearly defined pulp cavities and infundibular cement layers. A lateral projection would be required to evaluate fully the degree of displacement, but this could probably have been determined clinically.

discharge. Involvement of the more rostral teeth (PM 2 and 3) is the commonest cause of lateral facial swelling and discharging tracts in the maxillary region between the facial crest and diastema. Periapical infection of 108 or 208 may produce either or both clinical presentations. Standing lateral radiographs occasionally give an indication of dental involvement (see Fig. 11.24), but oblique views are almost always required for diagnostic confirmation. Signs to look for on lateral films are localized, ill-defined areas of increased radiopacity surrounding affected teeth, with coarsening of the texture of the overlying bone. This appearance is an indication of proliferative change associated with osteitis of the maxilla adjacent to infected tooth roots. In Figure 11.22 (a) shows such

changes and (b) confirms that the problem originates in 107. In horses in which periapical infection has led to maxillary sinusitis, a diffuse increase in radiopacity of the whole sinus cavity may be seen on standing radiographs (Fig. 11.23) and fluid levels may also be present (Fig. 11.24). However, these findings are non-specific and occur in other types of paranasal sinus disease. The ease with which teeth with periapical infection can be identified on oblique radiographs is variable. A study carried out in 1987 showed that independent observers failed to identify affected teeth correctly in over 50 per cent of cases,[11] but since that time, rigorous efforts to improve radiographic technique, increased experience and training have markedly increased accuracy of identification (Gibbs;

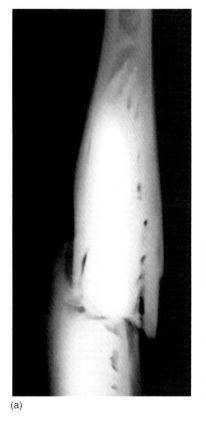
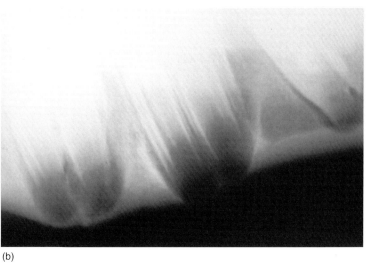

(a)                      (b)

**Figure 11.19.** Fractured mandibular ramus with dental involvement. (a) Ventrodorsal intra-oral and (b) ventro-45°-lateral–lateral radiographs of the right mandibular ramus of a 5-year-old horse. The ventrodorsal projection shows a slightly oblique fracture just caudal to 407 with minor axio-caudal displacement. In this view, the tooth appears to have been spared. However, on the oblique projection, the slightly over-ridden fracture line, which is seen from the ventral aspect, runs between the radicles of 407. 406 is excluded from the radiographic field.

unpublished data; 1997). The most consistent radiographic sign of periapical disease is an area of increased lucency around the affected apex or apices, referred to as a 'halo'. There may also be loss of the lamina dura, but as this structure is an inconsistent feature on radiographs of normal horses, its absence is not a reliable indicator of pathological change. In many cases the roots are damaged. They may be partly destroyed or distorted, increased in density and 'clubbed'. In cases in which infection is a result of displaced fracture or fragmentation of the crown, the radiographic effects are graphically displayed. Deposits of cement, appearing as fragments of unstructured mineralized tissue are sometimes seen adjacent to infected roots. The presence of maxillary osteitis may obscure radiographic

detail of affected teeth, making interpretation more difficult. Examples of maxillary periapical infection showing the above features are illustrated in Figure 11.25. Use of the ventrodorsal projection with offset mandible to demonstrate low-grade periapical infection, alveolar disease and chronic osteitis is shown in Figure 11.26. This technique should be considered if the findings on standard oblique radiographs are inconclusive.

### 'Dental' rhinitis

Dental infection which causes erosion of the internal wall of the maxilla can lead to severe rhinitis, which may be associated with dystrophic calcification of intranasal structures.[31]

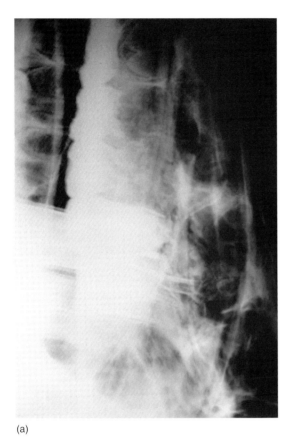

(a)

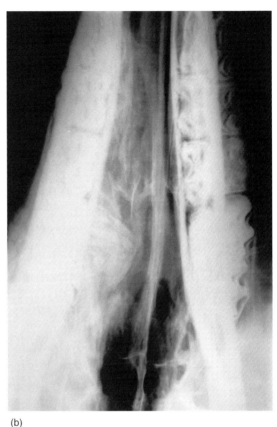

(b)

**Figure 11.20.** Facial and dental fractures. (a) Left dorso-30°-lateral–right lateral oblique and (b) ventrodorsal radiographs of a thoroughbred yearling taken after severe trauma to the head. In (a) the contents of the maxillary sinus are increased in radiodensity, giving a cloudy effect. Several free bone fragments can be seen within it. The dorsal portion of 209 is missing leaving a jagged border; several radiodense dental fragments lie adjacent to it. The rostral radicle of 210 is also disrupted. 66 and 67 are in wear and developing germs of 206 and 207 are present. (b) shows patchy increase in radiodensity of the right maxillary sinus and nasal chamber which extends rostrally to the level of PM 2. The nasal septum is deviated to the left. Bone and dental fragments can be seen in the maxillary sinus, including a large segment of M 1.

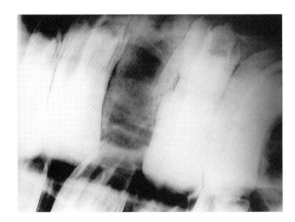

**Figure 11.21.** Iatrogenic dental fracture. Left ventro-30°-lateral–right lateral radiograph of the caudal left maxillary arcade of a 4-year-old thoroughbred horse. A large portion of the rostral border of the reserve crown of 210 has separated and another fracture line can be seen distal to it. The maxillary bone in the space originally occupied by 209 has a dense, woven appearance, indicating that in-filling is taking place. Note the elongation of the dental images as a result of the radiograph being taken with the affected side uppermost.

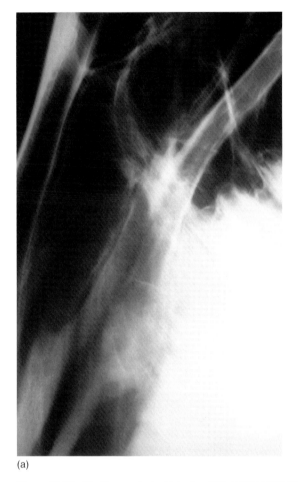

(a)

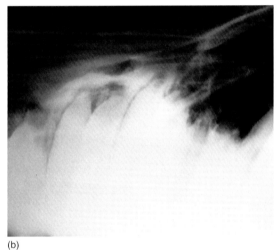

(b)

**Figure 11.22.** Maxillary periapical infection 107. (a) Standing lateral radiograph of the facial area of a 6-year-old hunter with a right-sided swelling rostral to the facial crest showing a localized, poorly defined area of increased radiopacity immediately dorsal to the roots of 106 and 107 and well rostral to the normal condensation of bone which marks the rostral border of the maxillary sinus. (b) Left dorso-30°-lateral–right lateral oblique radiograph of the same animal, showing a poorly marginated radiolucent halo around the roots of 107, the caudal radicle of which is short and blunted. The radiopacity of the surrounding maxillary bone is increased giving a cloudy, granular appearance.

Premolar teeth are most likely to be involved. Such a case is illustrated in Figure 11.27.

### Mandibular periapical disease

The radiographic features of mandibular periapical infection vary according to the age of the tooth or teeth involved and the severity and degree of activity of the septic process. In immature and recently erupted teeth (Figs 11.28a and b) the outline of the dental sac is usually distorted and irregular with deposition of smooth, well-organized new bone peripherally, some-

times in large amounts. In highly active infections, the proliferative bone may be fluffy and irregular. In well-established cases the affected roots become distorted and may be partly destroyed. Discharging tracts are often visible as radiolucent defects in the mandibular cortical bone. Congenital malformation or maleruption may predispose to periapical infection in young teeth (Fig. 11.28b).

In cases of infection involving mature teeth, radiographic changes tend to be more chronic, with bone proliferation predominating over alveolar destruction (Fig. 11.28c). Root deformity

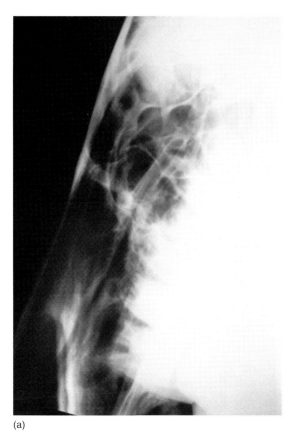

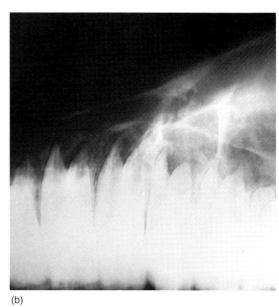

(a)                                                      (b)

**Figure 11.23.** Maxillary periapical infection 109. (a) Standing lateral radiograph of an 8-year-old part-thoroughbred horse with chronic, malodorous right-sided nasal discharge and no visible defects of the exposed crowns of the cheek teeth. There is a patchy increase in opacity of the contents of at least one of the maxillary sinuses, but no obvious increase in bone density. (b) Left dorso-30°-lateral–right lateral oblique radiograph of the right maxillary arcade of the same horse. The increase in opacity of the maxillary sinus is more intense and homogeneous in this projection. The root of the caudal radicle of 109 is rounded and an indistinct, non-marginated radiolucent halo can be seen around the whole root. There is no evidence of gross maxillary osteitis.

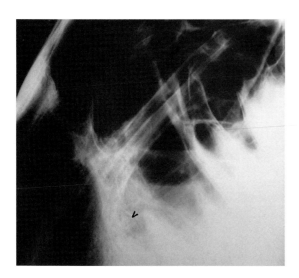

**Figure 11.24.** Maxillary periapical infection 208 with sinusitis. Standing lateral radiograph of an 8-year-old polo pony with a painful, antibiotic responsive, left facial swelling and recent onset of left-sided nasal discharge. Two fluid levels can be seen in the rostral compartment of the maxillary sinus, but there is no obvious increase in the density of the overlying bone. A small cement 'pearl' (arrowed) can be seen adjacent to the rostral radicle of one 208. An oblique radiograph confirmed periapical infection of left 208.

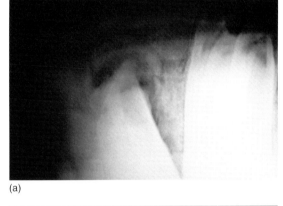

(a)

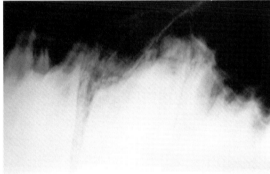

(b)

**Figure 11.25.** Maxillary periapical infections. Close-up images of dorso-30°-lateral–lateral oblique projections of the maxillary cheek teeth of four horses. (a) A 5-year-old hunter showing a distinct periapical halo with a thick, sclerotic margin around the caudal radicle of 106, which is more pointed than normal. Fragments of cement can be seen in the caudal part of the halo. The trabecular pattern of the surrounding maxillary bone is dense and coarse. (b) 9-year-old polo pony showing complete absence of the rostral radicle of 108 and an irregular cement 'pearl' superimposed on the caudal radicle. There is no obvious radiolucent halo or proliferation of maxillary bone and the sinus appears clear. (c) A 3.5-year-old thoroughbred horse with an ill-defined and poorly marginated radiolucent halo around the caudal radicle of 109. The normal rostral radicle has a narrower, clearly defined halo with a dense margin which represents the normal dental sac surrounded by lamina dura. There is a diffuse, cloudy increase in radiopacity in the area of the maxillary bone and sinus surrounding this tooth, which could be due either to osteitis or localized sinusitis. Note that the roots of 110, which is not yet erupted, are blunt and that the dental sac is represented by a wide periodontal membrane and ill-defined lamina dura. (d) An 8-year-old pony showing collapse and fragmentation of 109 with large cement fragments adjacent to its caudal root. There is marked but well-defined increase in density and trabecular coarsening of the adjacent maxillary bone, but no obvious opacification of the contents of the sinus. Note that adjacent teeth have migrated to decrease the gap between 108 and 110, indicating that the dental lesion is long standing.

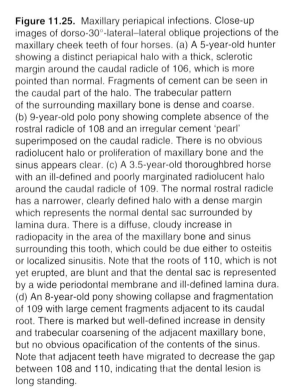

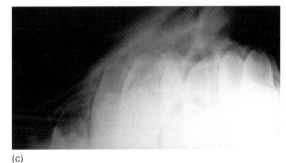

(c)

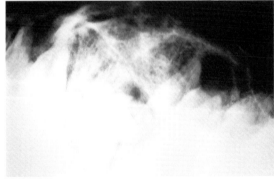

(d)

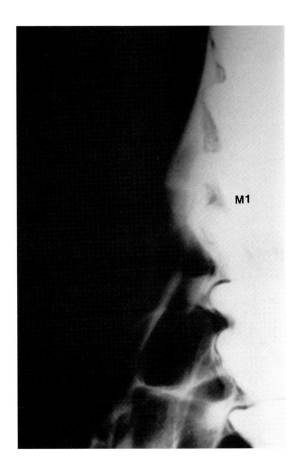

M1

**Figure 11.26.** Maxillary periapical infection 109 (M1). Ventrodorsal radiograph of a 12-year-old hunter, with the mandible displaced to the left and the head slightly rotated in that direction, collimated to show the buccal surfaces of the cheek teeth and adjacent maxillary bone. There is an indistinct radiolucent halo around the rostral radicle of 109 and the overlying bone is smoothly thickened. This horse presented with a chronic nasal discharge, quidding and facial swelling.

is the feature by which affected teeth can be identified (Fig. 11.28d).

The use of contrast sinography to delineate a discharging tract leading to an infected mandibular tooth root has been illustrated in a standard text[32] and may be worth considering if plain radiographic findings are equivocal.

## Periodontal disease

Radiography is not commonly indicated in the investigation of periodontal disease *per se*. but may be useful for demonstrating the effects of dental loss, displacement and malocclusion (Fig. 11.29).

## TUMORS AND CYSTS INVOLVING TEETH

Primary dental neoplasms are rare, but their clinical and radiological characteristics have

recently been reviewed in detail.[33] Amelo-blastomas (adamantinomas), which mainly affect the mandible, tend to be locally destructive, possibly cystic and expansile: ameloblastic and complex odontomas are expansile and contain mineralised material. Compound odontomas contain an orderly pattern of dental tissue and cementomas are composed of dense, mineralized material and are often associated with the root apices.

Cyst-like swellings of non-dental origin in the maxillae and mandibles of juvenile horses are well recognized. Teeth may be displaced and their development impaired. Numerous histological diagnoses have been claimed for such lesions, or they have simply been referred to as 'developmental cysts'. Some involve the maxillary sinuses.[5,6,7,9,11,13,32] The case shown in Figure 11.30 was classified as an ossifying fibroma.

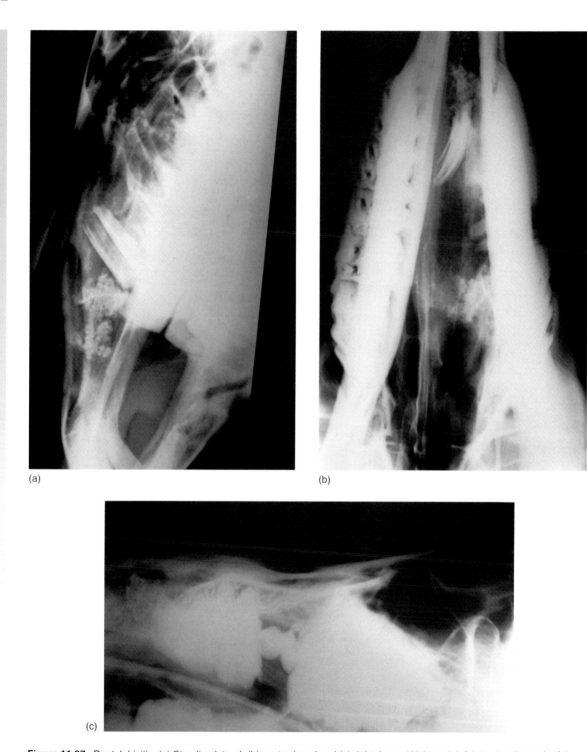

(a)

(b)

(c)

**Figure 11.27.** Dental rhinitis. (a) Standing lateral, (b) ventrodorsal and (c) right dorso-40°-lateral–left lateral radiograph of the facial area of a 13-year-old pony in good bodily condition with a purulent left nasal discharge of 6 months duration and absence of maxillary 108. Part of the missing tooth has been displaced into the right nasal cavity (b) in which there are also several large deposits of granular mineralized material. The normal contents of the cavity are severely disrupted and the nasal septum is displaced to the right. The contents of the maxillary sinus as shown on view (c) appear to be normal.

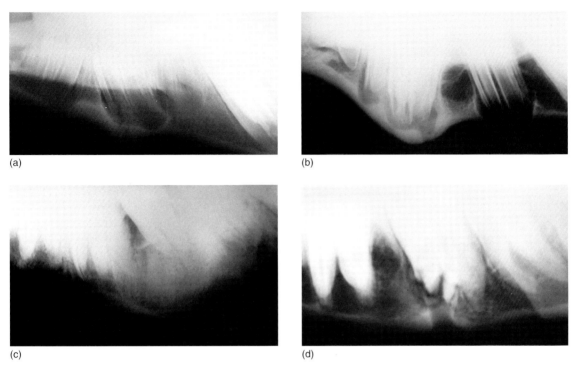

**Figure 11.28.** Mandibular periapical infections. Ventro-45°-lateral–lateral oblique radiographs of (a) a 2-year-old thoroughbred horse with a small ventral mandibular swelling and discharging tract. The dental sac of developing 307 is slightly irregular in outline, the overlying mandibular cortex is thickened, especially rostrally, and a linear, irregular radiolucent shadow leads from the rostral radicle to the exterior. The mineralized dental tissue does not appear to be disrupted. The image of the developing germ of 308 is partly superimposed on the caudal aspect of the affected tooth. (b) A 3-year-old thoroughbred horse with a prominent, hard, ventral mandibular swelling and discharging tract. 307 is deformed, the caudal radicle is large and appears to be duplicated. The apices are irregular in outline and convergent with somewhat ragged borders. The surrounding mandibular bone is grossly thickened and a large radiolucent tract runs through it. Adjacent 306 and 308 are within normal limits for their stage of development. (c) A 7-year-old hunter with a caudal mandibular swelling suspected of being neoplastic. The root of M 1 is surrounded by dense, floccular bone which appears to be retained by a normal cortex. The radicles of M 2 are short, rounded and convergent. Adjacent teeth are unremarkable. The small gray flecks represent chemical staining on the original radiograph. (d) A 10-year-old cob with a discharging tract and slight thickening of the ventral mandible of 2 years duration. The rostral radicle of 308 is grossly distorted. The apex is absent and the residual reserve crown is thickened and irregular in outline. A large, radiolucent shadow representing the tract passes from the diseased root through the thickened ventral cortex. An area of increased radiopacity of the interdental bone indicates diffuse proliferation due to osteitis.

Caudal cheek teeth may be displaced as a consequence of the expansile effect of maxillary sinus cysts. In a report of 14 cases, radiographic evidence of dental displacement was recorded in four of the ten adults in the series.[34]

Malignant tumors of osseous, connective and epithelial tissues tend to occur in older horses and are usually manifested by aggressive radiographic signs in which bone destruction predominates. If structures adjacent to teeth are involved, displacement is a likely consequence (Fig. 11.31). It should also be remembered that in the earlier stages, localized swelling caused by malignant neoplasms may be clinically similar to that associated with dental periapical infection, so that radiographic demonstration of bone destruction in the presence of normal teeth may be an important differentiating feature (Fig. 11.32).

# ALTERNATIVE IMAGING
## COMPUTED TOMOGRAPHY (CT)

In computed tomography, a minute X-ray beam scans a selected plane within the patient and the information derived from differential

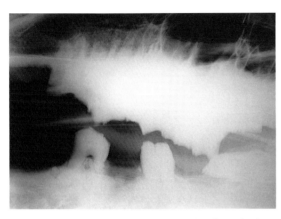

**Figure 11.29.** Periodontal disease. Lateral radiograph of an aged horse taken under general anesthesia. Loss and displacement of the mandibular cheek teeth as a result of periodontal disease has led to severe wear abnormalities in the maxillary arcades.

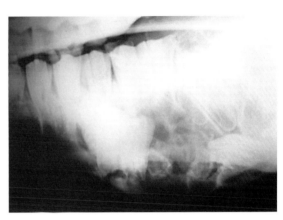

**Figure 11.30.** Ossifying fibroma. Lateral radiograph of the mandible of a 6-month-old foal with a large, hard swelling of one caudal horizontal ramus. 75–77 on the normal side are unremarkable and the unerupted 309 can be seen in a normal position. On the affected side, 75 and 76 are in place. 77 is normal in size and shape, but displaced ventrally. Small, distorted germs of 309, 310 appear to lie free in the soft tissue of the mass. Several smooth margined, amorphous clumps of mineralized material can be seen within the lesion.

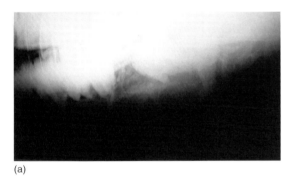

(a)

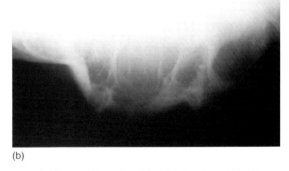

(b)

**Figure 11.31.** Anaplastic sarcoma. Two left ventro-45°-latera–right lateral oblique radiographs of the right hemimandible of an 18-year-old pony with a large, rapidly growing, firm ventral swelling. Oral examination was reported to show loosening and displacement of the fourth cheek tooth. (a) (high exposure) Shows that the displaced tooth is, in fact, 410. The more rostral teeth are in place, but the alveolar bone surrounding them has been destroyed. (b) (low exposure) Shows the massive, expansile swelling, composed mainly of soft tissue, but traversed numerous bone trabeculae. The mandibular cortex is thickened at the rostral site of origin of the mass.

absorption by the individual structures through which the beam passes is enhanced and displayed by computer-controlled electronic processes. Rapid technological advancement now allows highly sophisticated processing of the images produced, so that the area of interest can be represented in a variety of sectional orientations. Furthermore, by recording minor alterations in attenuation numerically, it is possible to make objective measurements of the radi-

ographic density of tissues and the changes associated with disease.[18]

To use CT in horses special facilities are required to permit accurate manipulation of the patient, and the scanner must have an aperture large enough to accommodate the part being investigated. Such examinations have been carried out in a few centers for some years and the essential requirements for space, environmental control, patient handling and access and

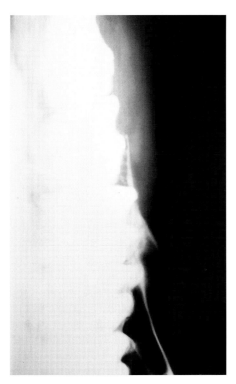

**Figure 11.32.** Undifferentiated sarcoma. Lesion orientated oblique radiograph of a 12-year-old pony with a 5 × 8 cm painless swelling over the infra-orbital canal. Standard projections showed increase in soft tissue radiopacity of the affected area but no evidence of dental disease. This radiograph shows the soft tissue outline of the mass and destruction of the lateral wall of the maxilla, which terminates abruptly at the level of 207. The teeth appear normal.

maintenance were reported as early as 1987.[16] Scanning protocols were also discussed. Since that time, refinements in equipment and computer software have led to a vast improvement in the quality of the scan images obtainable.

Computed tomography is particularly appropriate for examination of the equine facial area and dental structures, because of the high inherent radiographic contrast of the regions of interest. In dentistry, the need for clear, unobstructed images of the teeth is an additional powerful indication for this technique. Although availability of CT equipment in the average equine practice is unlikely to become universal, there is a steady increase in the number of specialist centers offering such services. Therefore, if correctly executed conventional radiography fails to give the information required to make a

properly informed decision on management of a dental problem and an appropriate facility can be reached, referral would be strongly justified.

The case shown in Figure 11.33 illustrates the use of CT to demonstrate a dental problem.

## NUCLEAR SCINTIGRAPHY

In nuclear scintigraphy, radioactive material is introduced into the body and its uptake by specific organs or lesions is measured using some form of photon counter, usually a gamma

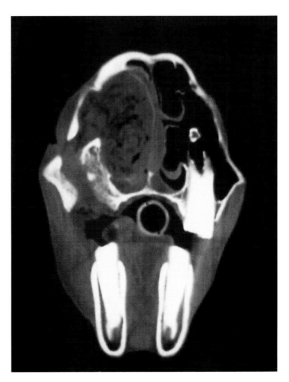

**Figure 11.33.** Computed tomography. CT image of a transverse scan through the head of a horse at the level of M 1. This animal showed persistent signs of maxillary sinusitis following extraction of right 109. Normal relationships between 209, the maxillary sinus, nasal cavity and ventral concha are shown on the left. On the right, 109 is absent, the alveolus is open and there is gross thickening of the maxillary bone on either side. The right maxillary and conchofrontal sinuses and nasal chamber are filled with material of mixed soft tissue density and gas lucency, representing ingesta which has entered from the oral cavity via the fistula. The nasal septum is displaced to the left and both dorsal and ventral conchae are virtually obliterated. There is a defect in the right outer maxillary wall and overlying soft tissue swelling (from Prof Dr K J Dik, University of Utrecht, with permission).

camera. The radionuclide is linked to a carrier substance which has an affinity for the tissue under investigation. In the case of bone, the carrier is a phosphonate compound and the isotope $^{99m}$Tc. This radiopharmaceutical is injected intravenously and after an appropriate time (approximately 3 hours for bone), the area under investigation is scanned, the emitted photons counted, processed by a computer and their distribution and intensity displayed electronically. Several display modalities are available, but the one commonly used for bone is microdot imaging (see Fig. 11.34).

The use of nuclear scintigraphy is increasing in popularity for demonstrating areas of high bone turnover in the equine skeleton. The technique is particularly indicated in cases in which conventional radiography gives negative or inconclusive results, or if the precise location of

a disease process cannot be established. As many dental disorders are associated with pathological changes in adjacent bone, scintigraphic images may provide useful information regarding the exact tooth or teeth involved.[19]

The advantages of nuclear scintigraphy over CT are that it can be performed in conscious animals and that as the imaging and recording equipment tends to be less expensive, facilities are more widely available. The disadvantages are potential radiation hazards, which entail strict control of isotope and patient handling and the fact that, as with conventional radiography, image interpretation contains a speculative element. Nevertheless, this technique is well worth considering as a supplementary imaging procedure for investigation of suspected periapical dental disease with a view to identification of affected teeth, but it must be remembered that although sensitivity for lesion detection is high, specifiicty for defining pathological changes is relatively poor. The application of nuclear scintigraphy is demonstrated by the case illustrated in Figure 11.34.

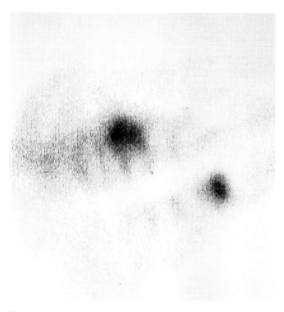

**Figure 11.34.** Nuclear scintigraphy. 5-year-old Cleveland bay mare presented with facial swelling and oral evidence of periodontal disease. Radiological findings were equivocal, with evidence of periapical disease around 107 and 108, which could not be related conclusively to either tooth. A scintigraphic image of the right side of the head made 3 hours after injection of $^{99m}$Tc-MDP shows localized increase in radionuclide uptake over the roots of 108. Increased uptake is also evident in the mandible at the level of 410. This was related to a small bony mass on the lateral aspect, believed to be associated with clinically insignificant trauma (from Jane Boswell, Royal Veterinary College, London, with permission).

### ACKNOWLEDGMENTS

**Geoffrey Lane,** Senior Lecturer Veterinary Surgery, University of Bristol, for providing the cases from which the radiographic illustrations were taken and for his cooperation and encouragement over many years.

**The radiographers** at the University of Bristol Department of Clinical Veterinary Science, for skill, patience and tenacity.

**John Conibear,** Photographic Unit, University of Bristol, Department of Clinical Veterinary Science for photographing the radiographs.

**Margaret Costello,** University of Bristol, Department of Clinical Veterinary Science for reading the script and helpful comments.

**Prof. Dr KJ Dik,** University of Utrecht, Netherlands, for case details and images illustrationg the use of computed tomography.

**Jane Boswell,** Royal Veterinary College, London, for case details and images illustrating the use of nuclear scintigraphy.

### REFERENCES

1. Kulczycki J (1936) Cited by Baker GJ (1971) *Equine Veterinary Journal*, 3, 46–51.

2. Becker E (1939) Cited by Baker GJ (1971) *Equine Veterinary Journal*, 3, 46–51.

3. Geres V (1962) A contribution to the pathology and diagnosis of dental disease in horses. *Veterinary Archives* 32, 258–261.

4. Habermann U (1963) Cited by Baker GJ (1971) *Equine Veterinary Journal*, 3, 46–51.

5. Cook WR (1970) Skeletal radiology of the equine head. *Journal of the American Veterinary Radiological Society*, 11, 35–55.

6. Baker GJ (1971) Some aspects of equine dental radiology. *Equine Veterinary Journal*, 3, 46–51.

7. Gibbs C (1974) The equine skull: its radiological interpretation. *Journal of the American Veterinary Radiological Society*, 15, 70–78.

8. Boulton CH (1985) Equine nasal cavity and paranasal sinus disease: a review of 85 cases. *Journal of Equine Veterinary Science*, 5, 268–275.

9. Wyn-Jones G (1985) Interpreting radiographs, 6: Radiology of the equine head. *Equine Veterinary Journal*, 17, 417–425.

10. Lane JG, Gibbs C, Meynick SE *et al.* (1987) Radiographic examination of the facial, nasal and paranasal sinus regions of the horse: I. Indications and procedures in 235 cases. *Equine Veterinary Journal*, 19, 466–473.

11. Gibbs C and Lane JG (1987) Radiographic examination of the facial, nasal and paranasal sinus regions of the horse. II. Radiological findings. *Equine Veterinary Journal*, 19, 474–482.

12. Dik KJ and Gunsser I (1990) In: *Atlas of Diagnostic Radiology of the Horse. Part 3: Diseases of the Head Neck and Thorax.* Schlutersche Verlagsanstalt and Druckerei, Hannover, pp. 13–69.

13. Butler JA, Colles CM, Dyson SJ, Kold SE and Poulos PW (1993) In: *Clinical Radiology of the Horse.* Chap. 8, Blackwell Science, London, pp. 313–333.

14. O'Brien RT (1996) Intra-oral dental radiography: experimental study and clinical use in two horses and a llama. *Veterinary Radiology and Ultrasound*, 37, 412–416.

15. Dixon PM (1997) Dental extraction in horses: indications and preoperative evaluation. *Compendium of Continuing Education for the Veterinary Practice*, 19, Equine 366–376.

16. Barbee DD, Allen JR and Gavin PR (1987) Computed tomography in horses. *Veterinary Radiology*, 28, 144–151.

17. Dik KJ (1994) Computed tomography of the equine head. *Veterinary Radiology and Ultrasound*, 35, 236.

18. Tietje S, Becker M and Bockenhoff G (1996) Computed tomographic evaluation of head diseases in the horse: fifteen cases. *Equine Veterinary Journal*, 28, 98–105.

19. Metcalfe MR, Tate LP and Sellett LC (1989) Clinical use of $^{99m}$TC-MDP scintigraphy in the equine maxilla. *Veterinary Radiology*, 30, 80–87.

20. HMSO (1988) *Guidance notes for protection of persons against ionising radiations arising from veterinary use.* Oxon. National Radiation Protection Board, Didcot.

21. Morgan JP and Silverman S (1993) In: *Techniques of Veterinary Radiography* (5th edn). Iowa State University Press, Ames, IA, (a) pp. 84–95, (b) pp. 355–365.

22. Schebitz H and Wilkens H (1978) In: *Atlas of Radiographic Anatomy of the Horse* (3rd edn) Paul Parey, Berlin, pp. 10–37.

23. Wyn-Jones G (1985) Interpreting radiographs. 6: The head. *Equine Veterinary Journal*, 17, 274–278.

24. Douglas SW, Williamson HD and Herrtage ME (1987) In: *Principles of Veterinary Radiography* (4th edn). Chap. 14, Ballière Tindall, Eastbourne, pp. 324–330.

25. Park RD (1993) Radiographic examination of the equine head. *Veterinary Clinics of North America. Equine Practice*, 9, 49–74.

26. Lattimer JC (1998) In: *Textbook of Veterinary Diagnostic Radiology* (3nd edn) ed. DE Thrall, Chap. 11, 'Equine Nasal Passages and Sinuses' WB Saunders, Philadelphia, pp. 112–124.

27. Sullins KE and Turner AS (1982) Management of fractures of the equine mandible and premaxilla (incisive bone). *Compendium of Continuing Education for the Veterinary Practitioner*, 4, S480–S489.

28. Dixon PM and Copeland AN (1993) The radiological appearance of mandibular cheek teeth in ponies of different ages. *Equine Veterinary Education*, 5, 317–323.

29. Kirkland KD, Baker GJ, Marretta SM *et al.* (1996) Effects of aging on the endodontic system, reserve crown and roots of equine mandibular cheek teeth. *Am J Vet Res*, 57, 31–38.

30. Edwards GB (1993) Retention of permanent cheek teeth in three horses. *Equine Veterinary Education*, 5, 299–302.

31. Richardson JD and Lane JG (1993) Metaplastic conchal calcification secondary to chronic peri-apical dental infection in seven horses. *Equine Veterinary Education*, 5, 303–307.

32. Stickle R (1998) In: *Textbook of Veterinary Diagnositic Radiology* (3nd edn) ed. DE Thrall, Chap. 10, 'The Equine Skull', WB Saunders, Philadelphia, pp. 105–112.

33. Pirie RS and Dixon PM (1993) Mandibular tumours in the horse: a review of the literature and seven case reports. *Equine Veterinary Education*, 5, 287–294.

34. Lane JG, Longstaffe JA and Gibbs C (1987) Equine paranasal sinus cysts: a report of fifteen cases. *Equine Veterinary Journal*, 19, 537–544.

# TREATMENT OF DENTAL DISORDERS

# EQUINE DENTAL INSTRUMENTATION

WL Scrutchfield, DVM, MS, Diplomate ACVIM, Texas A&M
University College Station, Texas 77845

## INTRODUCTION

This is an exciting time to be involved with equine dentistry. There is an ever increasing range of improved dental instruments and equipment available and, in particular, changes to float blades are a welcome addition. There is also an increasing number and variety of power instruments coming onto the market. Apart from a basic standard set, personal preference is the most important factor when selecting instruments and equipment for use in equine dentistry.

The names and addresses of current manufacturers of dental instruments discussed in this Chapter, equipment and supplies are listed on pp. 180–182.

## BASIC EQUIPMENT

A halter with a large noseband that will allow the horse to open its mouth widely is required (Fig. 12.1). A draft-horse halter with additional holes punched into the neck strap to fit smaller horses does nicely. A halter with an adjustable noseband can be helpful if, for example, hemorrhage develops due to some mishap, a compress can then be placed into the horse's mouth and the noseband tightened to hold the compress in place. The noseband can be opened and slipped off the horse's nose if a full mouth speculum has been placed over the halter. Some form of rigid dental halter can be useful to suspend the head of heavily sedated horses (Fig. 12.2). There are several different types of head supports for

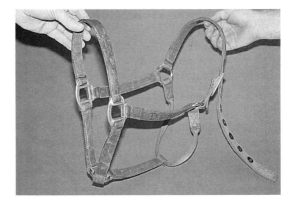

**Figure 12.1.** The halter must have a large noseband that allows the horse to open its mouth without restriction.

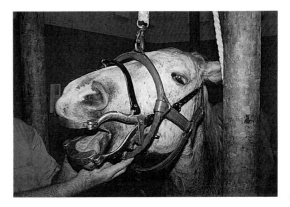

**Figure 12.2.** A rigid dental halter can be used to suspend the head of a sedated horse (Alberts Equine Dental Supply).

sedated horses including free standing models (Fig. 12.3). A crutch can be used to hold the sedated horse's head up if an assistant stabilizes

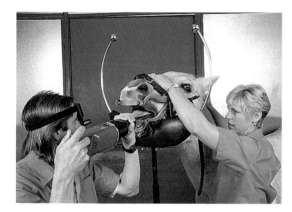

**Figure 12.3.** This is one type of free-standing head support that is available (Equi-Dent Technologies).

both the horse's head and crutch. Alternatively, the head can be supported from the ceiling utilizing a cotton rope and pulley with a quick release snap.[1] It is much easier to hold the head steady if one doesn't also have to hold the weight of the sedated horse's head.

A large plastic bucket with an attached nylon brush and filled with disinfectant solution is used to hold floats, dose syringe and other instruments. Traditionally, a steel bucket has been used but this may damage float blades more than a plastic bucket. Protective Tubes (Olsen and Silk Abrasives) or Bucket Buddies (Harlton's Equine Specialties) have been developed to protect expensive float blades when they are placed in buckets. The nylon brush is used to clean tooth material from float blades, S floats and other instruments. A dose syringe is used to flush feed material and hay from the mouth. A 6 inch nozzle with an enlarged flared distal end is less likely to damage the mouth if the horse jerks or swings its head while the mouth is flushed. Some type of disinfectant is required in the 'float bucket' to prevent the passing of microorganisms between horses. Chlorhexidine with glycerine (Nolvanson Teat Dip, Fort Dodge) has the additional benefit of lubricating hands and arms while palpating within the mouth.

A good light source is essential for examining the cheek teeth. Either penlights or head lights may be used. The use of a head light has the advantage of leaving both hands free while performing the examination and corrective pro-

cedures. Having both penlights and head lights available is desirable as both have their advantages. Many new improved models of both types are on the market, they may be battery operated, with or without rechargeable capacity or electrical lights.

## MOUTH GAGS AND SPECULA

Gags are normally placed between the cheek teeth on one side of the mouth to hold the upper and lower arcades apart to facilitate examination and corrective procedures. They have the advantages of being inexpensive, easy to insert and are out of the way for incisor procedures. Their disadvantages include limiting access to the mouth by taking up space, may cause injury to the teeth or palate, and it has been reported that heavily sedated horses may develop soreness on the opposite side from the gag. Apparently the soreness develops from excessive stretching of the temporomandibular joint fibers.

The gags of spool or coil design have fallen into disfavor as only one tooth of the upper and lower arcades is in contact with the spool or coil. This may cause the teeth to fracture. Further, these devices can slip off of the molar arcades into the palate and cause damage to the gums. Palate lacerations and injury to the palatine artery are also possible.[1] There are several gags designed in a short wedge or oval shape that seem much safer (Fig. 12.4). Some of these have rubber or nylon contact surfaces for additional safety. The types of mouth gags available today vary in size, shape and methods of retention. Some of the more common gags are the Schoupe mouth gag, Jeffery gag, Landmesser wedge, Bayer mouth wedge, Jupiter Spool and Meiers dental wedge. It is possible to use two of these type of gags (one on each side) while doing incisor procedures. Using two gags may prevent soreness in the temporomandibular joint that can develop in heavily sedated horses when only one gag is used.

The easiest and safest way to visualize and palpate all cheek teeth is by the use of a full mouth speculum. These types of specula are, as a rule, larger, heavier and more cumbersome than gags and there is a greater need for chem-

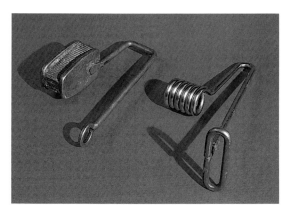

**Figure 12.4.** Two different dental gags are shown. The spool or coil speculum is on the right and a Landmeisser speculum on the left. The Landmeisser speculum is rectangular in shape (the coil speculum is round).

ical restraint when using a full mouth speculum. A full mouth speculum allows the practitioner to adjust the opening of the mouth, but care must be exercised to ensure that the horse's mouth is not opened beyond a comfortable limit. The speculum should not be left in the open position for extended periods of time without allowing the horse to relax. Whenever the mouth is opened wide, the buccal mucosa is pulled in against the edges of the upper cheek teeth. It is therefore advisable to remove sharp buccal enamel points from the upper teeth before forcing the mouth open.[1] There are numerous full mouth specula on the market today ranging in cost from inexpensive to a relatively large amount of money. The author usually uses a McPherson or Hausmann type

full mouth speculum (Fig. 12.5). There are specula available that are based on the old McAllen design and these are preferred by some dental practitioners (Fig. 12.6). A screw type speculum using a single threaded bolt that can be swung from side to side allowing more access to the mouth has recently been developed (Stubbs Equine Innovations) (Fig. 12.7). Flat gum plates are available with the Hausman type speculum which can also be used on cattle. This gum plate can be placed caudal to the upper incisor table to allow oral examination and palpation of horse with a parrot mouth.[1]

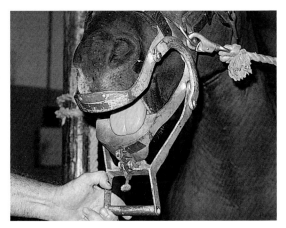

**Figure 12.6.** A MacAllen full mouth speculum is in place.

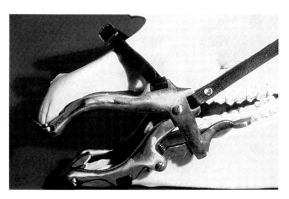

**Figure 12.5.** A McPherson type speculum is in place.

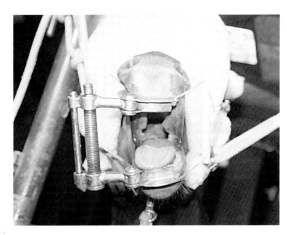

**Figure 12.7.** This shows a recently developed full mouth speculum that uses a single threaded bolt to hold the mouth open. The threaded bolt can be positioned to either side for greater access to the mouth (Stubbs Equine Innovations Inc.).

## MISCELLANEOUS EXAMINATION EQUIPMENT

Other equipment necessary for an oral examination includes a good light source – a hand held light or head lamp is essential. A flexible cable fiberoptic light can be used to illuminate the deep recesses of the oral cavity and buccal spaces. Various types of cheek retractors can allow better visualization in the buccal spaces. A long handled mechanics mirror or fiberoptic scope may be useful in visualizing the interproximal spaces. Dental picks and probes are available in various lengths and blade shapes. These devices provide tremendous aid in evaluating pockets between and around teeth that cannot be reached with a digit.

Moisturizing hand lotion will help lubricate and seal the hands from moisture and dirt. Gloves can be used to protect the hands from abrasions and debris. Soap and a nail brush are necessary to clean up properly after performing dentistry.[1]

## FLOATS

Floats come in all different shapes and lengths. The hand float consists of three basic parts – the handle or grip, the shaft and the rasp head. The handle can be of various sizes, shapes and materials. The shaft can be round, flat or three quarters round. The shaft stiffness is variable as is the length. Shorter shafts are used for work in the front of the mouth while longer shafts are used for the more caudal molar teeth. The horse's size may also dictate the length of shaft desired. Special smaller dental floats have been manufactured to make dental work on small ponies and miniature horses easier. Some draft breeds and warmbloods have very large heads making it difficult to reach the caudal recesses of the mouth with conventional floats. The float head can be set at various angles and positions on the end of the shaft. The head can vary in size and shape to accommodate various areas in the mouth.[1] Float selection is also a matter of personal preference and one needs to try many different float types to determine what would be the most comfortable and effective to use.

The solid carbide float blades are an improvement over the older style carbide chip blades (Fig 12.8). Recent metallurgic advances have greatly improved the abrasive surfaces of simple steel files that would rapidly rust and dull. Carbide chips braised onto a steel removable blade or directly on the head, are the first improvements evident in today's floats. Carbide grit instruments may be resurfaced. These rasps are sharp and durable and come in various sizes and shapes. The blades cut teeth in both directions so the files can be used on the push or pull stroke. The solid tungsten carbide float blade is the product of powder metallurgy. This hard, wear resistant material is obtained by mixing tungsten carbide powder with cobalt powder. The mixture is compacted under high pressure and sintered in a furnace that exceeds the melting point of steel. The result is the hardest metal made by man. This material requires diamond wheels to cut and sharpen it. Blades made of this material retain their sharpness ten times better than the best steel blade. These blades are made in various sizes and with different abrasive surfaces. The depth and pattern of the abrasive edge determines the amount of cut and resistance that the blade provides. These blades only cut in one direction so they are only used on either the push or pull stroke.

The blades are variably designed to file the many different tooth arrangements and vary in

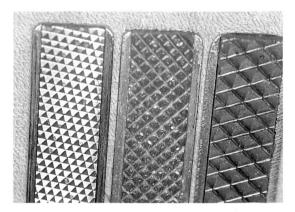

**Figure 12.8.** Three solid carbide blades with different degrees of aggressiveness or coarseness. The fine blade is on the left, the medium blade is in the middle and a coarse blade is on the right.

aggressiveness from fine to extra coarse. These blades are very aggressive and it takes experience to realize how much downward pressure to apply to the blade. When first learning to use the solid carbide blades it is best to use fine to medium blades and not try the coarse to extra coarse blades. The coarser the blade the larger the defects that develop in the blade teeth when the horse bites down on the blade or if the blade is abused in some manner. Finer blades actually stay sharp longer than coarse blades and can be resharpened more times as less carbide is removed in the sharpening process of fine blades. The solid carbide blades are expensive and brittle resulting in defects developing from blade abuse, but they remove much more tooth with less physical effort, and as a result they are the most widely used type of blade today.

Three different floats (short upper obtuse, long upper/lower straight, lower offset) are considered the standard float set. The short upper obtuse float is used to remove points on the rostral upper molars, to shape the second premolars and to remove small rostral hooks. Next, the long upper/lower straight float is used to remove points from both the upper and lower caudal molars. Then the lower offset float is used to remove points along the lingual aspect of the lower arcades.

Usually, depending on personal preference, additional floats are also added to the basic set. The author routinely uses seven floats though not all the floats are used while doing corrective procedures on an individual horse (Fig. 12.9). The floats used are:

1  A long straight float with a solid carbide blade set to cut on the push which is used in removing enamel points in the upper cheek teeth and the rostral five lower cheek teeth (6–10).
2  A long straight float with a solid carbide blade set to cut on the pull that is used to remove sharp points and hooks on the caudal lower molars (311 and 411). This allows one to advance the float slowly and carefully past the caudal aspect of the third molars to prevent banging into the ramus of the mandible and then to pull

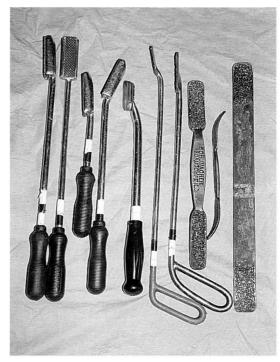

**Figure 12.9.** The seven different float handles and three S floats presently used by the author.

out forcefully to remove the point or hooks. It is somewhat of an extravagance to use two long straight handles, but certainly convenient to not have to change blades from push to pull and back. These first two floats are also used sometimes for leveling occusal tables.

3  A long angled (obtuse) float with a solid carbide blade set to cut on the push that is used to remove the sharp points on the outside of the upper rostral cheek teeth (106–8, 206–8) and in preparing the upper bit seats (106–206).
4  A short straight float with a solid carbide blade set to cut on the push. This float is used on canines, incisors and in preparing lower bit seats (306–406).
5  A medium length offset float with a short, oval solid carbide blade. This is a specialized float that is mainly used in the preparation of bit seats (106, 206, 306, 406).
6  A long back upper molar float that angles up to remove points and hooks on the

caudal aspect of the third molars (11s) with either a solid carbide blade or carbide grit blade. The upper third molars (111 and 211) tend to angle upward and this area is frequently missed by a straight float. There are several different types of upper back molar floats on the market.

7 A long straight float with a carbide grit blade built into the handle. These blades are much thinner than the solid carbide blades and are helpful when there is limited space between the upper and lower caudal molars (111–411 and 211–311).

## S-TYPE FLOATS

Three 'S'-type floats are available (Fig. 12.9). A medium to coarse S float is used in the final shaping of bit seats. A fine S float or steel file is used in the final smoothing or polishing of bit seats. A table float (a very large S float) is used to remove the sharp enamel edges on the palatine aspect of the maxillary cheek teeth and for some leveling of the occlusal surfaces. A table float can be used in areas where the teeth surfaces or edges are curved. An example would be an old horse with wave mouth.

## MOLAR CUTTERS

Undesirable results from using molar cutters include shattering or fracturing a tooth, cutting the tooth too short or cutting the tooth at an angle. Because of the possible complications that may result some people no longer use molar cutters, instead relying on various power instruments to shorten tall or long teeth. The author still uses molar cutters for cutting tall teeth and selected hooks. The blades of molar cutters should contact the sides of the tooth to be cut in a parallel manner. The blades should not contact the tooth with a scissor-like action because this increases the likelihood of shattering the tooth. A D-head compound action cutter is usually needed to cut maxillary teeth. A D-head simple action cutter is usually used to cut mandibular teeth (Figs 12.10 and 12.11). A C- or B-head simple action cutter is used to cut third

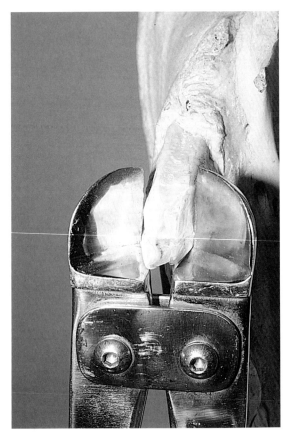

**Figure 12.10.** A D compound cutter being used to cut a mandibular tooth. A D cutter is the correct cutter for this tooth as the blades are in contact with the sides of the tooth in a parallel manner. Figure used by permission of the AAEP, 1996 AAEP Proceeding.

molar hooks (311 and 411). The second premolars (6s) tend to be pointed and would normally be the only teeth where an A-head cutter would be indicated.

If molar cutters are to be used then at least four cutters (D compound, D simple, C simple, and B simple) should be available so the cutter to be used fits against the tooth as described in Chapter 13 (Fig. 12.12).

## CHISELS

Captive bolt percussion chisels can be used to remove the maxillary second premolar hooks (106 and 206) mandibular third molar hooks (311 and 411) and even sharp enamel points. Their use will be discussed in Chapter 13.

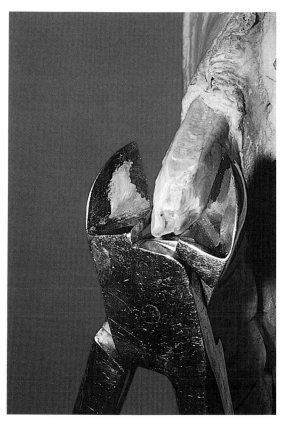

**Figure 12.11.** An A simple cutter in place on the same mandibular tooth as seen in Figure 12.10. It would be dangerous to use an A cutter on this tooth as it would result in a scissor-like cutting action with all the pressure at the rostral aspect of the tooth greatly increasing the likelihood of shattering the tooth. Figure used by permission of the AAEP, 1996 AAEP Proceeding.

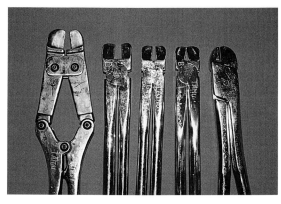

**Figure 12.12.** The five standard molar cutters are pictured with the compound 'D' cutters on the left. The four simple cutters are D, C, B and A from left to right. There are several specialized molar cutters available.

## CAP EXTRACTING INSTRUMENTS

Caps (retained deciduous premolars) are removed using maxillary and mandibular cap extracting forceps, forceps such as wolf tooth forceps or slightly sharpened screwdrivers. There are many different cap extractors on the market.

## WOLF TEETH EXTRACTING INSTRUMENTS

There are numerous wolf tooth elevators and forceps available. Personal preference dictates which instruments are used. The author prefers to have a variety of wolf tooth instruments available including a milk tooth elevator, an adjustable wolf tooth elevator, a Burgess wolf tooth extractor set and a wolf tooth forceps.

## PICKS AND MOLAR FRAGMENT ELEVATORS

Dental picks are used to determine if dental defects or periodontal pockets are present and to explore sagittally fractured teeth and other defects. Molar fragment elevators (World Wide Equine Inc.) are used for removal of molar root fragments and may also be used to determine the nature and extent of cheek teeth defects.

## POWER INSTRUMENTS

There is a growing variety of power instruments available for dental work and some practitioners have evolved to the stage where they only use power instruments (Fig. 12.13). It is exciting that instruments are being developed that allow good dentistry to be carried out with less physical exertion. However, the use of power instruments does not enable a practitioner to be effective without sufficient experience and knowledge. The use of power instruments will only result in much greater damage to the patient if they are used without proper skill. Power instruments can be divided into reciprocating and rotary types used to drive both burrs and disks.

Most of the reciprocating floats are produced by modifying reciprocating saws. There are

TREATMENT OF DENTAL DISORDERS

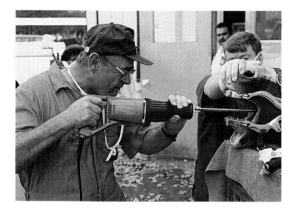

**Figure 12.13.** The author is using a reciprocating float with a $1\frac{1}{4}$ inch (3.2 cm) stroke (Equi-Dent Technologies).

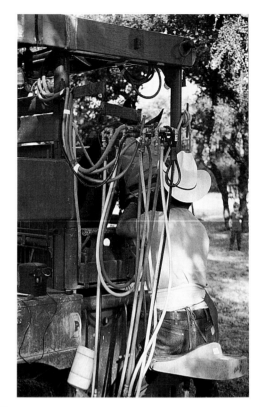

**Figure 12.14.** Portable stocks (crush) with airhoses mounted to run air-driven floats (Stubbs Equine Innovations Inc.).

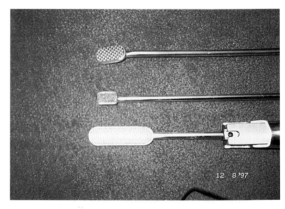

**Figure 12.15.** Some of the shafts and blades used with the air-driven floats. (Stubbs Equine Innovations Inc.).

differences between the various models. Stroke length varies from $\frac{5}{32}$ inch to $1\frac{1}{4}$ inch (0.4–3.2 cm) (Fig. 12.13). These floats may have a variable or fixed speed. Battery operated units are usually of fixed speed as variable speed units deplete batteries in a relatively short time.

The short stroked floats are fairly ineffective in the author's hands although liked by some practitioners. Care must be taken in using the long stroked floats as the ramus of the mandibles could be hit. One supplier suggests that only hand floats be used on the third molars (11s) due to the close proximity to the cranial aspect of the ramus of the mandible (Equi-Dent Technologies). The greatly increased efficiency of the long stroked floats make the less expensive carbide grit blades more effective.

Air powered reciprocating floats are now available (Fig. 12.14). These have a no-load speed of more than 9000 oscillations per minute and approximately a $\frac{3}{8}$ inch (0.5 cm) stroke. The author has limited experience with these floats but was impressed with their potential. The developer believes that four different float heads in air powered floats could replace hand floats, rotary tools, molar cutters, canine cutters and chisels (Fig. 12.15).

There are several different flexible shaft rotary grinders on the market (Fig. 12.16). These grinders usually need to be used with a foot speed control. In the past grinders have been used mainly for incisor procedures. As guards have been developed to protect soft tissue the use of grinders has greatly expanded to include reducing all teeth (Figs 12.17 and 12.18).

Various shaped burrs of either solid carbide or carbide grit are available. Normally cylindrical burrs are used to reduce incisors and cheek

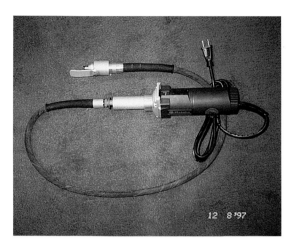

**Figure 12.16.** A type of rotary grinder used in dental procedures. There are several different makes of rotary grinders used for dental procedures.

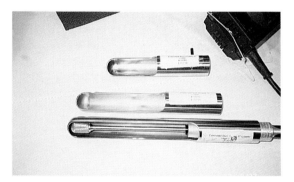

**Figure 12.17.** Guards developed by Harlton's Equine Specialties to be used with Dremel instruments for both cheek teeth and incisor procedures.

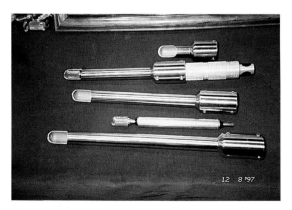

**Figure 12.18.** Guards developed by Carbide Products Co. to be used with Dremel instruments for both cheek teeth and incisor procedures.

teeth. Ball burrs are used to reduce second premolar hooks 106 and 206 and to shape bit seats. Some practitioners prefer to use rotary grinders with burrs in reducing tall teeth in old horses as they feel the burrs will loosen the teeth of old horses less than hand or power reciprocating floats. Diamond cut-off wheels are used to score incisors before cutting and are used by some practitioners to reduce canines.

Some of the rotary grinder units developed or modified for dentistry have provisions for irrigation (World Wide Equine Inc.; Equi-Dent Technologies; Jupiter Vet. Products) (Fig. 12.19). This is done from the concern that thermal damage may occur from burning, though evidence of thermal damage to horses' teeth has not been observed. One should only use sharp burrs and diamond cut-off wheels that are cleaned frequently. To reduce heat build up, the burr or diamond cut-off wheel should be moved continuously and not held in one place. Research is required in this area so that guidelines may be established.

Power instruments will allow some dental procedures to be carried out with less physical exertion and, in some instances, with more precision. They will however also allow the unskilled operator to make more serious mistakes and accidents. There is certainly a learning curve in using power instruments and practice on cadaver material is recommended. Protective

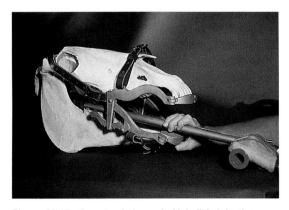

**Figure 12.19.** An extended guard with built in irrigation system to be used with a Dremel instrument to reduce any cheek tooth, but especially useful for M 3 hooks (3–411) (Equi-Dent Technologies, PO Box 5877, Sparks, NV 89432–5877).

eye glasses and a mask should always be worn when power tools are used and dental thermal injury avoided by the use of water sprays.

A good way to see what instruments are available and how they are used is to attend a seminar or wet laboratory where sales representatives are present. One can observe what instruments are used by the instructors and fellow participants. Ask the sales representatives what instruments they recommend for different corrective procedures and, if they will allow you to, exchange instruments that do not work for you. Visiting colleagues that are practicing good dentistry will provide exposure not only to what instruments are available but also how they are used.

## EQUINE DENTAL EQUIPMENT AND RELATED SUPPLIES

Alberts Equine Dental Supply
Box 11–174
Londonville, NY 12211
1–800-DENTAL-8

General line of dental equipment

Arnolds Veterinary Products Ltd
Cartmel Drive
Harlescott, Shrewsbury
Shropshire, SY1 3TB, UK
+441743 441632/+441743 462111

General line of dental equipment

Brassler USA Inc. Dental Instruments
800 King George Blvd
Savanah, GA 31419
1–800–841–4522

Burrs and diamond cut-off wheels

Carbide Products Co.
Equine Division
22711 Western Ave.
Torrance, CA 90501
1–800–64–BLADE

Carbide float blades, float handles, burrs, diamond cut-off wheels

DLM Tool Works
PO Box 216
Simorton, TX 77476
281–346–2355 or 533–9699

Carbide float blades, float handles, speciality items

Eisenhot-Vet AG
Sandweg 52, CH-4123
Allschil, Switzerland
061 307 9000/061 307 9009

Rotary power tool supplier

Enco Machinery, Tools and Supplies
1–800–873–3626 (a call to this number is routed to the nearest branch)

Burrs, diamond cut-off wheels, power grinders

Equi-Dent Technologies
PO Box 5877
Sparks, NV 89432–5877
(702) 358–6695

Reciprocating electrical floats, hand floats, rotary equipment, head supports

| | |
|---|---|
| Equi-Tech<br>8902 West Second Ave.<br>Stillwater, OK 74075<br>405–624–3318 | Full mouth speculum |
| Harlton's Equine Specialties<br>792 Olenhurst Court<br>Columbus, OH 43235–2163<br>1–800–247–3901 | General line of equine dental equipment |
| Identech Inc.<br>Right Light-Head Light<br>PO Box 4071<br>Wheaton, IL 60189<br>708–231–3665 | Head lights |
| Jorgensen Laboratories<br>1450 North Van Buren Ave.<br>Loveland, CO 80538<br>303–669–2500 | Limited – general line of equine dental equipment |
| Jupiter Veterinary Products<br>3635 North 6th Street,<br>Harrisburg, PA 17110 | Limited – general line of equine dental equipment |
| Kruuse<br>DK-5290 Marslev<br>Denmark<br>1-65-95-15-11 | Equine products |
| Kruuse UK Ltd<br>14A Moor Lane Industrial Estate<br>Sherburn in Elmet<br>North Yorkshire<br>LS25 6ES, UK<br>+441977 681523/+441977 683537<br>Email: *kruuse@jkruuse.dk* | General line of dental equipment |
| Light-Tech Inc.<br>8900 West Josephine Road<br>Sebring, FL 33872<br>1–800–462–5542 | Head lights |
| Meister Co.<br>Meister Equine Speculum<br>Bar 67<br>Hampton, CT 06247<br>860–455–9737 6– 9 pm EST | Full mouth speculum |
| Milburn Distribution Inc.<br>PO Box 42810<br>Phoenix, AZ 85080–2810<br>1–800–279–6452 | General line of equine dental equipment |

| | |
|---|---|
| Novalson teat dip solution<br>Fort Dodge<br>800 5th Street NW<br>Fort Worth, IA 50501<br>800–685–5656 | Chlorhexidine with glycerine |
| Olsen and Silk Abrasives<br>c/o The Shoe<br>181 Elliott Street, Box 610<br>Beverly, MA 01915<br>508–744–4720 or 508–922–0613 | Float handles and blades, S floats, incisor rasps |
| Pelican Products Inc.<br>23215 Early Ave<br>Torrance, CA 90505<br>310–326–4700 | Head lights |
| Stubbs Equine Innovations Inc.<br>HC3, Box 38<br>Johnson City, TX 78636<br>830–868–7544 | Air power tools and accessories, full mouth speculum |
| Surgical Holdings<br>Parkside Centre<br>Temple Farm Industrial Estate<br>Southend-On-Sea<br>Essex, SS2 5SJ, UK<br>+441702 602050/+441702 460006 | Custom-made equipment and general dental equipment |
| Western Instrument Co.<br>4950 York Street<br>PO Box 16428<br>Denver, CO 80216<br>1–800–525–2065 | Limited general line of equine dental instruments |
| World Wide Equine Dental Supply Company UK<br>'Brooklands'<br>Bells Hill Road<br>Vange, Basildon<br>Essex SS16 5JT, UK<br>+441268 555411 (Home)/0831 127537 (Mobile)/<br>+441268 555505 | Wide general line of dental equipment |
| World Wide Equine Inc.<br>PO Box 1040<br>415 East 4th<br>Glenns Ferry, ID 83623<br>1–800–331–5485 | General line of equine dental instruments |

### REFERENCES

1. Eisley J (1998) Dental care and instrumentation. *Veterinary Clinics of North America Equine Practice*, WB Saunders, Philadelphia.

# 13

# DENTAL PROPHYLAXIS

WL Scrutchfield, DVM, MS, Diplomate ACVIM, Texas A&M
University College Station, Texas 77845

## INTRODUCTION

In all aspects of equine medicine and surgery the concept of prophylaxis, that is the ability to use a practice that will prevent the development of subsequent serious disease, is the foundation of any health maintenance program. Dental prophylaxis – the examination of the oral cavity and the use of corrective procedures to arrest disease processes, for example the removal of sharp edges that may lead to dysmastication and periodontal disease – has been reaffirmed as an important part of the veterinary health care program for all horses.

Taking the time to educate owners of the value of complete examination and the indicated corrective procedures, and the professional fees for these services is necessary to prevent misunderstanding. Dental forms or charts should be used to record the abnormalities present, what procedures are performed initially and what procedures will need to be done in the future. Dental forms will also help in providing an estimate of professional fees before procedures are performed and in itemizing the bill after the procedures are done.

It is best to have new clients present when performing dental examinations and corrective procedures. The client can be shown any abnormalities that are present and what is to be done to correct them. This will give the client a much greater appreciation of equine dentistry and an understanding of the professional fees involved.

## FLOATING PROCEDURES

Floating (rasping or filing) is the most common dental procedure performed. While floating is performed mainly to remove the sharp enamel points from the buccal edges of the maxillary cheek teeth and from the lingual edge of the mandibular cheek teeth, it involves more than this. The rostral surfaces of the second premolars (106, 206, 306, 406) are rounded, small hooks, ramps, beaks and arcade irregularities are removed, and the normal 10–15° angle to the cheek teeth occlusal surfaces are restored. Take care *not* to level the arcades occlusal surfaces from side to side. The goal of floating is to maintain the symmetry and balance of the arcades and to allow a free elliptical chewing motion.[1] The author's techniques are also changing over time as he continually strives to make floating easier and more comfortable for both the horse and himself. Readers should develop their own floating technique and constantly think of ways to improve their method. One way to improve your own technique is to work with colleagues experienced in dental procedures to evaluate the efficiency of your technique and modify it if necessary. The author is not ambidextrous so all descriptions are for right-handed floating. The descriptions may be reversed for left-handed persons. It would be good to develop expertise with one's 'off-hand' as it would allow one to float more before developing fatigue.

The author no longer has a set routine, but several different routines that are used

185

TREATMENT OF DENTAL DISORDERS

depending upon the individual horse. These include the age of the horse, whether or not it is accustomed to having a bit in its mouth, whether very sharp enamel points are present on the buccal aspect of the maxillary teeth, if there are tall, sharp canines and the types and severity of the abnormalities present. A full mouth speculum is seldom used when floating the sharp enamel points of weanlings, yearlings and unbroken 2-year-olds. A full mouth speculum is usually used while performing dental examinations and corrective procedures in horses over 3 years old. Nearly all horses accustomed to a bit tolerate a full mouth speculum. If tall, sharp canines are present then they are cut and blunted first to reduce the likelihood of lacerating one's hand, wrist and arm (Figs 13.1 and 13.2). If the horse has very sharp enamel points on the buccal aspect of the upper maxillary teeth they should be floated off before inserting a full mouth speculum, as the cheek skin and buccal mucosa are tightened when the speculum is opened and this may cause discomfort if sharp enamel points are present. Tall, long teeth may need to be reduced before floating of sharp enamel points can be done.

The solid carbide planing blades on floats manufactured by several companies are much sharper than file or chip blades and enable quick and easy removal of sharp enamel points. When using sharp carbide blades, care must be taken to not remove the occlusal surface by over-floating. Types of floats and their uses are discussed in Chapter 12.

In nearly all floating the left hand is on the shaft near the blade to hold the float in place and to apply more pressure. While floating the right maxillary teeth either the left hand is in the interdental space lifting up and out on the shaft of the float (Fig. 13.3) or the noseband is grasped with the left fingers and the shaft of the float is lifted up and out with the thumb (Fig. 13.4). While floating the left maxillary teeth either the left hand is placed across the interdental space pushing the shaft of the float out and up (Fig. 13.5) or the left wrist is laid on the bridge of the horse's nose and the fingers held in a 'J' position lifting the shaft of the float out and up (Fig. 13.6). In floating the sharp points of the

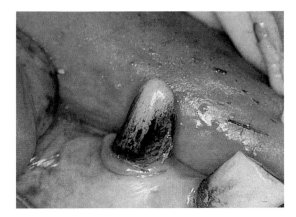

**Figure 13.1.** A tall, sharp canine is present.

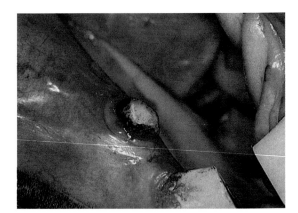

**Figure 13.2.** The tall, sharp canine in Figure 13.1 has been reduced and blunted or smoothed.

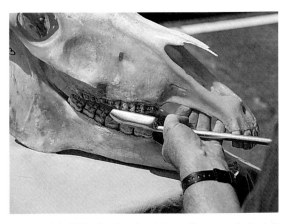

**Figure 13.3.** While floating the right maxillary arcade the left hand lifts the shaft of the float up and out. Contact with the cheek brings the float blade into the proper position for floating.

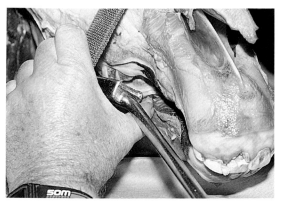

**Figure 13.4.** This is a different technique for floating the right maxillary teeth to that shown in Figure 13.3. The left fingers are hooked over the noseband and the shaft of the float is lifted up and out with the thumb.

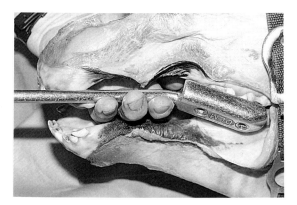

**Figure 13.5.** While floating the left maxillary arcade the left hand is across the interdental space with the fingers pushing the shaft of the float up and out.

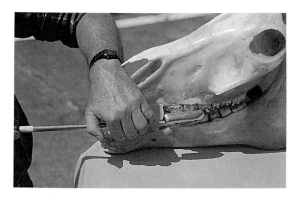

**Figure 13.6.** This is a different technique for floating the left maxillary arcade to that shown in Figure 13.5. The left wrist is laid on the horse's nose and the fingers hooked under the shaft of the float to lift it up and out. The wrist on the horse's nose helps control the horse's head movement.

maxillary teeth, do not try to push the float blade into the sharp points. Instead, concentrate on lifting or pushing the float out and up into the cheek. The cheek will bring the blade into the proper position for floating if you are holding the blade at the correct angle in relation to the sharp enamel points. The anisognathic jaw configuration (wider between the maxillary arcades than between the mandibular arcades) results in it being easier to float the upper arcades than the lower arcades because the horse cannot bite down on the float if the float is held in the proper position.

The rostral maxillary cheek teeth are floated first with the angled upper molar float (30° angle). The right and left caudal maxillary teeth are floated with the long straight float after the rostral aspect of the arcades are floated with the angle float in the same manner as previously described. Most of the strokes are done with the float blade positioned at a 45° angle to the buccal side of the tooth. The float does need to be rolled somewhat to round the edges of the teeth. Some horses have pronounced cingula (cusps) on the buccal surface of their maxillary teeth that may cause discomfort when a noseband presses the cheek against them. Sharp enamel points develop from the cingula, so if the cingula are reduced it will be longer before sharp enamel points develop. The cingula need to be removed or at least reduced by holding the float blade flat against the buccal side of the teeth for a few strokes. The caudal aspect of the maxillary third molars (111 and 211) commonly curves upward causing straight floats to miss this area (Fig. 13.7). A back upper float that curves upward is used to float this area (Fig. 13.8). This is important as it is not unusual for there to be sharp projections on the caudal aspect of the maxillary third molars (111 and 211). These sharp projections seem to cause discomfort in some performance horses. The use of two or three back upper molar floats angled up in different degrees enables the caudal aspects of the maxillary third molars (111 and 211) to be smoothed more effectively.

Usually the mandibular sharp enamel points of weanlings, yearlings and unbroken 2-year-olds are floated without the use of a full mouth

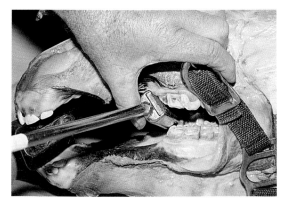

**Figure 13.16.** After the 206 is floated as shown in Figure 13.15, the fingers of the left hand are hooked over the noseband of the halter while the left thumb stabilizes and pushes the float blade into the tooth as the float is moved in a buccal to palatine direction.

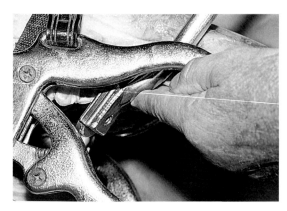

**Figure 13.17.** Some individuals create 'bit seats' with a full mouth speculum in place using a short, offset float on the upper teeth.

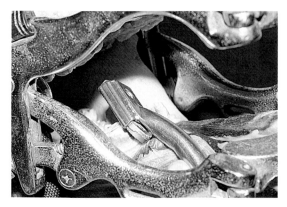

**Figure 13.18.** Creating a 'bit seat' with a full mouth speculum in place using a short, offset float Alberts on the lower teeth.

A short, straight float is used to shape mandibular bit seats. The tooth is beveled by floating as parallel to the rostral surface of the tooth as possible using short strokes. Some horses have excessive or loose tissue between the tooth and the cheek that may be injured while floating. A right-handed floater can abduct the cheek with the left hand while shaping the right mandibular second premolar. The horse's left mandibular second premolar can be beveled by gripping the head of the float and sticking the index finger into the cheek to push the excessive tissue out of the way. After shaping the teeth with a solid carbide float, a coarse S float and then a fine S float or file is used in the final shaping and polishing. It may be necessary to place the bit that is normally used into the horse's mouth and observe the relationship of soft tissue, bit and bit seat. Exaggerated beveling back will be needed in some horses to prevent soft tissue being pinched between the bit and the rostral surfaces of the mandibular second premolars (306 and 406).

The author creates bit seats without a full mouth speculum in place, but some practitioners leave the speculum in place while rounding and smoothing the second premolar. The shaft of an offset float is placed over the upper incisor plate while working on the upper second premolar (Fig. 13.17) and under the lower incisor plate while working with the lower second premolar (Fig. 13.18).

There are many other instruments and procedures used in shaping bit seats. An increasing number of practitioners shape bit seats using Dremel-type instruments (Fig. 13.19).[3] Either a cylinder burr or ball-shaped burr may be used. Some practitioners use different S floats for all the shaping and polishing by starting with coarse grit S floats and finishing with small grit floats or fine steel files. Using a lower molar roller float with an offset head is preferred by some in beveling back mandibular second premolars.

The bit seats should be balanced and of uniform shape and size. The upper right and left bit seats should be the same (if the original premolar tooth structure allows). This also applies to the lower bit seats. Regardless of what instru-

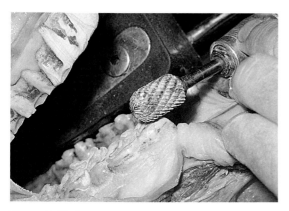

**Figure 13.19.** Some individuals use Dremel-type instruments with various burrs to create 'bit seats'.

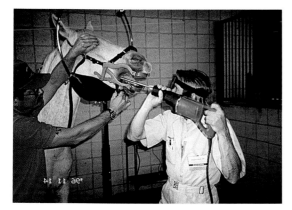

**Figure 13.20.** Some individuals have evolved to the point where they only use power (or motorized) instruments in their dental practice (Dr. Scott Greene).

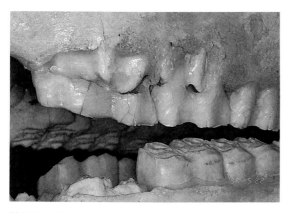

**Figure 13.21.** A late two-year-old horse that has shed the left 75 cap and still has the upper left PM 2 and PM 3 caps (65 and 66). A line of demarcation can be seen between the caps and permanent teeth.

ments are used, it is very important to visualize and palpate the bit seats to ensure that no sharp areas remain.

There are a variety of power floats on the market. These are discussed in Chapter 12. The short stroke floats are ineffective in the author's experience but liked by some practitioners. The $1\frac{1}{4}$ inch stroke float is effective in reducing waves and sharp enamel points on the rostral mandibular teeth. Care must be taken in floating the caudal mandibular teeth to not hit the ramus of the mandible.

It takes practice to become proficient with the different power floats. It is good to seek instruction from the vendor or distributor, or a practitioner that uses power floats and has developed good expertise. Some practitioners have evolved to the point that they use power instruments primarily or solely for performing corrective procedures (Fig. 13.20) (Greene SK; Stubbs RC – Personal Communication, 1996).

## RETAINED DECIDUOUS PREMOLARS (CAPS)

Retained deciduous premolars may cause inadequate mastication, anorexia, poor performance and malocclusion (step mouth). If a demarcation between the deciduous and permanent premolars can be seen or palpated the deciduous premolar should be extracted (Fig. 13.21). The permanent premolars can be damaged if the deciduous premolars are extracted too early. Most references give the shedding times for the second premolars (06s) as 2.5 years, for the third premolars (07s) as 3 years and the fourth premolars (08s) as 4 years. The author has found 2 years 8 months for second premolars, (06s), 2 years 10 months for the third premolars (07s), and 3 years 8 months for fourth premolars (08s) to be more accurate shedding times although still only a rough guide as there is quite a bit of variability (Moriarity L – Personal Communication, 1996).

There are several different upper and lower cap extracting forceps available. The 106 and 206 caps can be extracted with wolf tooth forceps or upper cap extractors. The author usually uses a slightly sharpened screwdriver to pry off the maxillary third premolar and fourth premolar caps (107 and 108; 207 and 208). The sharpened blade is worked into the space between the cap and permanent tooth from the rostral medial aspect and the cap is pried off. Some practitioners believe using a sharpened screwdriver may put too much pressure on the permanent tooth resulting in damage. The author has not observed any complications from the use of a screwdriver, but the reader should be aware of others' concerns. Mandibular cap forceps are used to extract mandibular caps. Caps are rolled medially during extraction so that if root spicules are broken off they are located medially where the horse might be able to work the spicules out with its tongue. Occasionally, caps may extend above the occlusal surface of the adjacent teeth and yet cannot be extracted without using excessive force. These caps should be floated down level with adjacent occlusal surfaces and extracted 6 to 8 weeks later.

Caps, and especially partial caps, can be difficult to identify at times. Careful examination of the premolars of late 2- and 3-year-old horses is indicated so that caps are identified and extracted if indicated (see Chapter 15).

## WOLF TEETH

There seems to be a trend to try to determine if a wolf tooth will or will not cause problems. This is done by determining the size and location of the wolf tooth, what the horse is used for, what tack is used and the ability of the rider. This author is not knowledgeable enough to do that and follows the advice in an old book 'no wolf tooth does any good, may do harm, so extract them all' (Fig. 13.22). That is not quite true as the wolf teeth of winning performance horses may not be extracted until the horse stops winning or the owner or trainer believes the wolf teeth are causing problems.

There are numerous types of wolf tooth elevators and instruments. The reader needs to try different types to see what is most effective for them. The author selects the elevator and instruments to be used depending upon the size and location of the wolf tooth. If the maxillary wolf tooth is rostral to the second premolars 106 and

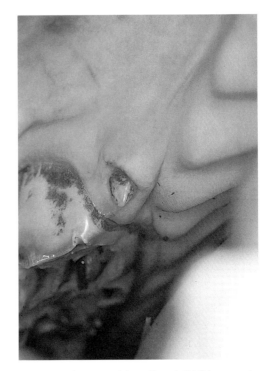

**Figure 13.22.** An upper right wolf tooth (105) is present.

206 with a space between them, an appropriately sized Burgess wolf tooth instrument is used to cut the gum away from the wolf tooth. Then a dental elevator is used to further loosen the tooth in the alveolus. (Fig. 13.23). After the wolf tooth is loose, it is either elevated out by placing an adjustable wolf tooth elevator between the wolf tooth and the second premolar (106 and 206) and prying or extracted with a wolf tooth forceps. If the wolf tooth is tight against the second premolar (106 or 206) or medial to the second premolar (106 or 206), then a milk tooth elevator is used to cut the gum and loosen the tooth in the alveolus. It is then either elevated out or extracted with forceps. If the wolf tooth is tight against the second premolars (106 and 107), forcing a Burgess instrument or elevator between the wolf tooth and the second premolars (106 and 107) will frequently result in the wolf tooth being broken off.

No matter how carefully one attempts to extract wolf teeth, some will be broken off. The root fragment will seldom cause complications. Any sharp edges and points should be smoothed

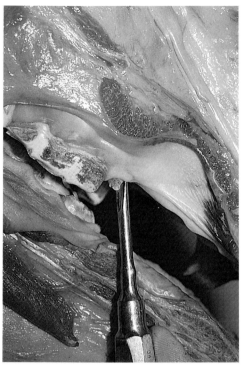

**Figure 13.23.** A dental elevator is useful to loosen the wolf tooth (05s) in the alveolus before extraction by elevator or forceps.

and the dental record should indicate that the wolf tooth was broken off.

If no maxillary wolf teeth are seen, the maxilla rostral to the second premolars (106–206) should be palpated for the presence of an unerupted (impacted or blind) wolf tooth. Unerupted wolf teeth should be removed from performance horses as the horse may have discomfort when the mucosa over the tooth is knocked by a bit.

The mandibles should also be examined for the presence of wolf teeth (305 and 405). Mandibular wolf teeth (305 and 405) are fairly common in some lines of standardbreds and are rarely found in horses of other breeds. The author has seen alveolar infections develop after extracting mandibular wolf teeth (305 and 405). This has not been a problem when owners lavaged the extraction site for a few days postoperatively.

Not all wolf teeth (05s) cause problems, but because some do and because proper shaping of the maxillary second premolars (06s) cannot be

done with wolf teeth present, wolf teeth should be extracted (see Chapter 15).

## CANINE TEETH

Tall or sharp canine teeth (104, 204, 304, 404) need to be cut and blunted before performing corrective dental procedures to reduce the likelihood of injuring one's hands and wrists. Other benefits of reducing and smoothing the canines include decreasing the chances of the horse being injured by catching a canine on some fixed object, less damage is caused if fighting, insertion and removal of the bit is easier and there is less tartar build up on the shortened canine teeth. Reducing the canines to near the gum line may increase the horse's comfort by alleviating constriction of the tongue between tall canines and the bit.

The canines may be shortened and smoothed using a variety of methods. The mandibular canine can be cut with canine or incisor cutters, or with nail cutters (used by farriers to cut off horseshoe nails (Fig. 13.24). Mandibular canines are flat from side to side so the cutter is placed

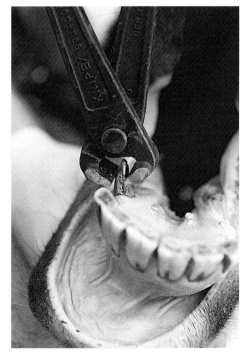

**Figure 13.24.** Canines can be reduced with a nail cutter.

to cut from medial to lateral (not rostral to caudal). Do not try to do all the reduction with the cutters as the tooth might shatter into the gum. The sharp remaining surface of the canine can be further shortened and rounded by rasping with a float. Final smoothing and polishing is done with an S float or steel file. The maxillary canines are seldom cut off, but reduced and smoothed with floats, S floats and steel files. A Dremel-type instrument with burr will reduce and round canines very rapidly. Some practitioners use a utility knife handle with hacksaw-type blades to cut off canines (Kelly LH – Personal Communication, 1996).

Usually the canines of young horses can be reduced to the gum without invading the pulp cavity. This is not true of the canines of older horses.

The small rudimentary canines of some mares may cause discomfort. These canines can be floated to the level of the gum or removed with rongeurs. If the mucosa over unerupted canines of either sex appears to be painful, the mucosa should be removed with rongeurs to allow the canines to erupt.

## TALL OR LONG TEETH

Most tall or long teeth have developed from the lack of occlusion which has resulted from the loss of the opposing tooth (Fig. 13.25). Quite a few horses have slightly tall or long teeth that are often missed on evaluation. A ramp may only be 2–3 mm in height or a maxillary second premolar (106 or 206) may only be 2 mm longer than normal. These may be missed until they become so tall or long that it would be difficult to reduce the tooth by hand floating. Using an adequate light, a full mouth speculum and careful palpation help to identify slight abnormalities and allow early correction.

Tall or long teeth may be either cut (or more accurately fractured) with molar cutters, ground down with various power instruments or rasped down with floats. The method chosen to reduce the tall or long tooth depends upon the size and location of the tooth, what instruments and equipment are available and what method the operator is comfortable performing.

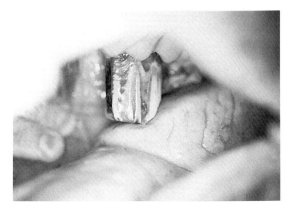

**Figure 13.25.** Most tall (long) teeth develop from being unopposed.

Some practitioners will not use molar cutters for fear of shattering a tooth or causing some other complications. There are several precautions to heed when using molar cutters. To decrease the likelihood of shattering a tooth, the tooth should be mature (i.e. in wear for 2 years or more) and the blades of molar cutters should contact the tooth to be cut in a parallel manner (not with a scissor-like action). A scissor-like action is to be avoided. The horse should be sedated, a full mouth speculum in place and the presence of good assistants is essential; in addition a head light is helpful in allowing both of the operator's hands to be free. An assistant should hold the tongue in such a manner that it is not injured when the cutter handles come together. The cutters should be held level with the table surface while cutting. One must not lift the handles up while straining to cut a tooth or an uneven table surface will be the result. Floating is required to remove the sharp edges left after cutting and to return the new occlusal surface to the correct angle.

It is impossible to use one cutter for the different teeth as the cutter blades need to close onto the sides of the tooth in a parallel manner. Compound D head cutters are required to cut most maxillary cheek teeth while a single D head cutter can be used to cut most mandibular cheek teeth. A simple cutter with either a C or B head is used to cut hooks on the mandibular third molars (311 and 411). Normally, A-headed cutters are only used to cut second premolars (06s) as these are the only pointed teeth.

Cutters vary greatly in quality and, when purchasing cutters, select the best quality possible. They will be expensive but should last a practice lifetime. There are practitioners that use various power instruments for major tooth reductions and never use molar cutters due to their concern of possibly creating complications (Greene SK; Stubbs RC – Personal Communication, 1996).

## HOOKS, RAMPS AND BEAKS

Teeth (or any part of a tooth not in occlusion) continue to erupt and become tall or long. Incomplete occlusion occurs most frequently between the maxillary and mandibular second premolars (06s) and results in the formation of hooks or beaks on the rostral portion of the maxillary second premolars (106 and 206). It is not uncommon for hooks to develop at the caudal aspect of the mandibular third molars (311 and 411). Care must be taken to not confuse the normal upward slant of the table surface of the mandibular third molars (311 and 411), due to natural curvature of the mandibles of horses with short heads, with actual hooks. One must palpate to determine the distance from both the rostral and caudal occlusal surfaces to the gum. If the distance from the caudal occlusal surface to the gum is the same as the distance from the rostral occlusal surface to the gum, no hook is present. If the upward curvature at the caudal aspect of the mandibular third molars (311 and 411) is mistaken for a hook and the tooth is cut with molar cutters, up to one half the tooth might be removed taking the table surface out of occlusion and possibly shattering the tooth or exposing the pulp. There have been several cases of infected mandibular third molars (311 and 411s) following inappropriate cutting. Many horses have long maxillary second molars (110 and 210) and short mandibular second molars (310 and 410). The examiner may believe the mandibular third molars (311 and 411) are too tall when they are of normal height. Hooks may be removed with a chisel, power instrument or float. The horse's age, height of the hook, space in the mouth and instruments avail-

able determine the approach taken to remove hooks.

Tall hooks on the mandibular third molars (311 and 411) can be cut with simple molar cutters. Usually a C head simple cutter is used for large hooks, but if the C head gap is too wide to cut the hook, then a B head cutter is used. Sharp enamel points rostral to the hook are removed by floating first. The cutter is advanced along the arcade with the blades closed until the hook is reached. The blades are opened and the cutter is advanced. The cutter is then closed cutting off the hook. Care must be taken to not lift the handles of the cutter in an effort to get a better grip on the hook with the blades. This would result in removal of too much tooth and increase the likelihood of shattering the tooth (Fig. 13.26). An assistant should restrain the tongue in such a manner that it is not injured when the cutter handles come together. Using a full mouth speculum and a head light is helpful, but it is still difficult to visualize the hook with the cutter in place. The teeth of horses under 9 years of age may be too immature to be safely cut with molar cutters. Several precautions should be taken in using molar cutters. After the hook is cut the remaining sharp edges must be smoothed by floating.

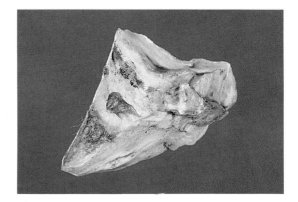

**Figure 13.26.** This is an example of an excessive amount of tooth that has been cut off with molar cutters while attempting to cut off the hook. This improper cutting of lower M 3 hooks (3–411s) may result in a shattered and/or infected tooth. Figure used by permission of the AAEP, 1996 AAEP Proceeding.

An Equichip chisel is handy to remove hooks that are not too large. The chisel is advanced down the arcade with a full mouth speculum in place and hooked over the hook. The captive bolt is then pulled out cutting off the hook. The chisel handle must be held as high as possible to ensure that only the hook is cut off. Holding the chisel handle level with the occlusal surface of the arcade can result in up to two thirds of the tooth being removed which is undesirable.

Several practitioners are using Dremel-type power instruments with guards to remove the hooks on the mandibular third molars (311 and 411) as well as for creating bit seats. There are very specialized power instruments available which have a long extension and a guarded rotary burr just for reducing the caudal aspect of the mandibular third molars (311 and 411).

The hooks or beaks from the rostral aspect of the maxillary second premolars (106 and 206) can be reduced by chisels, molar cutters, power instruments or floating. Care must be taken if using a chisel as too much tooth may be removed if the chisel is held too high on the tooth, or the chisel is not held at a sufficiently steep angle. Having a full mouth speculum in place will help in getting the proper angle to the chisel and prevent it from damaging any mandibular teeth. The chisel is placed over the upper incisor plate and against the rostral surface of the maxillary second premolars (106 or 206) at the point where the hook is to be removed. A score line can be made at the point where the cut is to start, by using a utility knife with a hacksaw blade, to keep the chisel from slipping up to the gum line and removing too much tooth.

The maxillary second premolars (106 and 206) can be loosened and even removed by excessive banging with a chisel. The author still removes a few 106 and 206 hooks or beaks with a chisel, but prefers to remove small hooks by floating and large hooks with a rotary-type power instrument.

Hooks or beaks can be removed with molar cutters but care must be taken not to shatter the tooth. Having angle headed cutters with the correct size gap would be helpful. A Dremel-type instrument can be purchased for less than an angle headed cutter and can do many more procedures than the angled headed cutter.

Dremel-type instruments are increasingly being used to remove hooks or beaks from maxillary second premolars (106 and 206) as well as to create bit seats. Some practitioners use guards with cylinder-type burrs and others ball burrs with no guards. Usually some type of buccal retainer is needed to protect the buccal mucosa from injury. The use of a Dremel-type instrument is the author's preferred method of removing hooks and beaks as it eliminates removing too much tooth or loosening the tooth (as a chisel may) and does not shatter teeth (as molar cutters may). Also, as the tooth is reduced a bit seat can be created.

Hooks or beaks can be removed by floating if no other instruments are available. With a full mouth speculum in place, the float is inserted over the upper incisor plate of the speculum and into the mouth under the hook. The solid carbide float blade should be set on the pull. By placing one hand under the blade a large amount of pressure can be placed on the blade and the hook or beak reduced fairly quickly.

## DENTISTRY FOR OLD HORSES

Although some old horses have relatively good teeth and only routine floating and minor incisor adjustments are indicated, horses of 20 years and older frequently have severe wave mouth and incisor abnormalities (Fig. 13.27). The teeth of many old horses have reached the stage where they can be helped but not 'fixed'.

The cheek teeth of old horses may be accidently extracted or loosened during corrective procedures because the reserve crown is so greatly reduced. This possibility should be explained to owners before corrective procedures are performed on the teeth of old horses. It is helpful to have skulls of young and old horses with sections of the bone removed to demonstrate the different length of reserve crown and root in each age group. It is better for the owner to be aware that teeth may be accidently extracted or loosened before starting corrective procedures.

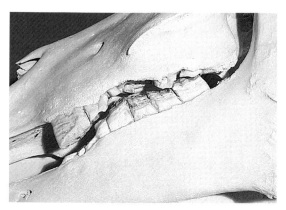

**Figure 13.27.** An example of severe wave mouth seen in some old horses.

Some old horses may have medical problems that should be evaluated before corrective dental procedures are performed. It would be embarrassing to have an old horse die of pre-existing medical problems or stress following corrective dental procedures.

The author has taken a conservative approach to correcting severe dental abnormalities of old horses. Tall or long teeth that reach into the opposite gum or that are opposed by worn out teeth are shortened to the level where they are out of occlusion. Teeth that have been worn down to the point that they no longer have any enamel left wear much faster without the hard enamel. Shortening is done using molar cutters, floats or rotary-type instruments. Sharp points, hooks and any other sharp areas are smoothed using floats on rotary-type instruments. After finishing with corrective procedures, all the cheek teeth must be palpated to determine if they are still solidly embedded. It can be difficult to determine if a tooth is loose or not. One cannot just push out on the tooth to determine loose-ness. Each tooth should be grasped between thumb and fingers and rocked vigorously. Some teeth that are only slightly loose may in time tighten and should be allowed to do so. Excessive loose teeth, teeth with a bad odor and loose or odiferous root fragments should be extracted. Root fragment extractors are helpful in removing parts of old teeth and root fragments.

When teeth are extracted from old horses or the horse has periodontal disease, antimicro-bials should be administered. These horses, as well as other horses lacking good occlusion of the cheek teeth, need to be given a pelleted or extruded feed especially formulated for old horses. Some clients maintain their old horses by soaking pellets and alfalfa cubes and feeding them from deep, plastic tubs. Corn oil added to the diet will increase the caloric intake and will help to maintain some horses with very bad teeth.

It is difficult to know how much shortening should be done on the incisors of old horses. It is good to bring the cheek teeth into greater occlusion, but may be deleterious if the increased occlusion causes discomfort in the remaining cheek teeth. Incisor reduction is discussed later in this chapter.

## INCISORS

Many horses have abnormalities of the incisors that may cause difficult mastication and decreased performance. The incisors are easy to observe and can be evaluated with less difficulty than the cheek teeth. Most abnormalities can be corrected or at least greatly improved with relatively simple procedures and equipment. Stalled horses that are fed high-grain diets seem to have more incisor abnormalities than pastured horses.

The deciduous central (01s), intermediate (02s) and corner (03s) incisors are normally shed at 2.5, 3.5 and 4.5 years of age respectively. Deciduous incisors are occasionally retained. A deciduous incisor is retained and should be extracted if the contralateral incisor is permanent and in wear and/or the opposing incisor is permanent and in wear, or if a permanent incisor is erupting behind the deciduous incisor. If the permanent incisor is erupting directly beneath the deciduous incisor, the retained incisor will consist of exposed crown and a short unexposed crown (incisor cap) only.

These short retained incisors (caps) will require minimal elevation and can be removed with forceps. If the permanent incisor has erupted behind the retained deciduous incisor, the crown (or cap) is easily removed with forceps in most cases. However, the deciduous root or partial root usually remains beneath the gingiva and may keep the permanent tooth from moving forward into normal position. An incision is made over the part of the root left in place and the gingiva reflected. The root fragment is then elevated and removed. The gingival flaps are trimmed. If a central (01) or intermediate (02) retained incisor has been extracted, frequently the space available for the permanent tooth is too narrow. To allow the permanent incisor to move into its proper location, the edge of the deciduous incisor lateral to the space is removed with a file or rasp until the space is wide enough to allow the permanent incisor to move rostrally.

Incisor reductions are performed with Dremel-type grinding instruments using carbide burrs, grit drum burrs, and diamond cut-off wheels Figs 13.28 and 13.29. Small reductions can be done with instruments such as a simple hoof rasp or ordinary file. Incisors cannot be safely cut with molar cutters or nippers unless deeply scored by using a cut-off wheel, hacksaw blade, file or similar instrument. Most incisor reductions are done with some type of power instrument, but can also be done manually. Diamond cut-off wheels are very effective when a large amount of incisors must be removed and when it is easy to determine how much incisor is to be removed. They can be very dangerous to the horse and operator if not used in a careful, safe manner. The operator needs to have the fingers of the hand which is not holding the handpiece braced against some part of the horse's mouth. Then the thumb or some part of this hand is braced against the handpiece to steady it and help prevent cutting the horse or operator's hand if the horse moves during the procedure. This principle of having the free hand act as a brace between the horse's mouth and handpiece applies to all Dremel-type instrument procedures whether using a diamond cut-off wheel or various burrs.

The author prefers carbide burrs for small reductions, for smoothing and finishing procedures, and when it is difficult to determine how much incisor needs to be removed. Others prefer the fine grit burrs (Greene SK – Personal Communication, 1996). Thermal injury to the incisors is a concern.[4] Burrs and diamond cut-

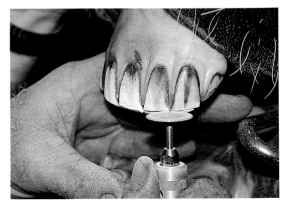

**Figure 13.28.** Diamond cut-off wheels are very effective in reducing incisors. Care must be taken in their use as they can injure the patient and operator.

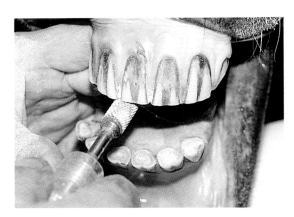

**Figure 13.29.** Various types of burrs are used in reducing incisors.

off wheels should be sharp and kept free of built-up tooth material to reduce the amount of heat created. It has been suggested that running diamond cut-off wheels at speeds of 2000 to 5000 rpm will result in minimal heat produced (Greene SK – Personal Communication, 1996). The author does not know of any incisors or cheek teeth injured by heat build-up, but the precautions of using sharp burrs and diamond cut-off wheels, keeping them clean, using low speeds and continuous movement should be followed, as is the use of systems to irrigate the tooth's surface while using Dremel-type instruments for tooth reduction. These measures are all aimed at reducing thermal damage (Fig. 13.30).

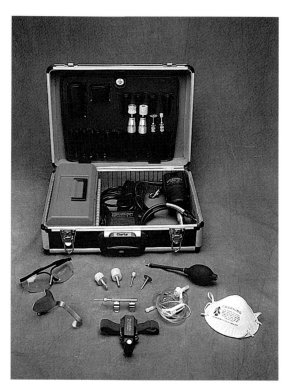

**Figure 13.30.** A commercially available dental kit that includes a system that allows irrigation during corrective procedures (Equi-Dent Technologies Inc., PO Box 5877, Sparks, NV 88432–5877).

The most common cause of an incisor becoming tall or long is that the opposing incisor is missing. These tall or long incisors should be reduced by rasping, burring with a cylindrical burr or cutting with a diamond cut-off wheel to level the incisor arcades. Reducing the tall incisor will help keep the cheek teeth from being forced out of occlusion during the grinding phase of mastication. Reducing tall incisors may also enhance performance by 'unlocking' the incisors allowing unrestricted lateral movement of the mandibles.

Incisor abnormalities have been separated into four classes, these are grinning, tilted, stepped or irregular and frowning (Fig. 13.31).[4] Grinning incisors probably develop when the upper central incisors (101 and 201) erupt before the lower central incisors (301 and 401) and become long, extending below the occlusal surfaces of the lower left and right intermediate

and corner incisors (302, 303 and 402, 403). The normal lateral movements of the mandible during eating wears the incisors into a 'grin'. Grinning incisors are fairly common. Frowning incisors develop when the lower central incisors (301 and 401) erupt first and become tall. Frowning incisors are rare.

Tilted (diagonal or slanted) incisors may develop when some cheek tooth abnormality is present preventing bilaterally symmetrical excursion and mastication. The mandibles may be offset to the side with the tallest incisors (Fig. 13.32). Tilted incisors are fairly common and may develop with no discernible cheek teeth abnormalities. Trauma has been suggested to be the cause of stepped, missing or misshapened teeth.[4]

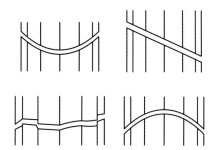

**Figure 13.31.** Four different incisor abnormalities are shown – grinning, tilted or diagonal, stepped or irregular and frowning.

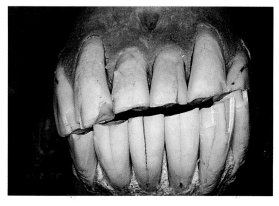

**Figure 13.32.** This is a tilted or diagonal incisor abnormality.

It may be impossible to correct these types of abnormalities in one session. If the amount of incisor reduction required to level the incisor occlusive surfaces from side to side would leave a gap between the upper and lower incisors, then the correction should be done in multiple sessions over time. It has also been suggested that no more than 6 mm of incisor reduction be done in one session to allow the soft tissue structures of the temporomandibular joint to adjust to the change in the length of the incisors (Greene SK – Personal Communication, 1996). Other practitioners may remove up to 10 mm in one session (Rucker BA – Personal Communication, 1996).

The author starts correction of grinning incisors by leveling the lower incisors. Leveling of the upper incisors is only done if it is determined that reducing them will not create a gap between the upper central (101 and 201) and lower central incisors (301 and 401) in the central or neutral position. Frowning incisors are treated in the opposite manner to grinning incisors. Stepped incisors may be 'locked' with the horse unable to move the mandibles laterally without opening the mouth, and this reduces cheek teeth occlusion. The incisors are leveled from side to side by reducing tall/long areas as much as possible without creating a gap between the upper central (101 and 201) and lower central (301 and 401) incisors.

Slightly tilted incisors can be corrected by shortening the upper and lower long or tall incisors. It may be impossible to completely level the more severely tilted incisors without creating a gap between the upper central incisors (101 and 201) and the lower central incisors (301 and 401). Continue the corrective shortening of the tall incisors every 4 to 6 months until the incisor occlusal surfaces are level from side to side.

There are instances where the incisors have become excessively long resulting in malocclusion of the cheek teeth. There is normally no premolar or molar contact (upper and lower cheek teeth not in contact) when the teeth are in centric occlusion, that is the upper central incisors (101 and 201) are directly above the lower central incisors (301 and 401). If the horse has normal cheek teeth occlusive angles of 10–15° (from side to side) and good cheek occlusion, the upper and lower incisors will separate as the mandible is moved laterally. It has been shown that there is a range of normal mandibular excursion to molar contact from 2 to 20 mm.[4] Since it usually takes years for lack of incisor wear to result in them becoming long enough to interfere with molar occlusion, incisor reduction for excessive length is seldom indicated in horses less than 9 to 10 years of age (Rucker BA – Personal Communication, 1996).

There are several methods of estimating the length that the incisors should be shortened. Rucker suggested determining the lateral excursion to molar contact (move the mandible laterally and see when the upper and lower incisors start to separate) and then remove half of this length.[4]

Another method of determining the amount of incisor length to be removed has been described by Greene (Greene SK – Personal Communication, 1996). The interocclusal space (defined as the distance between the occlusal surfaces of the upper and lower arcades) is estimated by elevating the sedated patient's head, retracting the cheek and using a pen light or transillumination to visualize the distance between the cheek teeth occlusal surfaces. The central incisors (01s) should be in contact and in complete occlusion. This estimation is performed after all cheek teeth corrective procedures are completed. If hooks or ramps on the second premolars (06s) have been corrected then the interocclusal space between the third premolars (07s) and fourth premolars (08s) will be used as a guide to the length of incisors to remove. If no more incisor is removed than visualized interocclusal space, no gap will be created between the upper and lower incisors. Once the amount of incisor to be removed has been determined, a line is drawn on the incisors with a permanent marker as a guide.

The author usually uses both of these methods to estimate the amount to shorten the incisors as well as clinical judgment involving the animal's condition in relation to its nutritional state and the work it performs. It has been shown that there is a wide range of normal cheek teeth occlusion. More incisor reduction is done in the horse which is not maintaining its body condition in relation to its daily food ration and the work it performs compared to the horse which is maintaining its weight. Usually the author shortens the incisors to where the lateral excursion to molar contact (the distance the mandible is moved laterally before the upper and lower incisors start to separate) is between 5 and 10 mm but never removes more than 6 to 10 mm at one time.

When the author first described bite rehabilitation procedures in 1991 it was believed that a gap should be created between the upper and lower incisors to ensure that the cheek teeth were brought into maximum occlusion.[6] In 1995 it was reported that creating a gap between the upper and lower incisors produced difficult or painful chewing for 2 to 12 months.[5] Possible reasons for the complications included (a) severe changes in tension on the temporo-mandibular joint capsule, (b) alteration of chewing pattern and therefore muscle usage and (c) lack of normal rostral or caudal motion of the mandible as the horse lowers and raises the head.[5]

In the author's experience the creation of a slight gap between the upper and lower incisors seldom causes any problems. If a horse does have difficulty eating after a gap has been created there have usually been inadequate corrective procedures performed on the cheek teeth. When problems of the cheek teeth have been corrected, the horses have returned to eating normally. However, because of the concerns expressed in the report it is best to stop the shortening of incisors before the gap is created.[5]

The incisors can develop a variety of abnormal conditions that interfere with eating and performance. The incisors can be examined fairly easily since they are at the front of the mouth. Common sense should be used in correcting the abnormalities detected (Fig. 13.33).

## SAFETY

For the most part dental prophylaxis in the horse is carried out in the standing, sedated animal. At all times the practitioner must be

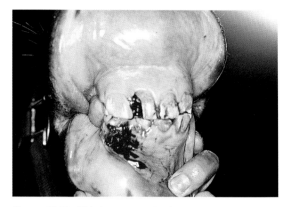

**Figure 13.33.** This is an example of how incisors may be damaged if corrective procedures are not performed correctly. This incisor fractured while being nipped without proper scoring first.

cognitive of signs of fright pain and discomfort that may result in a flight reaction from the patient bringing risks of injury to itself, assistants and the veterinarian. In some cases general anesthesia may be required.

Working with dental floats, including power equipment, requires some strength, dexterity and mastery of technique. Do not hesitate to rest to relieve strain on the horse and yourself. Try whenever possible to avoid working with your elbows above the line of your shoulders, keep your elbows down and in (working on sedated horses with a 'head drop' helps this). Minimize gripping with the elbows and wrists extended and select float handles that suit your conformation. These simple tips will reduce the risk of repetitive stress injuries, for example carpal tunnel, tennis or tooth floaters elbow and rotator cuff impingement.

## A TIMETABLE FOR ROUTINE DENTAL EXAMINATION

The following timetable was prepared by Easley (1996).[7]

  1  Birth
     Examine for (a) congential defects of the lips or palate, (b) tongue motion and strength, (c) dental malocclusions and (d) evaluate all body systems. Recommended

procedures are to provide genetic and orthodontic consultation and perform corrective surgery if necessary. Look for other problem signs such as underdeveloped carpal or tarsal bones, ruptured extensor tendons and hernias.

2  6–8 months
Examine for (a) incisor and premolar occlusion all incisors should be erupted, (b) missing teeth, (c) sharp enamel points or hooks and (d) examine the tongue and buccal mucosa for ulcers. Recommended procedures are to provide orthodontic consultation and float teeth if necessary.

3  16–24 months
Check for (a) upper and lower wolf teeth eruption, (b) points and hooks on premolars and (c) bit lesions. Recommended procedures are to float teeth and round off the rostral corner of the second premolar. Extract wolf teeth.

4  2–3 years
Check for (a) upper and lower wolf teeth or blind wolf teeth, (b) deciduous tooth eruption – central incisors and premolars, (c) corners of the mouth and interdental space for bit injuries and (d) evaluate molars and premolars for points or hooks. Recommended procedures are to float outside of upper and inside of lower cheek teeth, remove caps if present and ready for removal, and extract wolf teeth. Also round off rostral corners of upper and lower second premolars upper (106–206), lower (306–406).

5  3–4 years
Evaluate (a) corners of the mouth and interdental space for bit injuries, (b) incisors for retained deciduous teeth or supernumerary teeth, (c) molars and premolars for points and retained third premolars (second cheek teeth) upper (107–207), lower (307–407), (d) size and shape of the lower jaw (e) check for blind wolf teeth and (f) percuss sinuses. Recommended procedures are to remove caps if present, float teeth and remove wolf teeth.

6  4–5 years
Check (a) all incisors for eruption, (b) canine teeth for sharp edges or eruption delays, (c) entire molar arcade for proper eruption and alignment fourth premolars (third cheek tooth) upper (108–208), lower (308–408), (d) visually the upper rostral and lower caudal cheek teeth for hooks from malocclusion, (e) digitally for points on sharp edges of cheek teeth and (f) percuss sinuses. Recommended procedures are as to remove deciduous teeth if ready, grind or rasp hooks if present, float teeth and remove mucosa over canines if gingival eruption cysts are present.

7  5 years and older
Perform the following: (a) examine mouth visually and digitally, especially noting hooks and uneven wear, (b) evaluate canines for sharp edges and tartar, (c) percuss sinuses (d) use olfactory senses to detect evidence of oral decay or gingivitis, (e) observe incisors for even wear and (f) evaluate lateral jaw excursion. Recommended procedures are to float teeth, remove hooks using a chisel or rasp and level or shorten the incisors if indicated.

The author would suggest that we educate our owners and trainers to have dental examinations and indicated corrective procedures performed before starting any horse in training.

## SUMMARY

A thorough visual and manual examination of the patient must be performed to identify any abnormalities. Sedating the patient and the use of a full mouth speculum facilitates both the examination and corrective procedures. The use of proper dental instruments makes it much easier for both the patient and veterinarian. A dental form can be used to maintain a record of what procedures were done, what will have to be done in the future and to itemize the charges.

## REFERENCES

1. Fischer D and Easley J (1994) Floating: Making equine dentistry a practice profit center. *Large Animal Veterinarian*, Nov–Dec, 16–22.
2. Scrutchfield WL (1996) Correction of abnormalities of the cheek teeth, in *Proceedings of American Association of Equine Practitioners*, 42, 11–21.
3. Shideler RK (1983) Dentistry for the snaffle-bit horse in Proceedings. *American Association of Equine Practitioners*, 301–312.
4. Rucker BA (1996) Incisor procedures for field use in Proceedings. *American Association of Equine Practitioners*, 42, 22–25.
5. Rucker BA (1995) Modified procedure for incisor reduction in Proceedings. *American Association of Equine Practitioners*, 41, 42–44.
6. Scrutchfield WL (1991) Incisors and canines in Proceedings. *American Association of Equine Practitioners*, 117–121.
7. Easley KJ (1996) Equine dental development and anatomy in Proceedings. *American Association of Equine Practitioners*, 42, 1–10.

TREATMENT OF DENTAL DISORDERS

# BASIC EQUINE ORTHODONTICS

Jack Easley, DVM, MS Equine Veterinary Practice PO Box 1075 Shelbyville, KY 40066

## INTRODUCTION

The prevention and treatment of dental malocclusions is the field of dentistry known as orthodontics. Orthodontics in its most basic form is the controlled movement of teeth through the alveolar bone. The purpose of equine orthodontics is to preserve oral function and periodontal health of the horse. This broad topic cannot be covered in detail in this text. However, this chapter is an attempt to outline some basic orthodontic principles and give examples of how they might be applied to equine dental practice.

## ORTHODONTIC PRINCIPLES

The broad category of orthodontics generally deals with tooth movement in mature animals. Interceptive orthodontic treatment encompasses procedures used in the adolescent horse with mixed dentition. Functional orthodontics is the area of dentistry that deals with tooth and jaw movement in the young, rapidly growing horse. Orthognathic surgery is the field of surgery that combines orthodontics with maxillofacial surgery to correct craniofacial deformities.

The general laws of biomechanics apply to all types of tooth movement. The alveolar bone is reabsorbed whenever the root, for a certain period of time, causes compression of the periodontal ligaments. New alveolar bone is deposited whenever there are stretching forces acting on the bone. However, these laws are subject to numerous variations and exceptions when factors such as magnitude, direction and duration of force are introduced.[1] The orthodontic principles of tooth movement are at work on adult horses that develop abnormal wear patterns on exposed dental crowns. These abnormal wear patterns place stresses on teeth resulting in movement of the teeth. Such movement affects mastication and oral health. The application of orthodontic wire, springs, coils, arch bars, bands, brackets and elastics have limited application in correction of common equine malocclusion problems. Dental floating and crown occlusal correction are forms of orthodontic correction used or applied to reduce abnormal forces placed on teeth and thus improve occlusion.

The extraction of deciduous teeth in an effort to guide the eruption of the permanent teeth into a favorable occlusion has been referred to as interceptive orthodontics.[2] It is necessary to have a thorough understanding of the growth and development of the dental and osseous structures to time deciduous tooth removal and avoid complications in attempting to guide teeth into proper occlusion. A lack of understanding and knowledge can create disastrous results including deterioration of dentition and facial balance. Interceptive orthodontics, when wisely and judiciously applied to well-selected cases, can enhance dental occlusion as well as prevent dental malocclusions that will cause functional problems with mastication and dental wear throughout the horse's life (Fig. 14.1) (see Chapters 13 and 15).

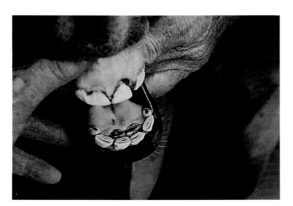

**Figure 14.1.** Crowded lower incisor arch with retained deciduous 701, 801 causing displacement (labiocclusion) of permanent 301, 401. Following the principles of interceptive orthodontics, the deciduous teeth were removed and the exposed mesial crown portion of 702 and 802 were filed widening the space for 301 and 401 to migrate forward.

Many dental malocclusions involve an abnormal skeletal relationship of the upper and lower jaws. General form and capacity for growth of bone are inherited characteristics. A basic understanding of the growth of the upper and lower portions of the head is important in diagnosis and treatment of many types of malocclusions. The mandible can be divided into a number of anatomical elements: a basic element, two subsidiary elements for the attachment of muscles, and an alveolar process or tooth bearing element.[3] Growth of the mandible occurs in two ways. There is appositional growth from endochondral ossification which occurs in all borders of the mandible, except the cranial border of the ramus, and there is epiphyseal-like growth of the condyles. The upper jaw is an integral part of the cranium in contact with other bones of the skull and its growth depends mainly on endochondral growth.

Bone is plastic and its external form and capacity for growth are affected and modified by environmental forces and factors.[4] A branch of orthodontic treatment first referred to as biomedical orthodontics has developed over the past century. Using the theories of bone plasticity traced back to Fouz and Wolff, several techniques have been employed to correct dentofacial deformities and malocclusions in the horse utilizing the principles of functional

orthodontics. A more descriptive term, functional jaw orthopedics, was popularized by Karl Haupl who refined the concepts and techniques used in this branch of human dentistry today.[5] Pressure, whether functional or artificially created, affects bone growth. Bone-cell growth is constantly taking place from an increase in size and change in form in the young horse to the replacement of dead cells in the adult. Bone metabolism remains constant whether forces acting on the bone are normal or abnormal in direction or amount, but bone grows in the direction of least resistance. Therefore, forces of occlusion, when acting incorrectly, become factors of malocclusion.

The concept of functional orthodontics is to use whatever appliance, device or technique possible to modify the forces placed on the jaws of young, growing animals. Such modification in youth encourages growth in a way that corrects, or at least limits the extent of, malocclusion in adulthood. Dental filing to reduce hooks and elongated teeth that interfere with normal jaw growth would be the simplest application. Fixed as well as removable appliances have been utilized with mixed results in an attempt to modify jaw growth and dental arch relationships (Figs 14.2 and 14.3).

Surgical correction of dental malocclusion and dentofacial deformities in the horse have seen limited application. The most severe types of deformities such as wry nose have been corrected successfully in a limited number of cases by following the principles of orthognathic surgery (Figs 14.4a, b and c. Fig. 4.11).[6–8]

Ideal occlusion rarely exists in nature and because of the wide range of variation between individuals we must base our diagnosis of abnormal occlusion, or malocclusion, on a highly arbitrary concept of the imaginary ideal. Malocclusion can be categorized in three etiological types: (a) congenital or genetic malocclusion, (b) eruptive malocclusion and (c) traumatic malocclusion. Fundamental to orthodontic diagnosis is understanding the concepts of normal occlusion.

The incisor table surface is in ideal occlusal contact when the horse's head is in the grazing position. The six upper and six lower incisor

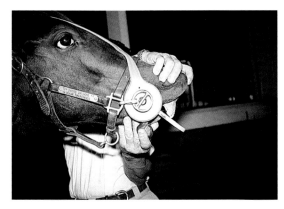

**Figure 14.2.** Removable functional orthodontic device in the mouth of a 5-month-old foal with a parrot mouth deformity. This device is used to improve the dental alignment and encourage jaw growth.

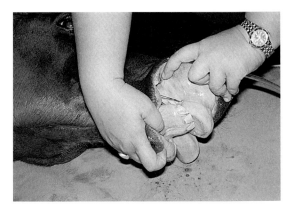

**Figure 14.3.** An attached functional orthodontic device applied to a 4-month-old parrot mouth foal. This appliance is formed from acrylic and placed in the roof of the mouth. The device incorporates a metal incline plane to encourage rostral movement of the mandible and prevent downward drift of the incisive bone and upper incisor teeth. Retention wires are placed behind 507 and 607 and brought forward around the upper incisor arcade to discourage rostral growth of the upper jaw.

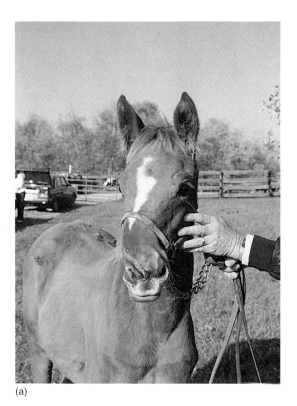

(a)

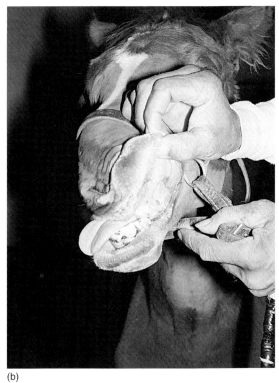

(b)

**Figures 14.4a–c.** Wry nose foal with the premaxilla deviated at a 60 degree angle to the maxillae. The nasal passage on the convex side was occluded due to deviation of the nasal septum. This foal was surgically corrected in a two stage procedure. The first surgery required moving the premaxilla allowing the upper incisor arch to come into normal contact with the lower. The second surgery to remove the nasal septum was performed 30 days after the first.

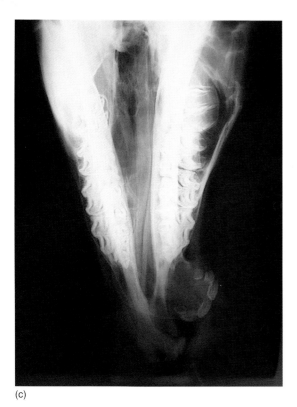

(c)

**Figures 14.4.** *continued.*

teeth are in mesiodistal contact at the occlusal surface with the teeth forming an arch at the front of the mouth. The eruption pattern of deciduous incisors is consistent with a full set of six deciduous incisor teeth coming into occlusion at 6 to 9 months of age when the jaw is wide enough to accommodate these teeth. The shedding of deciduous and the eruption of permanent incisors follows a standard sequence and pattern. Continuous crown attrition and tooth eruption maintains a continually functional exposed crown. The exposed crown length and angle of inclination increases slightly with age, but occlusal contact between the upper and lower arcades should remain consistent. The canine teeth erupt in most male horses between 4.5 and 6 years of age. The root of the upper canine should be positioned in the suture between the maxilla and premaxilla. The lower canine erupts further forward making for a longer lower diastema or interdental space. The upper first premolar teeth (wolf teeth) normally erupt just rostral to the second premolar teeth. The first premolars are rarely present in the lower jaw.

The horse is anisognathic with the lower jaw and molar arcade being narrower than the upper. The hypsodont molarized cheek teeth in each arcade are in mesiodistal contact at the occlusal surface, so that each arcade appears as one large tooth. The attrition or abrasion of the upper and lower molar arcades is dependent on full rostral caudal occlusal contact of the arcades during normal mastication. The 10 to 15 degree angle of inclination of the molar tables is the result of attrition resulting in more wear of the palatal aspect of the upper and buccal aspect of the lower arcades. The angle of the root and reserve crowns allow the exposed crown to maintain good occlusal contact throughout the life of the horse. This has been referred to as mesial drift. During function, teeth move individually in their sockets under the heavy stresses associated with mastication. Where adjacent teeth are in contact and constantly erupting and as the crowns are being worn, mesial drift causes shortening of the dental arcade.[9] The length and angle of the dental arches varies between breeds and head types. The general shape of the equine skull, its length, height and contours are determined by and allow for the shape of the eyes, upper respiratory system and teeth. The shape of the head varies among breeds but should be in proportion with the body. In 1905, JW Axe proposed a general rule of proportions for head and body size[10] basing his work on measurements by French hippotomists of the nineteenth century in which the head was used as the basis of proportion for all other body parts. More recent work by Willoughby (1975) has shown that there are breed differences in the proportion of head to body size.[11]

The thoroughbred head usually has a straight line from the ears to the muzzle. and is the shortest of all breeds measured when taking the length of the head as a percentage of the withers' height. The Arabian head has an undulating profile with a bulging forehead and a dish below the eyes. Arabians and quarterhorses have shorter heads with the quarterhorse having less of a dish in its face and larger jowls than the Arabians. The Standardbred typically has a larger head with a slightly arched face or 'Roman nose'. The Draft breeds and Shetland ponies (cold blooded breeds) have heads that are disproportionally large compared to the light horse breeds. Cheek teeth of Arabian horses are said to be only two thirds as long and broad as those of cold blooded horses.[12] It would stand to reason that the more massive the teeth, the more powerful, coarse and common looking the head must be. As we breed horses to 'refine' the head we reduce the space to accommodate teeth. The relationship of the upper and lower jaws and the dental occlusal paths have a dramatic effect on masticatory function. In the horse with hypsodont dentition, continuous crown abrasion and attrition makes dental occlusion have a dramatic affect on dental crown wear. Abnormal dental wear patterns are a major contributing factor to dental disease.

Malocclusion in the horse can involve single teeth in an arcade or involve the entire dental arch relationship (Figs 14.5a and b). Severe malocclusion is often accompanied by disproportion of the face and jaws. These problems are referred to as dentofacial deformities.[7] Many types of malocclusion are not pathologic but simply equine morphologic variation. Most horses with reasonable dentofacial alignment

and occlusion with normal jaw function should be considered to have normal occlusion. While very small abnormalities in occlusal contact can affect dental wear, the impact on function cannot be predicted in all cases from morphology. Equine veterinary literature has given limited space to any type of dental malocclusions with the simple exception of parrot mouth. This condition has been inaccurately stated as the most common malocclusion encountered in equine practice.[13] If the oral examination is limited to the incisor arcades this would appear to be so. However, the fact is, many types of malocclusion occur in the equine species.[14] Colyer (1935) and Joest (1970) described many variations seen in equine teeth that lead to various types of dental malocclusion.[15,16] Hypsodont teeth that are not properly aligned in the dental arcade suffer from severe abnormalities of wear. Abnormal tooth wear has been shown to be the leading cause of dental disease and to adversely affect proper mastication.

To date no research has been done in the equine species to determine what normal craniofacial development and growth entails. Cephalometric studies need to be undertaken to determine normal head and jaw relationships. This chapter intends to present the types of malocclusions seen in clinical practice. Correlations as to the cause, and treatment options available

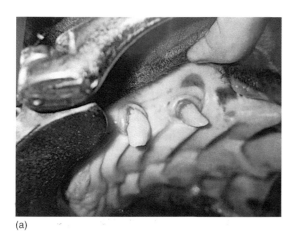

(a)

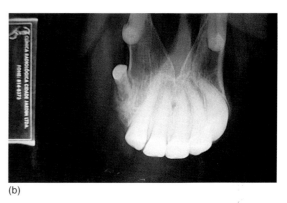

(b)

**Figures 14.5a–b.** Two caniniform teeth in the maxillary interdental space. A radiograph shows bilateral canine teeth in the normal position. The tooth in the diastema, while having the crown and root shape of a canine tooth, appears to be a displaced corner incisor tooth (from C Omura, with permission).

are based on information extrapolated from studies carried out in other animal species including humans. It is hoped that the information presented here will stimulate interest at the academic research level to provide further information and better tools in order to progress in breeding horses with good dental occlusion, also to provide better management of those animals unfortunate enough to be born with or develop various types of dental malocclusions.

Surveys on equine dental patients have shown a high percentage of horses with significant dental malocclusions.[14,17] Many of these cases were severe enough to cause clinical problems and a certain per cent were classified as a handicapping unsoundness.[14] Historically, treatment has been aimed at correcting dental overgrowth by shortening long incisor teeth and correcting cheek teeth hooks.[18] More recently, orthodontic techniques have been introduced to equine practitioners to correct some of the more severe problems.[19,20] Poor understanding of biomechanical principles of orthodontics has led to poor clinical results and even severe complications. Dentofacial deformities involve both the dental complex and the facial skeleton. Hopefully, the future will yield a better understanding of the use of combined maxillofacial surgical and orthodontic procedures to correct malocclusions and facial abnormalities.

## FACTORS AFFECTING HEAD SHAPE AND DENTAL CONFORMATION

It is widely acknowledged that most malocclusions have a genetic component.[21–23] It is difficult, if not impossible, to quantify how much of a problem is caused by genetics and how much is due to prenatal and postnatal environmental factors. Due to the polygenetic inheritance of craniofacial and dental characteristics, it is extremely difficult at present to identify the cause of most genetic malocclusions. Human studies have concluded that the heritability of skeletal characteristics is high, but that of dental characteristics is low.[24] Studies have shown that cross-breeding dogs of different skull shapes (dolichocephalic, mesocephalic and brachycephalic) reproduces most of the craniofacial

and dental malocclusions seen in clinical practice. Tooth malposition without jaw malocclusion has not been documented in these studies.[25] Independence of genetic control of the size of the teeth from both maxilla and mandible was demonstrated. Jaw length and shape, and tooth bud position appear to be under genetic control. Tooth form (whether shaped like incisor, canine, premolar or molar) was found to be the most stable characteristic of the canine skull. It has been shown that upper and lower jaw conformation and tooth position are independently determined of each other.[25–27]

The genetic nature of some jaw defects seen in horses and cattle has been associated with generalized diarthrodial joint abnormalities (Figs 14.6a and b).[28–32] Incisor occlusion in various breeds of cattle has been studied and it has been concluded that incisor relationship is heritable but the mode of inheritance could not be established.[33] Work by Wiener and Gardner concluded that a longer suckling period customary in dairy calf management may reduce the incidence of incisor overjet.[33] Meyer and Böker observed overjet in thirty-one calves at birth, found that the anomaly disappeared by months of age.[34] Observations in different breeds of sheep have shown that certain skull shapes predispose to certain types of malocclusions. Ovine breeding experiments have alluded to a genetic propensity to malocclusion, but there is some possibility that these conditions can be produced by non-genetic causes such as maternal malnutrition and aging.[35] Goats belonging to the Nubian breeds have strongly convex facial profiles and are predisposed to incisor underjet.[36] The same predisposition has been observed in equine breeds with a dished face.

All domestic horses are of mixed wild origin with widely varying head sizes and types. The size of the teeth and the type and size of the jaw are the legacy of different ancestral types.[12] The genetic determination of the length of upper and lower jaws as well as tooth size are located in three different chromosome sectors (alleles) each of which may be inherited independently of one another.

The genetic and functional environment work closely in the resulting growth.[37,38] The

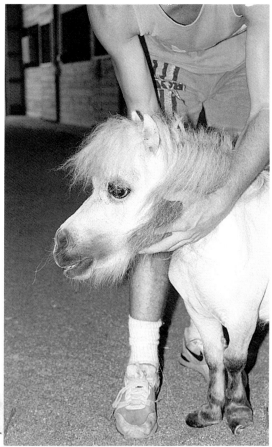

(a)

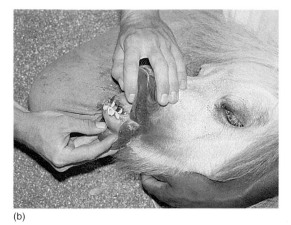

(b)

**Figures 14.6a and b.** Achondroplasia is a heritable condition in which there is defective development and growth of primordial cartilage. The ancestry of the miniature horse incorporated achondroplastic dwarf mutants into the breed. The genetics are usually partially expressed and only rarely will the head and limb defects as expressed in this case be seen.

intrauterine environment has a known effect on facial growth and development. Intrauterine molding, when pressure during intrauterine growth distorts the developing face, has been documented in humans and may be the cause of some facial and skeletal limb deformities seen in foals.[39] Postnatal environmental factors include all non-genetic influences brought to bear on the developing individual. These include the environmental effects of muscle function and neuromuscular adaptation.[40,41] In the growing horse, forces placed on the teeth and jaws from abnormal wear patterns on the exposed dental crowns are another factor to consider.

The scientific basis of environmental causes of malocclusion rests primarily in experimental findings with animals.[38] Under certain experimental conditions growth can be modified quite extensively and, in certain circumstances, growth can be stimulated or stunted. The duration rather than the magnitude of soft tissue pressure has a greater effect on growth. Environmental factors that are recognized as leading to dentofacial abnormalities include: (a) habits of long duration such as sucking, (b) the influence of posture of the head, mandible, tongue and lip (posture determines the resting soft tissue pressures), (c) the influence of tooth eruption and crown wear, and (d) trauma (osseous, soft tissue, articular or dental). The current theory for determining craniofacial bone growth states that growth of the face occurs as a response to functional needs and is mediated by the soft tissue in which the jaw is embedded.[42] The soft tissues grow and both the bone and cartilage follow this growth. Function plays an important role in normal jaw growth and is closely related to inherited growth patterns. Jaw growth perturbation be induced by trauma to the soft tissues. sed lip pressure results in increased cranio dis-proportion. In response to the disturb of optimal occlusal relationships, growth of the jaw can be modified to a new functional environment. In humans, it is known that in order to modify inherited jaw growth, the functional disturbance must be of sufficient magnitude and duration (more than 6 hours per day for thumb sucking in children).[5]

In horses that develop abnormal crown wear patterns on their teeth, functional orthodontics can correct the problems allowing the horses to realize more fully their genetic potential. Epidemiological studies are needed in order to establish breed or family predisposition to malocclusion. The system presently being used in human and small animal dentistry for classification of malocclusion is not well adapted to use in the horse.[2,43,44] A well-designed classification system and use of this system by a broad base of well-informed observers is necessary to draw meaningful conclusions. Cephalometric studies as well as studies of jaw interrelation during craniofacial growth in the horse are needed.

## SEQUELAE TO MALOCCLUSION

Horses have hypsodont erupting and wearing teeth and malocclusion leads to abnormal wear patterns. Mechanical forces placed on abnormally wearing teeth can lead to tooth movement in the alveolus. This movement can be tipping, rotating or shifting depending upon the angle of force. Most malocclusions cause teeth to wear in such a fashion as to apply abnormal forces on the teeth and jaws that exacerbate the malocclusion. These abnormally worn teeth alter the masticatory pattern in some animals. They can also lead to secondary abnormalities of wear such as altered angle of the molar tables and limited wear of the buccal edges of the upper and lingual edges of the lower arcades. The most severe form of this type of altered wear pattern is referred to as shear mouth. Shear mouth is a condition whe... one or both molar arcades wear at a...... ...mely steep angle resulting in lim... ...ovement.

## EXAMPLES OF ALTERED WEAR CAUSING A SHIFT IN TOOTH MOVEMENT

Rostral or caudal hook formation can place forces on the tooth crown with the protuberance forcing it away from the arcade. This will lead to periodontal pockets with feed material becoming packed between the teeth. Periodontal

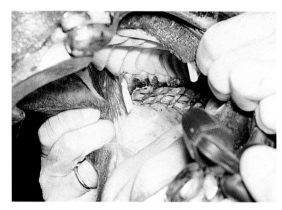

**Figure 14.7.** Prominent hooks on 106 and 206 due to malocclusion of the upper and lower dental arcades. The rostral pressure placed on this tooth has moved it forward causing a space or diastema between 106 and 107. This condition can lead to severe periodontal disease and eventual tooth loss.

disease which is left uncontrolled will eventually lead to abscess formation, loosening of the tooth in the alveolus and eventually its expulsion (Fig. 14.7).

Long enamel points or ridges form in the arcade between teeth in the opposing arcade due to malalignment of the upper and lower jaws. These long ridges of enamel act as a wedge between the teeth in the opposite arcade. The enamel wedge forces the teeth apart creating a periodontal pocket into which food will become packed.

Misplaced teeth lead to abnormal crown wear on the occlusal portion forcing the crown out of alignment with the remaining arcade. The unopposed portion of the crown becomes protuberant and develops an excessive crown angle (Figs 14.8a and b). Mechanical forces placed on the protuberant crown force the tooth further out of alignment and can cause a tipping or increased malalignment of the crown. This leads to periodontal packing of feed around the displaced crown. The tooth in the opposing arcade will not wear normally and may become protuberant or develop excessive enamel points or ridges that mirror the defect in that arcade.

A missing or displaced tooth in one dental arcade will lead to abnormal wear of the opposing teeth. The opposite teeth then become protuberant. The mesial and distal teeth in the same

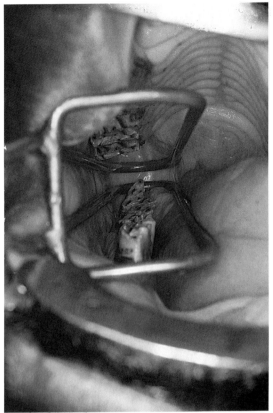

(a)

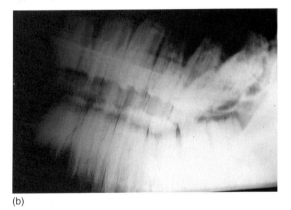

(b)

arcade tend to drift into the space that is unoccupied. This drifting can open spaces between successive teeth in the same dental arch leading to periodontal pockets forming between teeth and inspiring sequential drifting. This is not a consistent feature and at times the entire dental arch will move together and close the gap. This closure shortens the dental arch and predisposes dentition to abnormal wear patterns (hooks) on the ends of the opposite arcade.

Rostral and caudal hook formation can also apply mechanical forces on the jaw that affect the mechanics of growth, mastication, deciduous tooth shedding, head carriage and temporomandibular joint function. As the protuberant crown becomes more prominent at the end of the dental arcade, it can limit rostrocaudal jaw motion and place mechanical forces on the jaws. In the young, growing foal with a premolar malalignment that predisposes to hook formation, the protuberant tooth crown works mechanically to alter jaw forces and restricts the growth of the shorter jaw. In the young horse with mixed dentition, mechanical forces placed on the jaws and teeth from hooks inhibit growth of the shorter jaw and compress the deciduous tooth crowns thus limiting the space for shedding deciduous teeth (Fig. 14.9). This condition also predisposes erupting permanent teeth to impaction. In the adult horse, hook formation

**Figures 14.8a–b.** A 4-year-old Appaloosa mare presented for weight loss and quidding hay. Lingual inclination or mesioversion of the lower second molars 310 and 410. These teeth are crowded because 311 and 411 have erupted in the curve of the mandible (Curvature of Spee) and are mesially inclined. This has also led to an impaction of the upper 111 and 211. The problem resolved over a 2 year period with frequent crown reductions on lower teeth 10 and 11, keeping them out of occlusion with the uppers. By removing the abnormal masticatory forces from these teeth crowns they drift into normal functional occlusion.

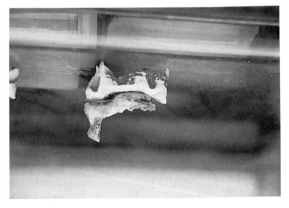

**Figure 14.9.** Deciduous premolar 606 and 706 caps removed from a 3-year-old Quarterhorse with a swelling on the mandible just below 707. The distal pressure placed on the crown of 706 by the rostral hook on 606 caudal causing crowding and impaction of 707.

can lead to several pathological processes depending upon the size, shape and position of the hook and the performance demands placed on the horse which affect the mouth.

When a horse's head moves up and down, the jaw position changes slightly. When the head is elevated the lower jaw retracts caudally in relation to the upper jaw. This can be demonstrated by elevating the head high in the air and noticing the occlusion of the incisor teeth. The cheek tooth arcades also shift with head position. Some speculate this as being the reason for a higher incidence of rostral 06 hooks on horses that eat hay from a rack or net elevated on the stall wall as opposed to the horses that eat hay or grass in the normal position off the ground.

With flexion of the neck, a horse lowers its head and the lower jaw tends to move forward in relation to the upper jaw. This becomes important when dealing with horses that are asked to perform with the neck bent in collection. Such incidences would occur in dressage horses, gaited horses or harness horses worked in an overcheck with their neck forced into flexion. Rostral upper or caudal lower hooks inhibit the forward motion of the lower jaw with the mouth closed. We see horses that tend to open their mouths when collected. Trainers use various nosebands to force the mouth closed thus preventing relief from the forces placed on the jaws and limiting the amount of flexion the horse can exhibit. Secondary problems such as soreness in the temporomandibular area or in muscles of the neck or back are associated with this problem.

## DOCUMENTATION OF MALOCCLUSION AND CRANIOFACIAL DEFORMITIES

The clinician should document the history and clinical findings of all cases that may require any type of orthodontic treatment. A complete history including the horse's pedigree and an occlusal examination of its parents is helpful in the genetic counseling of the client. Historical information will also allow the clinican to determine whether the condition was noticed at birth or soon after and if it is becoming progressively worse as the horse grows and develops. The

proposed use of the horse and breed information are necessary to ethically manage the cases where a hereditary component may be responsible for the deformity.

The clinical assessment should begin with a general physical examination of the patient and a complete, detailed oral examination. Photographs and skull measurements are useful in monitoring clinical progress. Radiographic evaluation of the skull allows for more complete assessment of the problem and is another source of permanent, measurable documentation for monitoring changes over time. Dental impressions and stone castings are helpful in the documentation of deformities as well as in treatment planning (Figs 14.10a and b). Stone castings can also be

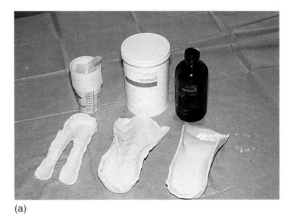

(a)

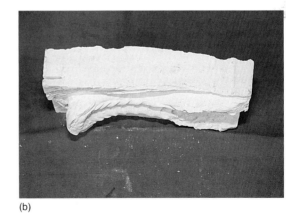

(b)

**Figures 14.10a–b.** Dental impressions can be taken and stone castings made of all or any portion of the dental arcade. Impression trays are custom made to fit the area of the horse's mouth. Stone castings are used to document abnormalities and monitor treatment progress.

used in the fabrication and fitting of removable or fixed appliances. Bite registrations using base plate wax allow for proper alignment of upper and lower stone models as well as for following treatment progress in the live animal.[2]

## PARROT MOUTH

This condition is seen in most animal species including humans. It is commonly thought of as an overjet of the incisor teeth. The syndrome in horses can involve the incisor portion of the arcade alone or occur in combination with varying degrees of malocclusion of the upper and lower cheek teeth arcades. The mismatch in arcade length can be either a brachygnathism of one jaw or a prognathism of another.[15] Breeding studies on cattle show the incidence of parrot mouth is 2 to 13 per cent in animals inspected for breeding soundness. This is in line with the incidence reported in several equine studies of 2 to 5 per cent.[14,17] The degree to which this condition is expressed at birth and the progression of the problem throughout growth and development of the horses needs to be worked out.

It is my impression that few foals are born with the full expression of parrot mouth. Mandibular brachygnathism has been reported with other congenital deformity syndromes involving the musculoskeletal system.[29] Without cephalometric norms, it is impossible to categorize these defects as either a short lower jaw or a long upper jaw. This condition is most often the result of the breeding of two animals with normal dental occlusion but extremely different head types. The classical thoroughbred cross would be the result of a stallion with a sprinter's build and short, wide head crossed with a lean built distance mare with a narrow, refined, long head.

The mixing of different head conformation types is seen to produce problems with malocclusions in other breeds. Dish-faced Arabians crossed with narrow, straight-faced American saddlebreds have produced foals with both overjet and undershot jaw conformation. The degree of malocclusion seems to depend upon many factors. Some horses are only affected in the cheek teeth area, others only in the incisor area

while some are affected in both. Biomechanically, the horse, having hypsodont teeth that depend on normal occlusal contact for wear, is more seriously affected at all stages in life than most other species.

The foal born with a slight incisor overjet will soon develop an overbite. As the upper incisors elongate, the palate and incisive bones are pulled downward by gravity. The lower incisors become trapped as they begin to contact the palate behind the uppers. This places caudal pressure on the mandible inhibiting growth and creating a cascade of events that worsen the deformity. As the lower jaw growth is stunted, the cheek teeth malocclusion worsens causing rostral hooks to form on the upper first cheek teeth 506 and 606. The unopposed incisor teeth continue to erupt but are not in wear and become elongated. These elongated incisors interfere with the normal masticatory cycle limiting free lateral motion of the cheek teeth. This can further lead to abnormal wear of the cheek teeth.

Foals with minor incisor overjet with no overbite or cheek tooth malocclusion have benefited from occlusal wiring of the upper teeth.[19,20] This technique is used to inhibit rostral growth of the upper jaw from the second cheek tooth forward while allowing the normal growth of the mandible to catch up. This wiring technique is biomechanically unsound for use in animals with incisor overbite or cheek teeth malocclusions.

More severe malocclusion problems have been improved or corrected by the use of functional orthodontic devices early in the horse's life while it is in the rapid stage of growth and development. Orthognathic surgery has been attempted in a few cases but with limited success.

When advising owners about how to manage horses with occlusal abnormalities, keep in mind that it is unclear how malocclusion is inherited. It is a complex conformational trait and the outcome of multiple genes (polygenetic). Each breeding animal has a different propensity to pass the deformity on to its offspring. It is always risky to breed from animals which have defects, or to breed from animals that have previously produced offspring with defects. The breeder's long-term goals and philosophy should dictate breeding decisions. What are the animal's good traits? How serious is the defect? Breeding from horses with any type of defect will probably increase the incidence of that defect and eventually lead to an intolerable level. An extreme approach would be to neuter animals with defects and remove their sires and dams from the breeding population. While this would prevent animals with a defect from passing it on, it would also prevent them from reproducing their good conformational, performance and behavioral traits. One good strategy would be to not remate two animals that have previously produced defective offspring. Another approach would be to remate these animals and only retain offspring in the breeding program that do not exhibit the defect. It is a good practice to mate animals with similar virtues and different faults.

Any orthodontic management of parrot mouth should follow four basic principles. (a) Prevent or reduce abnormal wear of the teeth, (b) prevent or correct downward gravitation drift of the incisive bone and upper incisor teeth, (c) inhibit rostral growth of the maxilla and premaxilla, (d) stimulate rostral growth of the mandible.

The most important management tool in the correction of parrot mouth is to correct and/or prevent the abnormal dental wear. All abnormal dental wear patterns inhibit rostral and lateral movement and growth of the mandible. Rostral hook formation at 106 and 206 and caudal ramping and hook formation on 311–411 should be reduced. Excessive transverse ridge formation on the cheek teeth should be reduced and excessive enamel points or vaulted ceiling of occlusion corrected. Excessive incisor length from lack of wear should be reduced to bring the lower incisors out of contact with the soft tissues of the palate. The upper and lower incisors should be reduced to allow free lateral motion of the jaw.

Foals born with no contact between the upper and lower incisor teeth, have an incisor overjet. Within the first 3 to 6 months of life, gravity and soft tissue tension on the upper lip cause the premaxilla and incisive bone to tip downward. This downward curve will be evidenced on an oral examination as a bow in the palate midway between the cheek teeth and the incisors. This downward movement of the upper incisors in combination with lack of attrition or wear, will lead to an overbite. Quite often the lower incisors will make contact with the palate caudal to the upper incisors. The combination of long incisor teeth and downward curvature of the upper jaw tends to trap the mandible, preventing rostral mandibular growth and normal lateral jaw motion. Incisor crown reduction can help decrease this trapping effect. Fixed or removal function orthodontic devices can be used to correct the overbite and allow free movement and rostral growth of the mandible.

In foals under 6 months of age, with sufficient growth left in the lower jaw, tension band wires have been used to inhibit rostral growth of the upper jaw. An 18 gage stainless steel wire can be used as a tension band device. Wires placed caudal to the second upper cheek tooth and brought forward around the upper incisors will inhibit growth in this portion of the upper jaw. The lower jaw continues to grow normally and the overjet is corrected.

If no contact is present between any portion of the upper and lower incisor arcade, a combination of tension band wires and a functional orthodontic device is used. Such a device in the most simple form consists of a removal plate attached to a bit, extending rostral between the incisor arcades. When the mouth is closed, upward pressure is placed on the upper arcade discouraging its ventral drift. A more sophisticated fixed appliance can be fashioned to fit in the roof of the mouth. This device can be molded from acrylic constructed on a plaster model or fashioned on a live animal in dorsal recumbency under general anesthesia. An incline plane can be incorporated in this device to place force on the lower jaw when the mouth is closed. The application of these devices cannot be 'cookbooked' because each case presents a slightly different set of anatomical and biomechanical situations that requires detailed evaluation and careful planning.

217

Some equine breed registries require horses possessing any undesirable trait or condition, commonly considered a 'genetic defect', to have this condition indicated on their registration certificate. It should be brought to the attention of the owner or breeder when a severe malocclusion is diagnosed for this reason. It would be considered unethical to attempt to correct a known genetic defect in order to allow an owner to misrepresent the animal in the show ring or breeding shed.

In human research, scientists are using elegant image processing, microscopic, physiologic, biophysical, biochemical and genetic engineering research procedures to study dentofacial deformities. Clinical observation and detailed documentation will further promote understanding of why and how malocclusions and interjaw malrelations appear and how they can be prevented or treated. The equine practitioner can benefit greatly from the new human biomedical discoveries. Genetic studies to detect the chromosomal factors that play a role in head shape, and genetic consultation and engineering in breeding planning in order to prevent problems will be seen in the next century.

## CONCLUSION

Equine orthodontic principles are at work in the horse's mouth starting early in life and continuing well into old age. Changes occur as the deciduous teeth erupt, the jaws grow and develop, deciduous teeth are shed, permanent dentition erupts and wear of the hypsodont teeth occurs.

The equine practitioner who is familiar with the principles of diagnosis and documentation of malocclusion is better able to use the controlled movement of teeth and adjustments of jaw growth for treatment. Knowledge obtained through observation, diagnosis, documentation and adjustments will provide the equine dental patient the best occlusion and help maintain proper oral health.

### ACKNOWLEDGEMENTS

J. Eugene Schneider, DVM, Head, Equine Section, Kansas State University. Retired. For personal communication and instruction on intra-oral wiring to correct Parrot mouth.

LH Skip Fischer, Simpsonville, Kentucky. For collaborations in development and manufacturing of a removal functional orthodontic device and methods for taking dental impressions.

Carla Omura, São Paulo, Brazil. For photographs and radiographs of abnormal dental cases and technical assistance.

Dan Fischer, Lincoln, Nebraska. For assistance in development of the attached functional orthodontic device.

## REFERENCES

1. Roberts EW (1994) Bone physiology, metabolism, and biomechanics in orthodontic practice. In: *Orthodontic Practice, Current Principles, and Techniques* (2nd edn) eds TM Graber and RL Vanarsdall, Mosby, St Louis, pp. 193–234.
2. Wiggs RB and Lobprise HB (1997) *Veterinary Dentistry Principles and Practice*. Lippincott-Raven, Philadelphia, pp. 435–481.
3. Osborn JW (1981) *Dental Anatomy and Embryology*. Blackwell Scientific Publishing, Oxford, pp. 255–260.
4. Scott EJ (1938) An experimental study in growth of the mandible. *American Journal of Orthodontics*, 24, 925–934.
5. Graber TM (1994) Functional appliances in orthodontics. In: *Orthodontic Practice, Current Principles, and Techniques*, (2nd edn), eds TM Graber and RL Vanarsdall, Mosby, St Louis, pp. 383–436.
6. Musich DR (1994) Orthodontics and orthognathic surgery. In: *Orthodontic Practice, Current Principles, and Techniques* (2nd edn), eds TM Graber and RL Vanarsdall, Mosby, St Louis, pp. 835–907.
7. Tucker MF (1993) Correction of dentofacial deformities. In: *Contemporary Oral and Maxillofacial Surgery* (2nd edn), Mosby, St Louis, pp. 613–656.
8. Valdez H, McMullen W, Hobson H, *et al.* (1978) Surgical correction of a deviated nasal septum and premaxilla in a colt. *Journal of the American Veterinary Medical Association*, 173, 1001–1004.
9. Gidley JW (1901) Tooth characters and revision of the North American species of the genus equus. *Bulletin of American Museum of Natural History*, 14, 91–141.
10. Axe JW (1905) *The Horse: its Treatment in Health and Disease*. Gresham Publishing, London.
11. Willoughly DP (1975) *Growth and Nutrition in the Horse*. AS Barnes, New York.
12. Shafer M (1980) *An Eye for a Horse*. JA Allen, London, pp. 103–107.
13. Orsini PG (1992) Oral cavity. In: *Equine Surgery*, ed. JA Auer, WB Saunders, Philadelphia, pp. 299–300.
14. Uhlinger C (1987) Survey of selected dental abnormalities in 233 horses. *Proceedings of the 33rd Annual Meeting of the American Association of Equine Practitioners*, 577–583.

15. Miles, AEW and Grigson, C (1990) *Colyer's Variations and Diseases of the Teeth of Animals*, (Revised edn), Cambridge University Press, Cambridge.

16. Joest E (1970) *Handbuck der Speciellen Pathogischem Anatomie der Haustere* (Vol. V/I), Paul Parey, Berlin and Hamburg.

17. Duke, A (1989) *Equine Bit Analysis*. Handout notes from Annual Conference of American Veterinary Dental Society, New Orleans.

18. Baker GJ (1985) Oral diseases of the horse. In: *Veterinary Dentistry*, ed. CE Harvey, WB Saunders, Philadelphia, pp. 220–221.

19. McIlwraith CW (1984) Equine digestive system. In: *The Practice of Large Animal Surgery*, ed. PB Jennings, WB Saunders, Philadelphia, pp. 558–560.

20. DeBowes RM (1990) Brachygnathia. In: *Current Practice of Equine Surgery*, eds AN White and JN Moore, JB Lippincott Co, Philadelphia, pp. 469–472.

21. Emily P (1990) The genetics of occlusion. *Veterinary Forum*, June, 22–23.

22. Goldstein G (1990) The diagnosis and treatment of orthodontic problems. In: *Problems in Veterinary Medicine (Dentistry)*, Vol. 2(1), pp. 195–213.

23. Kertesz P (1993) Orthodontics. In: *A Color Atlas of Veterinary Dentistry and Oral Surgery*, ed. P. Kertesz, Wolfe Publishing, London, pp. 63–72.

24. Harris EF and Johnson M (1992) Heritability of craniometric and occlusal variables: a longitudinal sibling analysis. *American Journal of Dentofacias Orthopedics*, 99, 258.

25. Stockard CR (1941) The genetic and endocrine basis of differences in form and behavior. *The American Anatomical Memoirs*, No. 19, Wister Institute Anatomy and Biology, Philadelphia.

26. McKeown M (1975) Craniofacial variability and its relationship to disharmony of the jaws and teeth. *Journal of Anatomy*, 119(3), 579–588.

27. McKeown M (1975) The allometric growth of the skull. *American Journal of Orthodontics*, 67(4), 412–422.

28. Jayo M, Leipold HW, Dennis SM and Eldridge FE (1987) Brachygnathia superior and degenerative joint disease, a new lethal syndrome in Angus calves. *Veterinary Pathology*, 24, 148–155.

29. Lear TL, Cox JH and Kennedy GA (1997) Autosomal Trisomy in a Thoroughbred Colt: *65, XY, +31. Equine Veterinary Journal*, 31(1), 85–88.

30. McLaughlin GB and Doige LE (1981) Congenital musculoskeletal lesions and hyperplastic goiter in foals. *Canadian Veterinary Journal*, 22, 130.

31. Myers VS and Gordon GW (1975) Ruptured common digital extensor tendons associated with contracted flexor tendons in foals. *Proceedings of the 21st Annual Meeting of the American Association of Equine Practioners*, 67.

32. Buton TE (1985) Spontaneous craniofacial malformations and central nervous system defects in an aborted equine fetus. *Journal of Comparative Pathology*, 95, 131–135.

33. Wiener G and Gardner WJF (1970) Dental occlusion in young bulls of different breeds. *Animal Production*, 12, 7–12.

34. Meyer VH and Becker H (1967) *Eine Erbliche Keiferanomalie Bein Rind*. Deutsche Tierarztliche Wochenschrift, 74, 309–310.

35. Purser AF, Wiener G and West DM (1982) Causes of variation in dental characters of Scottish blackface sheep in a hill flock and relations to ewe performance. *Journal of Agricultural Science*, 99, 287–294.

36. Epstein H (1971) *The Origin of the Domestic Animals of Africa*, Vol. 2. Africana Publishing, London, 296.

37. Petrovik AG (1984) Experimental and cybernetic approaches to the mechanism of action of functional appliances of mandibular growth. In: *Malocclusion and the Periodontium, Cranial Growth Series*, (ed. JA McNamara, monograph) 15.

38. Burdach J and Mooney MP (1984) The relationship between lip pressure following lip repair and craniofacial growth: an experimental study in beagles. *Plastic and Reconstruction Surgery*, 73(4), 544–555.

39. Crowe MW and Swerczek TW (1985) Equine congenital defects. *American Journal of Veterinary Research*, 46, 353–358.

40. McNamara JA (1973) Neuromuscular and skeletal adaptations to altered function in the orofacial region. *American Journal of Orthodontics*, 64, 578, 189, 136.

41. McNamara JA (1980) Functional determinants of craniofacial and shape. *European Journal of Orthodontics*, 2, 131.

42. Hennet PR and Harvey CE (1992) Craniofacial development and growth in the dog. *Journal of Veterinary Dentistry*, 9(2), 11–18.

43. Angle EH (1899) *The Angle System of Regulation and Retention of the Teeth and Treatment of Fractures of the Maxillae* (5th edn). SS White Manufacturing, Philadelphia.

44. Hennet PR, Harvey CE and Emily PP (1992) The angle classification of malocclusion: is it appropriate for use in veterinary dentistry? *Journal of Veterinary Dentistry*, 9(3), 10–12.

## 15

# EQUINE TOOTH REMOVAL (EXODONTIA)

Jack Easley, DVM, MS PO Box 1075 Shelbyville, KY 40066

## INTRODUCTION

Equine dental extractions have been performed and described in the veterinary literature for centuries.[1,2] Initially dental treatments were limited to the easily accessible teeth in the front of the mouth (incisor, canine and wolf teeth). In 1566 Blundeville stated that the horse had only sixteen teeth.[3] Wolf tooth removal was described in the seventeenth century as a method to remedy bitting problems.[4,5] Throughout the twentieth century exodontia has classically been the backbone of equine oral surgery.[6-10] However, the removal of teeth is only one branch of equine dental care.

The routine aim of equine dentistry is to preserve teeth, but in many cases exodontia becomes necessary.[11] There are a wide range of indications for tooth removal and most of these depend upon which tooth in the arcade is causing a problem. Some common indications for tooth removal are associated with one of the following:

1  retained deciduous teeth
2  interceptive orthodontics
3  severe periodontal disease
4  highly mobile teeth
5  supernumerary teeth
6  dental impactions
7  endodontic disease with secondary osteomyelitis
8  surgical consideration in oral fractures
9  severe disease or injury to the dental crown or root
10  malocclusions
11  disarming
12  occlusal trauma
13  neoplasia
14  bitting discomfort
15  sinus disease secondary to dental disease.

The decision to extract a tooth should be a cooperative determination between the veterinarian and owner or trainer. The veterinarian's knowledge will guide the procedure. Tooth removal should be a last resort after other methods to manage the diseased tooth or dental related problems have failed. The specific tooth or numbers of teeth involved, the dental disease process and the age of animal dictate the surgical technique employed and instruments utilized. The extraction can be simple or very time consuming, frustrating and fraught with operative and postoperative complications.[11,15,16]

Contraindications for extraction include a horse suffering from acute infection with cellulitis or acute infectious stomatitis. Also, horses suffering from disease in other major organ systems may be poor surgical candidates. The primary disease should be controlled with appropriate medical therapy prior to exodontia. Diseased teeth with high concentrations of bacteria present in the periodontal area may shed bacteria into the bloodstream when manipulated.[12-15] This makes the use of prophylactic antibiotics pre- and postoperatively necessary to prevent septicemia.[14] Routine dental corrective procedures should be performed prior to surgery. For example, the tooth or teeth in occlusion with the one being removed should have their crown height reduced, thereby taking the stress off the socket plug in the postoperative period.

The most common reason for cheek tooth removal is to eliminate a tooth which has suffered extensive dental disease or fracture of the tooth with concurrent infection. As a rule this tooth is the easiest to remove because there is usually some loss of periodontal attachments. Teeth with periapical infections and healthy alveolar attachments present more of a challenge, especially in younger patients. The most common tooth removed in the horse is the upper first premolar (wolf tooth) in young horses that wear a bit when worked. Deciduous teeth quite often require removal in horses between 2.5 and 5 years of age to allow proper eruption of permanent dentition. Incisor and/or canine teeth are often involved in injuries to the rostral mandible or premaxilla. These teeth should be saved and stabilized in the fracture repair if at all possible. If severely damaged, removal may be necessary.

Historically, equine cheek tooth removal has been thought of and referred to by veterinary surgeons as unsophisticated surgery, leaving the impression among many in our profession that this work is beneath their level of expertise.[17] This may, in part, account for the lack of progress in equine dental extraction techniques and the abhorrent rate of the postoperative complications reported in the literature.[12,13]

The equine dental surgeon must be well versed in the anatomy, physiology, embryological formation and development of the hard and soft tissue of the equine masticatory system. The surgeon must be aware of age-related changes in teeth and the impact this has on dental wear and disease. Finally, there must be good surgical support for anesthesia as well as intraoperative imaging to guide the surgeon in his work.

The process of completely examining the masticatory system and careful surgical planning cannot be overemphasized. Preoperative examination and postoperative treatment are critical to a desirable long-term prognosis. Good owner/veterinarian communication with proper understanding of the complexities of the procedures, the need for good short-term and long-term aftercare and follow-up are important to insure overall owner satisfaction.

Once a tooth is removed, the incisor or molar dental arch is disrupted and the long-term effect on the remaining teeth in the arcade must be considered. Serious long-term consequences of exodontia include drifting of the mesial and distal teeth in the same arcade leading to diastema between teeth and periodontal pocketing of feed and then disease. Other problems associated with abnormalities of wear are created by malocclusion of unopposed continually erupting hypsodont teeth. The surgical approach to dental extraction will depend on the tooth being removed and the disease process involved. This chapter will discuss the details of tooth removal from the front of the mouth to the back.

## INCISOR TOOTH REMOVAL

The deciduous incisors of the horse are often injured or avulsed in conjunction with fractures of the mandible or premaxilla. These teeth should be salvaged if at all possible and incorporated in the fracture repair. Retained deciduous incisors can be a cause of displacement or maleruption of permanent incisors. Malerupted or impacted deciduous incisors should be removed to allow permanent teeth room for normal eruption (interceptive orthodontics). The process of extraction in most of these cases is quite simple because the short deciduous tooth reserve crown and root complex is easily loosened and elevated from its alveolar attachment (Fig. 15.1). If in doubt, radiographic evaluation should be used to confirm the anatomy and position of the unexposed portion of the suspected tooth as well as surrounding unerupted teeth.

Damaged or diseased permanent incisor teeth should be managed periodontically or endodontically, if possible, to retain their function in spacing the incisor arch and wearing the opposing dentition as long as possible.[18] Permanent incisors requiring removal should be approached in a thoughtful way owing to the deep implantation and curvature of the

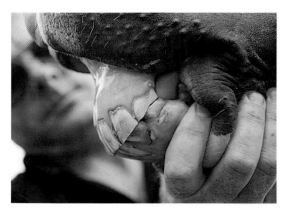

**Figure 15.1.** Root slivers from retained deciduous incisor teeth. These root fragments can be easily elevated and extracted.

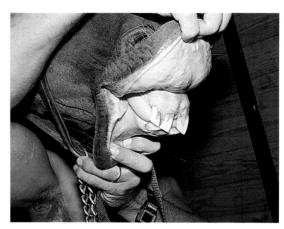

(a)

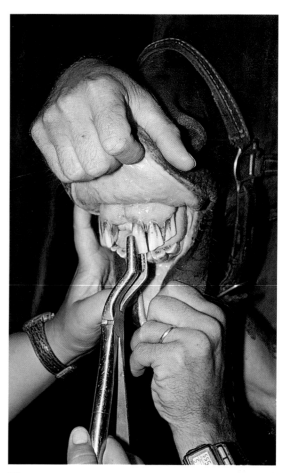

(b)

**Figure 15.2.** (a) A damaged upper incisor tooth that is clinically loose and has lost most of its alveolar attachment. (b) Extraction forceps positioned on loose incisor. The horse has been lightly sedated and restrained.

reserved crown. Incisors, unless already loose from periodontal disease or injury, cannot be readily extracted by any ordinary method except in extreme old age (Fig. 15.2). During youth and middle age their extraction can only be accomplished by removal of the anterior alveolar plate and then elevating the tooth out with a chisel or elevator.

Isolated incisors can be removed in the standing sedated horse using regional anesthesia. The labial mucosal is incised longitudinally down to and through the periosteum overlying the alveolar plate. The labial alveolar plate is removed with a $\frac{1}{4}$ inch wide osteotome or chisel and mallet exposing the reserve crown and root of the affected tooth. When the tooth is exposed throughout its entire length, it is pried out by driving the chisel under the root and elevating it. The alveolus should be irrigated and curetted removing all diseased or loose bone and dental fragments. The mucosal flaps are trimmed and the dental socket packed with gauze and healing allowed by second intention. Loose or damaged incisors may be extracted with forceps (Fig. 15.3a and b).

In cases where the entire arcade of incisor teeth needs to be removed, for example to disarm a vicious stallion, general anesthesia is required.[6,19] A single liberal horizontal incision can be made at the margin of the mucosa and the labial mucosa reflected vertically or dorsally over the bony covering of the incisor arcade.

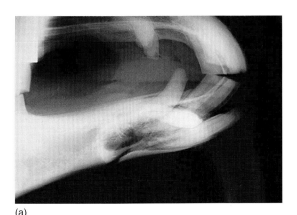

(a)

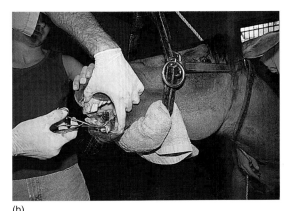

(b)

**Figure 15.3.** (a) Radiograph of a loose lower canine tooth associated with a fracture of the rostral mandible. (b) The tooth was removed with forceps because it interfered with fracture fixation.

The alveolar plate is then removed from each tooth with an osteotome and mallet or an oscillating orthopedic saw and the teeth elevated from the alveolus. Hemorrhage can be controlled with epinephrine-soaked gauze packing and pressure. Each alveolus is lightly curetted and care taken to remove all diseased or loose tooth or bone fragments. The coronal portions of the bony alveolar plate on the three remaining sides are reduced about $\frac{1}{4}$ inch with a bone rongeur and the surrounding mucosal margins elevated. The labial mucosal flap is then pulled back over the rostral edge of the bone, drains placed and the mucosa sutured. The horse should be on a restricted diet for several days after surgery. Keep in mind that removal of one or both incisor arcades will limit the horse's ability to graze forage. The lower incisors help keep the tongue inside the mouth. Chronic tongue protrusion will result with the complete removal of this arcade.

## CANINE TOOTH REMOVAL

Canine teeth are seldom diseased except from pulpitis or periostitis following injuries to the tooth or jaw. Canine teeth can be a source of tartar accumulation and subsequent periodontal disease in the older horse. Stallions have had canine teeth removed to disarm them but crown reduction is a less invasive and more practical method to handle this problem. Canines, if loosened from disease or associated with a jaw fracture, can often be removed with forceps (Fig. 15.3a). However, the long curved root of the canine is deeply embedded in the curved alveolar socket and this prevents forceps extraction or simple elevation of this tooth in most cases.

Canines seldom need to be removed if periodontally intact. If the dental disease process cannot be managed with medical or endodontic therapy, then surgical removal may be the only option. These teeth can be removed under general anesthesia by surgical removal of the lateral alveolar plate and elevation of the tooth, as in the case of incisor teeth (Fig. 15.3b). Care should be exercised when removing the lower canine with respect to the superficial branch of the mental nerve. Preoperative radiographs are helpful in planning the approach to the root of these teeth.

## WOLF TOOTH EXTRACTION

'Wolf tooth' is the common term used to describe the first upper premolar (Fig. 15.4).[20] These teeth come in various shapes and sizes. The appearance of the exposed crown is not necessarily a reflection of the size or shape of the root (Fig. 15.5). The number and position of these teeth are quite variable. Forty to eighty per cent of domestic horses erupt upper wolf teeth, but it is not unusual to only have one.[21] These teeth usually erupt at 6 to 18 months of age but this is also quite variable. These teeth are usually

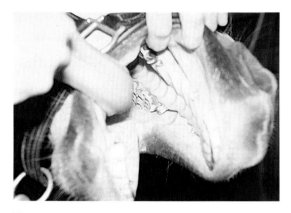

**Figure 15.4.** Normal upper wolf teeth in a 6-year-old gelding. Notice the newly erupted canine teeth with sharp crowns rostral to the diastema.

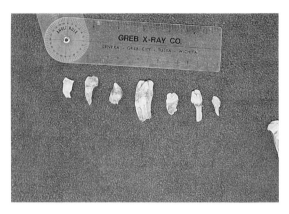

**Figure 15.5.** Wolf teeth extracted from seven different horses. Notice the variation in crown and root size and shape.

positioned just rostral to the upper PM 2, but they can be positioned on the buccal side of the first cheek tooth or up to 1 inch rostrally (Fig. 15.6). Double wolf teeth have been seen as well as teeth displaced in the interdental space (Fig. 15.7). Unerupted wolf teeth, referred to as 'blind wolf teeth', can be detected as firm nodules under the buccal mucosa rostral to the first cheek tooth (Fig. 15.8a–d). These are often painful and at times covered with ulcerated mucosa.

Wolf teeth can cause bitting problems from several standpoints. First it is difficult, if not impossible, to properly round the rostral edge

of PM 2 to accommodate bitting with a wolf tooth in place (see Chapter 13). Displaced or sharp-crowned wolf teeth can cause buccal pain and ulceration when bitting pressure is placed on the cheeks. Some wolf teeth do become loose or diseased and have been shown to be a cause of head shaking or bitting problems.

Because of the potential for problems, it is customary practice to extract wolf teeth in young horses that are used for performance. In most cases, these single-rooted teeth can easily be extracted from the socket in total with proper restraint, equipment and practice. Horses should be sedated and given analgesia

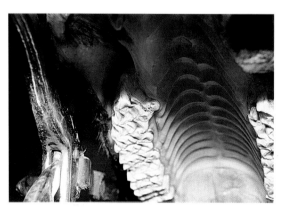

**Figure 15.6.** Palatally displaced upper wolf tooth.

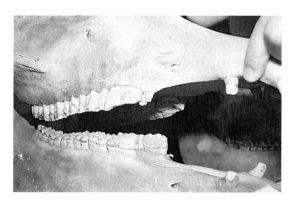

**Figure 15.7.** Equine skull demonstrating a set of double wolf teeth.

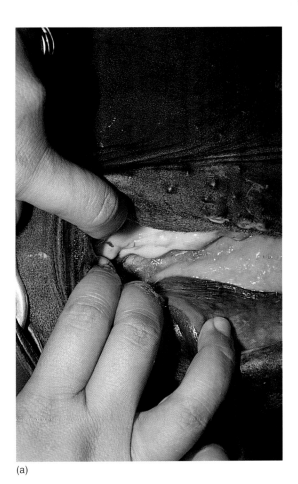

(a)

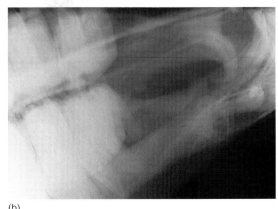

(b)

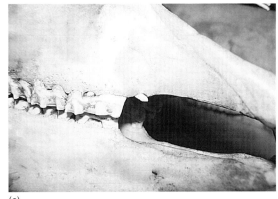

(c)

**Figure 15.8.** (a) An unerupted blind wolf tooth under the oral mucosa rostral to 06. (b) Radiograph showing an unerupted wolf tooth as a radiopaque nodule in the rostral maxilla. (c) A cadaver specimen showing a blind wolf tooth. Notice the tooth has tilted and migrated rostral. (d) A blind wolf tooth being removed with the cone end of a Burgess elevator.

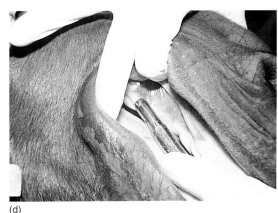

(d)

or a local anesthetic before these teeth are removed.[22] Usually minimal physical restraint is required.

Various dental elevators, gouges and extraction forceps have been developed to loosen and extract these teeth. Bone rongeurs and small curettes may be needed to remove root fragments. Gel foam can be used to pack the open socket of lower wolf teeth to prevent feed from being packed into this area leading to alveolar osteitis (dry socket). A complete set of wolf tooth instruments to allow uncomplicated tooth removal would include a Burgess or Musgrave elevator set, a gouge dental elevator no. 34, a half moon wolf tooth elevator, wolf tooth extraction forceps, fragment forceps (Alberts), dental extraction forceps no. 62, and a bone rongeur (Mead or Bane) (Fig. 15.9).

A cylinder type punch extractor (Burgess) can be placed over the crown of the tooth to excise the mucosa and allow the root elevator to have an area for seating. A curved root elevator should be introduced into the alveolus and gentle pressure placed on the root circumferentially. When the elevator has reached the bottom of the dental socket, pressure on the tooth and a quick downward flick of the wrist will usually extract the tooth from its socket. If a crown is broken the alveolus should be palpated for loose retained fragments. If remaining slivers are detected they should be removed with a curette or a small rongeur. Small root fragments firmly embedded in the alveolus can be left with no detrimental effects. Loosened wolf tooth root fragments have been known to work to the surface in 7 to 14 days after partial tooth extraction. They can become a source of inflammation and irritation and should be removed.

Care should be taken when extracting wolf teeth to avoid having a sharp elevator slip under the palate. The palatine artery can be accidentally injured leading to profuse hemorrhage. If this should occur, pressure applied to the area with a sponge or towel will usually control the hemorrhage. Attempts at ligating the palatine artery can cause more harm as it is difficult to reach the artery which is buried in a groove of the palatine bone.

Blind or unerupted wolf teeth can be evaluated by radiographs if one is uncertain about their presence or position. The best way to remove them is to place a Burgess or cone type wolf tooth elevator over the mucosa at the most rostral aspect of the tooth crown. The cone is pushed through the mucosa, over the crown of the tooth and the entire piece of tissue pried from the bone. These unerupted teeth are usually small and completely covered with cementum.

Rarely a wolf tooth will be encountered that is quite large and looks as if it has become molarized like the other cheek teeth.[23] These should be evaluated radiographically and if unopposed, they need to be shortened or extracted. These may prove to be supernumerary teeth in some cases.

Lower first premolars are occasionally detected in the mandible rostral to the first cheek tooth. These are usually quite small and may only be a small tooth sliver detected soon after the deciduous teeth have shed. However, they can be large with sharp crowns. Lower first premolars have caused problems in bitted horses. Their presence should always be noted during an oral examination on a performance horse. They can be difficult to see on the oral examination because they may be partially covered by a loose fold of buccal mucosa at the lip commisures. Digital palpation just rostral to the first lower cheek tooth is the most accurate way to detect these short-crowned teeth. Unerupted lower wolf teeth are rare and can only be detected radiographically (Fig. 15.10). These teeth can be elevated using the same techniques as the uppers. The empty alveolus should be packed with gel foam to prevent feed from accumulating in the open dental socket.

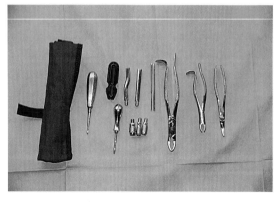

**Figure 15.9.** Set of wolf tooth instruments showing (1) nylon storage bag, (2) small bone curette, (3) cylinder type elevator set, (4) gouge dental elevator, (5) wolf tooth forceps, (6) dental extraction forceps and (7) fragment forceps.

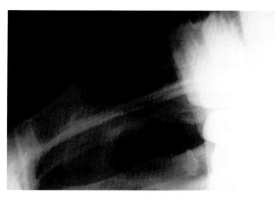

**Figure 15.10.** A radiograph demonstrating an unerupted or blind lower wolf tooth. This horse exhibited severe bitting problems that resolved when the tooth was removed.

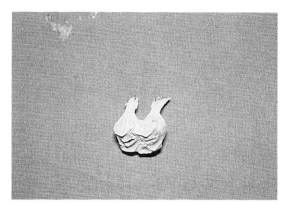

**Figure 15.11.** Deciduous premolar 3 cap with two long buccal root slivers.

## DECIDUOUS PREMOLAR EXTRACTION

In the 2.5- to 4-year-old horse, deciduous premolars and incisors are replaced by permanent teeth. As the developing permanent tooth pushes to the surface it presses on the roots of the worn deciduous tooth, gradually cutting off its nutrition. The worn crown of the deciduous tooth (cap) becomes loose and eventually dies whereby it is displaced or shed into the mouth. The alveolar walls adjust to these changes by bone production and reabsorption to provide a new socket for the embedded portion of the developing permanent hypsodont tooth. This wafer-thin portion of deciduous tooth crown, called a cap, can have a variable number of root slivers (Fig. 15.11). The caps appear much like a table with four legs laying over the top of the permanent tooth. Gingivitis and periodontal disease can result if these root slivers are broken off and remain in the subguigival space after the cap is shed.

The eruption pattern of permanent molarized dentition follows a sequence that predisposes to entrapment (impaction) of deciduous PM 3 and 4 (Fig. 15.12). Delayed shedding of deciduous premolars can predispose to gingivitis, periodontal irritation or infection (Fig. 15.13a–c). Retained, split or displaced deciduous premolars can be distracting to the training process of a young horse (see Chapter 13). In some cases they have been recognized as a factor in dorsal displacement of the soft palate.[24] Impacted caps

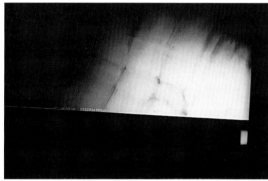

(a)

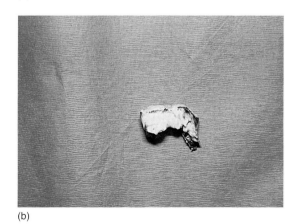

(b)

**Figure 15.12.** (a) Radiograph of an impacted lower premolar 4. This tooth has become wedged between the first molar and the third premolar. The horse had a painful enlargement on the affected mandible that resolved 60 days after the cap was removed. (b) The entrapped cap after removal. The crown is flattened on its distal occlusal surface where it had been wedged under the first lower molar tooth.

TREATMENT OF DENTAL DISORDERS

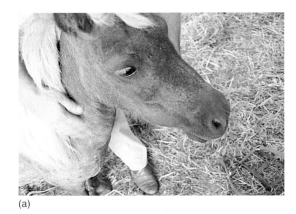

(a)

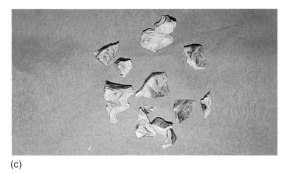

(c)

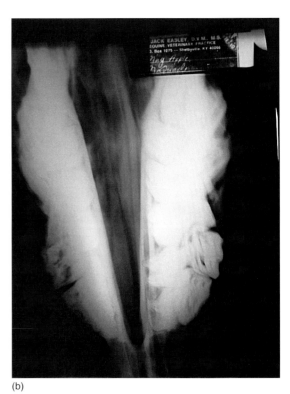

(b)

**Figure 15.13.** (a) A 5-year-old miniature mare with feed packed in the buccal recesses adjacent to the upper cheek teeth. Oral examination revealed a wide sheared upper occlusal surface on the premolar arcades with very sharp buccal enamel points. (b) A radiograph showing wide upper dental arcades with all three deciduous premolars displaced buccally and the permanent premolars erupted in their normal position. (c) The cap fragments removed from this mare. She ate normally within days of having the problem corrected but continued to pack feed in the buccal space for 5 to 6 months. This was due to the recessed gingival margins on the buccal sides of the permanent premolars.

manifested as bony enlargements on the ventral mandibular ramus or maxilla rostral to the facial crest can cause lingual displacement or delay eruption of permanent teeth. Facial swellings are only cosmetic in most cases. However, they can become pathological if eruption is severely inhibited or blood-borne bacteria inhabit the inflamed dental pulp (Fig. 15.14a–b). This can lead to anachoretic pulpitis and facial swelling with a draining tract on the mandible.[25] Caps should be evaluated by palpation, visual inspection and in some instances radiographic interpretation may be required.

Various forceps, elevators and dental picks are available to aid in the diagnosis and treatment of retained deciduous teeth (Fig. 15.15a–b). These include equine molar forceps 17 inch, Reynolds cap extractors, upper and lower, Alberts molar

forceps 11 inch, a 7 inch and an 11 inch modified screw driver, a no. 34 gouge dental elevator and dental extraction forceps no. 69.

To remove the cap of deciduous premolars two and three, small wolf tooth extraction forceps work well. On the fourth premolar cap, open head molar extraction forceps possess a better angle on which to clamp the cap. The forceps are clamped firmly on the base of the cap and pulled lingually across the arcade and the tooth extracted. Care should be taken not to place the forceps below the level of the gums as the palatine vessels along the upper arcade could be disrupted upon clamping, resulting in severe hemorrhage. Rolling the cap toward the lingual surface will reduce breakage of the buccal roots, which can leave slivers of the cap and will allow only the lingual cap roots (lingual

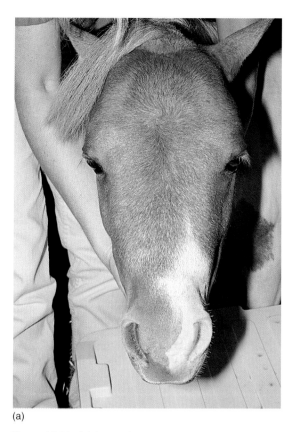

(a)

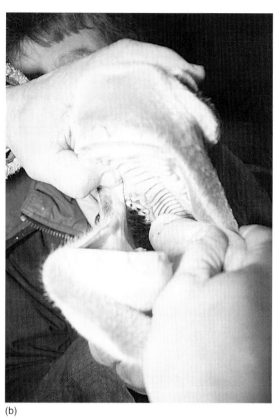

(b)

**Figure 15.14.** (a) Severe facial swelling in a 3-year-old miniature horse. The horse experienced severe respiratory distress when exercised. (b) Oral examination revealed a partially erupted permanent second premolar crown rostral to the deciduous tooth (appeared at first glance to be a large wolf tooth).

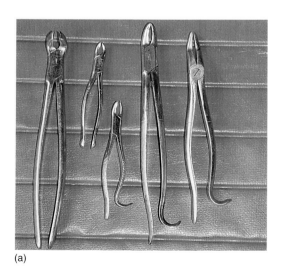

(a)

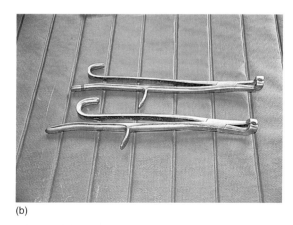

(b)

**Figure 15.15.** (a) Set of deciduous premolar extraction instruments showing (1) premolar extractor, 12.5 inches long, (2) closed head cap forceps, (3) open head cap forceps, (4) liatard style forceps and (5) Wolf tooth, cap or incisor extraction forceps, 12 inches long. (b) A Reynolds premolar cap extractor set. The jaws are wide and at a 10° angle on the forceps to remove upper premolars. The jaws are closer together and straight to fit on the lower premolars.

slivers) to break. The lingual slivers can be easily removed by the horse with its tongue or by the veterinarian with a root elevator. If slivers do exist on either the lingual or buccal sides of the premolars, they can be worked out of the gum with a dental pick or plucked out with a set of closed head rongeurs. When caps are removed, the underlying permanent tooth will erupt and should be in wear in 3 to 4 months. Sharp enamel edges will be present on these teeth in 3 to 6 months and the horse should be rechecked and floated at this time. Radiographs may be necessary to diagnose retained deciduous premolars. If one cap has shed, all other caps in that corresponding quadruplet should be removed.

## CHEEK TOOTH REMOVAL

### ORAL EXTRACTION

Permanent cheek teeth have been extracted from horses ranging in age from 4 years to 40 years with a wide range of dental pathology. The earliest method to remove diseased cheek teeth in the horse was via the oral route. This method has been practiced by veterinary surgeons for centuries on severely diseased or loose teeth. Molar extraction forceps have been available for well over 100 years and until very recently have changed little in design.[26] Along with the advent of equine general inhalation anesthesia which made working in the mouth around a mask or endotracheal tube difficult, this technique lost popularity. The late-twentieth-century veterinary literature has reserved oral tooth extraction to teeth that are loose, or to teeth in old horses with short dental crowns.[27]

With improvement in sedatives and analgesics, standing surgical procedures have become more popular. The use of nasotracheal intubation and development of better quality screw type oral specula have made oral access during general anesthesia practical. These factors have lead to the resurrection of oral cheek tooth extraction and the development of a wide range of better quality instruments to perform extractions.[28,29]

Intraoral tooth extraction should be the primary method of tooth removal employed by the veterinary surgeon. Even though a retrograde approach to the sinus or periradicular area may be necessary to reach an existing secondary condition, extraction should be attempted first. Proper extraction technique based on sound dental surgical principles minimizes postoperative discomfort and encourages rapid healing of associated soft tissues.

Oral extraction can be performed on any tooth but special consideration must be given to teeth with gross caries as those crowns may disintegrate during extraction. Diseased caudal maxillary teeth are often associated with secondary sinusitis and surgical drainage of the sinuses is required in this situation. The more caudally situated teeth are more difficult to access through the mouth making instrument placement and maneuvering more challenging.

Careful preoperative examination of the patient is important and all aspects of the approach to therapy should be planned before surgery is undertaken. Special consideration should be given to the age of the horse, type of dental pathology, position and number of root apices, and to the structural integrity of the tooth crown. Radiographic and endoscopic examinations should be carried out pre- and postoperatively to support the clinical findings. In aged animals with short reserved crowns or in the case of advanced periodontal disease which has resulted in loosening of the tooth, extraction may be carried out digitally (Fig. 15.16a–b). In young horses with apically diseased teeth and long reserved crowns firmly attached in the deep alveolus, extraction will require more effort and expertise.

A set of dental extraction instruments, shown in Figure 15.17a–d, can include:

1. Molar spreaders or separators with the proper size blade and angle of handle to fit between the mesial and distal margins of the tooth to be removed.
2. A set of molar extraction forceps to fit the crown of the tooth being removed
   (a) an open head molar extractor
   (b) a closed head molar extractor
   (c) right and left upper molar claw forceps
   (d) serrated forceps.
3. Dental fulcrum

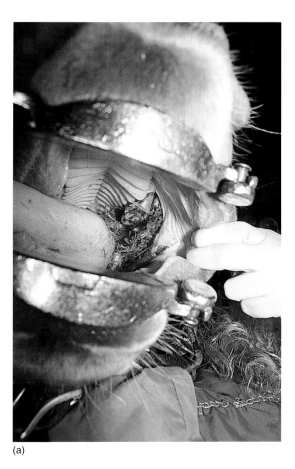

(a)

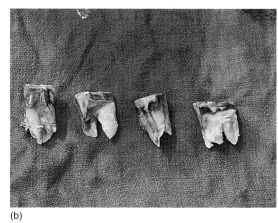

(b)

**Figure 15.16.** (a) An aged horse with severe periodontal disease with feed-packed deep alveolar pockets around the tooth crown. (b) The first two upper cheek teeth in each arcade were loose on digital palpation. The teeth were easily extracted with short cap forceps.

4   Molar cutter sized to fit tooth crown.
5   Set of dental chisels.
6   Set of dental elevators and curettes.
7   General orthopedic instruments
   (a)   bone curettes
   (b)   rongeurs
   (c)   bone cutters
   (d)   osteotome
   (e)   mallet
   (f)   bone file.
8   Material to pack or cover dental socket, such as acrylic or base plate wax.

Intraoral tooth extraction is best performed on the standing horse. This is contrary to previous literature which recommended general anesthesia on a horse in lateral recumbency.[30] Sedative analgesics are administered and the horse's head restrained in a steel frame dental halter or head stand.[31] Regional anesthesia can be performed and is helpful in gaining patient cooperation.[32] A full mouth speculum is needed to gain good access for working in the oral cavity. A head light or fiberoptic light is essential for visualization of instrument placement.

Teeth can be extracted in the reluctant or fractious horse under general anesthesia. A cuffed endotracheal tube passed through the down nostril will assure a patent airway during surgery and recovery. This prevents aspiration of blood or lavage fluids into the trachea. A screw type full mouth speculum allows good access to the oral cavity without having the horse lying on the cheek plates of conventional specula. Care must be exercised when using a mouth speculum in an anesthetized horse not to open it too wide and fracture the jaw or to hold it open for a prolonged period of time as this could lead to postoperative soreness in the muscles of mastication or the temporomandibular joints.

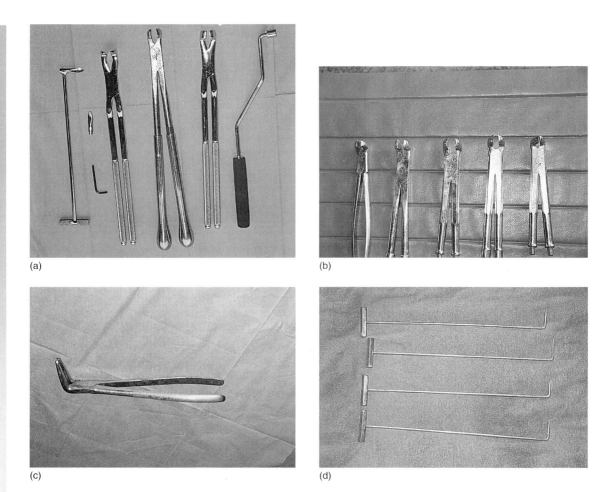

**Figure 15.17.** (a) A basic molar extraction set, (1) equine dental chisel or osteotome with interchangeable blades, (2) molar spreader, (3) concave long jaw molar forceps, (4) serrated short jaw molar forceps and (5) equine dental fulcrum. (b) Five different sized concave long jaw extraction forceps. It is important that the forceps be of the correct size to fit tightly on the tooth crown. (c) Long nosed root fragment forceps. This instrument is helpful in removing thin crown or root fragments left in the dental socket after extraction. (d) Set of root fragment elevators and picks. The instruments are designed to loosen and elevate the crown and root fragments from the dental socket.

The extraction technique described is a modification of that described by Merillat (1906).[6] It takes 400–500 kg of force to extract a cheek tooth from a fresh cadaver skull (S Sears, personal communication, 1998). Therefore, oral extraction cannot be performed without first loosening the tooth. Teeth with split or damaged crowns can be loosened with an equine dental osteotome and forceps (Fig. 15.18a–b). A tooth with a healthy crown is loosened by placing a spreader between the mesial and distal interdental spaces of the involved tooth (Fig. 15.19a–b). The spreader blades are carefully placed between the teeth at the gingival margin and the handles closed bringing the blades partially together. Just enough force should be placed on the spreader to slightly move the tooth. The blades are held in this position placing pressure on the periodontal ligaments, stretching them beyond the elastic limit over a 5 to 10 minute period. The spreader is removed and replaced on the opposite interdental space and the handles again closed, prying the teeth apart. This process is repeated until the spreader blades are easily closed, both mesial and distal to the affected tooth. Next, the gingival mucosa is separated from the buccal and

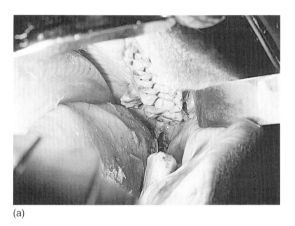

(a)

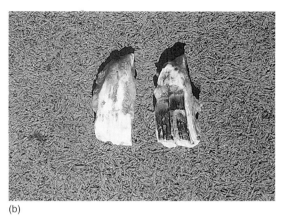

(b)

**Figure 15.18.** (a) Split upper first molar in an 18-year-old horse. This tooth was loosened and orally extracted with a closed head extraction forceps. (b) the extracted fragments.

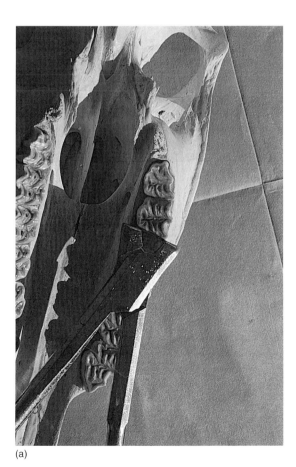

(a)

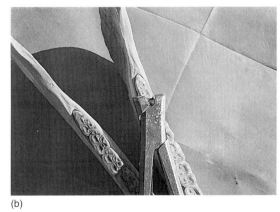

(b)

**Figure 15.19.** (a) The molar spreader blades placed between the upper first and second molar teeth. Notice the angle of the handles with the blades in the proper position. (b) Molar spreader blades placed between the second and third lower molars. The interdental spaces are not perpendicular to the dental arcade making proper instrument placement more difficult.

lingual edges of the tooth crown with a sharp dental elevator or osteotome. This will expose enough crown to allow forceps placement. It may be advantageous to remove a collar of alveolar plate on the buccal and/or lingual edge of the tooth crown to allow a more secure forceps placement. Care should be exercised when elevating on the palatial side of the upper teeth not to damage the palatine artery.

The proper sized extraction forceps are placed on the tooth crown and secured with a length of rubber or elastic tied around the handles. The forceps are then rocked from side to side. Torsion is placed on the tooth until it is felt to loosen in its socket. Undue haste or too great a force must be avoided and care must be taken to prevent crown damage from sudden movement of the horse's head. When the tooth begins to loosen a sucking sound can be heard. Tooth looseness can be checked by removing the forceps and palpating the crown. Keep in mind that the tooth is like a post in a hole. A great deal of movement must be placed on the portion of the post above ground to be reflected in even a small amount of movement at the bottom of the post hole. In a young animal with the ratio of exposed crown to reserved crown and root favoring the latter, more movement of the exposed crown is needed to result in any movement at the bottom of the alveolus. Conversely, in an old horse with almost all of the crown being exposed even a slight movement in the crown would put great pressure on the roots. A normal tooth is locked in place because the irregular shape of the reserve crown and roots mirrors the shape of the alveolus. However the thin alveolar plate is relatively easy to deform into the spongy surrounding bone and it is the combined process of disrupting the periodontal ligament and deforming the contour of the alveolus that is essential in order to completely loosen the tooth.

Once the tooth is loose the forceps should be repositioned to get a firm grip on the crown. A fulcrum block is placed near the head of the forceps. Gradual firm traction will readily bring the tooth from its socket (Fig. 15.20). The tooth should be examined to make sure it has been removed in its entirety and no root fragments or

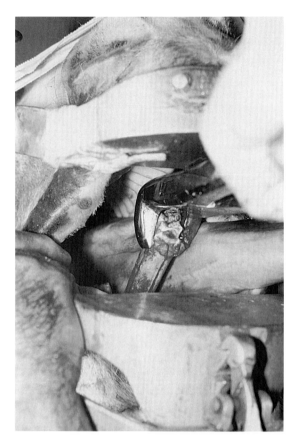

**Figure 15.20.** Lower cheek tooth being extracted with forceps.

slivers of crown have been left in the socket. The alveolus should be examined and any bone or tooth fragments removed. Operative radiographs will confirm that the correct tooth has been removed and the alveolus has been left clean and intact. In the caudal recesses of the oral cavity in a young horse with a long reserve crown, the tooth may require sectioning with a molar cutter to allow it to be delivered into the oral cavity.

Lower cheek tooth sockets that are chronically infected from oral debris may need to be drained ventrally. This can be done with a $\frac{1}{4}$ inch Steinmann pin or $\frac{1}{2}$ inch trephine hole made in the ventral lateral aspect of the mandible below the affected alveolus (Fig. 15.21). To protect the open alveolus, place several 4 × 4 gauze sponges tied in the center to a length of $\frac{1}{4}$ inch umbilical tape. The tape ends are passed

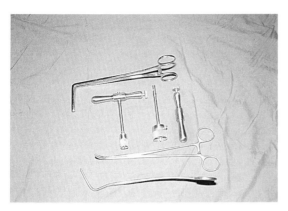

**Figure 15.21.** Instruments to approach the bottom of the dental socket including (1) trephine with $\frac{1}{2}$ inch diameter blade, (2) trephine with 1 inch diameter blade and (3) right angle forceps with long ends to reach the bottom of the dental socket.

into the empty alveolus through the oral cavity and out of the drainage hole. The gauze roll is wedged firmly into the space between the opposing teeth and secured in the socket with umbilical tape tied around another roll of gauze on the outside of the skin incision. The ends of the tape should be kept long enough to allow it to be replaced without having to thread another piece of tape each time the packing is changed. The gauze should be changed daily and the wound irrigated until the periphery of the dental socket is covered with healthy granulation tissue, about 5 to 10 days postoperatively.

The alveolus should be protected from oral contamination with a patch or plug of acrylic dental base plate wax or polymethmethacrylate (PMMA). Dental base plate wax is a satisfactory product for this purpose. Dental base plate wax has a melting point of 37.8°C (100°F), which is above the temperature of the mouth and remains solidified when placed in the oral cavity. After the tooth has been removed and the alveolus cleansed of fragments, two sheets of the wax, measuring $3 \times 6 \times \frac{1}{8}$ inch each, are submerged in hot water (95–100°C). Within a few seconds the wax becomes soft and pliable and can be molded roughly into the shape of the tooth just extracted. This should be done hurriedly so that the molded shape may be inserted into the alveolus before the wax has 'set'. As the soft wax plug is inserted into the alveolus, it conforms to the shape of the cavity and the little irregularities therein stabilize the plug and prevent its dislodgment during mastication.[33]

The entire plug should be about one quarter the length of the root of the removed tooth to allow room for the development of granulation tissue in the root socket. The plug should extend only slightly above the top of the gingiva so that it is not involved in chewing. After the wax is in place, its surface is molded carefully with a finger to build a slight flange over the gingival line to seal the alveolus (Fig. 15.22a–b). A similarly fashioned plug made from dental acrylic or bone cement has been found to be more successful in sealing the alveoli and preventing postoperative complications.[34] Bone cement (PMMA) can be combined with radiopaque contrast media or antibiotics if needed. Hoof acrylic should not be used for this purpose as this creates an endothermic reaction.

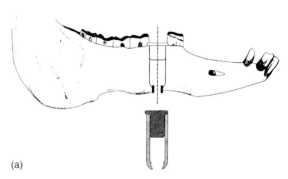

(a)

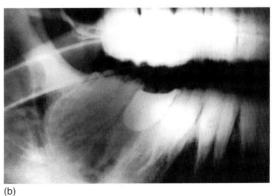

(b)

**Figure 15.22.** (a) Diagram of placement of dental plug. (b) Radiograph of gutta percha dental plug after extraction of 410. Taken from GJ Baker, RA Mansmann and ES McAllister. Equine Medicine and Surgery, 3rd ed. with permission.

## LATERAL APPROACH TO TOOTH EXTRACTION AFTER REMOVAL OF ALVEOLAR PLATE

Merillat in 1906 recommended the Williams operation for removal of the first three upper cheek teeth.[6,35] This technique involved removing the lateral alveolar plate through a horizontal skin incision over the roots of the affected tooth. The tooth roots and reserve crown are visualized and the tooth elevated from the alveolus in its entirety. This lateral approach was later modified by Evans to incorporate a lateral buccotomy to gain better exposure to the upper and lower rostral four cheek teeth.[36,37] Recently, a vertical buccotomy incision through the masseter muscle has been adapted by Lane for extraction of the fourth and fifth mandibular cheek teeth.[38]

The horse is placed under general anesthesia in lateral recumbency with the affected side up. Nasotracheal intubation through the down nostril will allow good oral access during surgery. An oral speculum is inserted and the oral cavity is lavaged with a dilute solution of chlorhexidine. The lateral aspect of the head is prepared for aseptic surgery. A ventrally curved incision is centered over the affected tooth, beginning at the level of the facial crest and extending ventrally to the occlusal surface of this tooth (Fig. 15.23a–j). The skin flap is reflected dorsally exposing the zygomatic muscle which can be sectioned or retracted out of the operative field. The dorsal buccal branch of the facial nerve should be identified and reflected. The initial incision does require accurate positioning and meticulous dissection to avoid the facial artery and venous plexus, the dorsal buccal branch of the facial nerve and the parotid salivary duct. This salivary duct erupts into the mouth on a caruncle adjacent to the second upper cheek tooth. The facial vein and salivary duct can be ligated and transected if necessary for good surgical exposure. To expose the fourth upper cheek tooth, a longitudinal incision is made through the masseter muscle 2 cm below the facial crest. This will require exposure of the facial vein which should be ligated and transected. The oral mucosa is incised vertically to expose the oral cavity. The buccal gingiva is incised rostral and caudal to the affected tooth and reflected dorsally. An oscillating saw or osteotome is used to sever the bony alveolar plate along the interdentium along each side of the affected tooth and a 2-cm-wide piece of bone is removed. In an old horse, care should be taken not to remove too much bone and enter the maxillary sinus over the third or fourth cheek tooth. A diamond cutoff wheel or burr can be used to divide the crown of the tooth longitudinally in two or three segments. The soft tissues should be protected to prevent injury by the cutoff wheel. A thin osteotome can be used to break the center portion of the tooth. Alternatively, the tooth can be loosened through the oral cavity with a molar spreader making sectioning unnecessary. Once the tooth is loose it can be elevated with a chisel, periosteal elevator or molar forceps. The alveolus should be inspected and cleaned with a dental pick and curette. Radiographs should be taken to check for osseous or dental fragments left in the alveolus. The buccal mucoperiosteal flap can be sutured to encourage primary healing and minimize contamination of the socket. If this is not feasible, the base of the socket is packed with sterile roll gauze led to the skin surface through a separate stab incision. A dental plug fashioned from dental base plate wax, acrylic, or PMMA is placed over the gauze to the level of the surrounding gingiva. This will prevent contamination of the healing socket. The buccal incision is closed with absorbable interrupted Lembert sutures. The masseter and buccinator muscles are apposed with simple interrupted absorbable sutures. The subcutaneous skin and fascia are closed in routine fashion. If paranasal sinusitis is present, the sinus should be irrigated. The horse should be allowed to recover from general anesthesia protecting the airway with a cuffed endotracheal tube during the recovery process. The gauze packing is removed in sections over a 72 hour period. The plug should be checked in 5 to 7 days. The area should have filled with granulation tissue in 14 to 21 days and covered with epithelium in about 30 days.

Buccotomy and alveolar plate removal should be recommended as the extraction technique of choice for rostral teeth in both jaws that

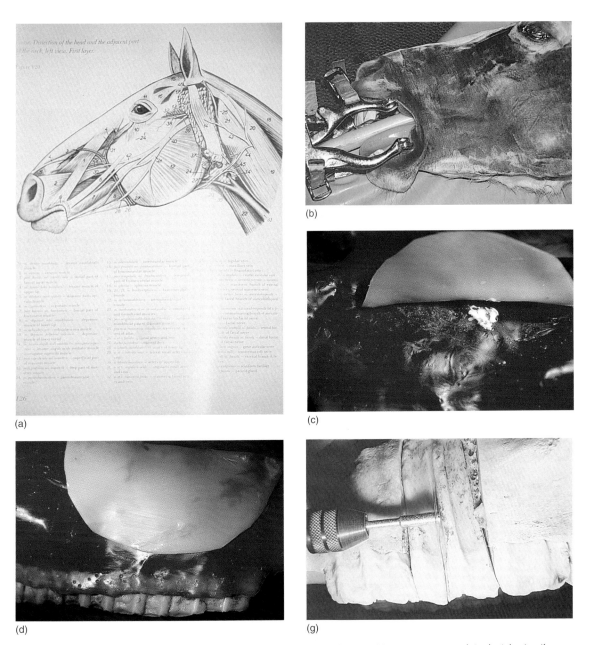

**Figure 15.23.** (a) Horse positioned in lateral recumbency being prepared for lateral buccotomy approach to dental extraction. The full mouth speculum is in place. An endotracheal tube is necessary to protect the airway during surgery but does limit access to the oral cavity. (b) The surgical anatomy of the buccal region should be studied prior to surgery. Nerves, blood vessels, salivary ducts, and muscles often obstruct a direct approach to the affected tooth. (c) Wax over a cadaver model demonstrating the lateral buccotomy approach to removal of the upper fourth premolar. A dorsal based skin flap is made and the buccinator muscle and oral mucosa incised. (d) The buccal mucosa is exposed. (e) A vertical mucoperiosteal incision is made mesial or distal to the affected tooth and the flap elevated exposing the alveolar plate. (f) The buccal alveolar plate is removed with a burr or osteotome. (g) In a young horse with a long reserve crown, sectioning the tooth longitudinally will aid in ease of delivery from the dental socket. (h) Post-extraction, the socket should be carefully examined and all tooth or bone fragments removed. Care should be taken not to damage the dorsal alveolar plate which makes up the floor of the maxillary sinus. (i) The mucoperiosteal flap should be sutured if possible to encourage healing and minimize contamination of the socket. The empty socket is packed with roll gauze that is gradually removed over several days postoperatively. (j) The buccotomy incision is closed in layers taking care to get a good oral seal. The skin wound healed by first intention leaving a minimal blemish.

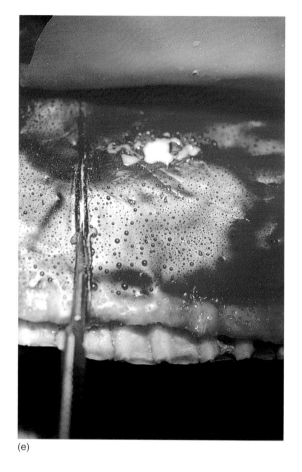

(e)

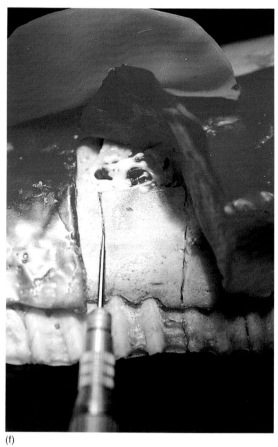

(f)

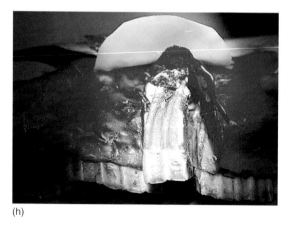

(h)

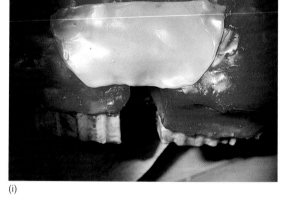

(i)

**Figure 15.23.** *continued.*

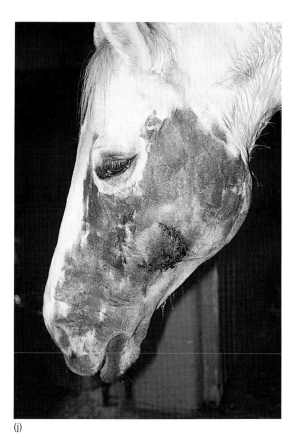

(j)

**Figure 15.23.** *continued.*

are not good candidates for oral extraction. This would include teeth with damaged crowns or teeth set in a socket surrounded by sclerotic bone that would not easily deform, thus not allowing the tooth to loosen in the socket. With this technique there is little chance that the wrong tooth would be removed or an adjacent tooth would be damaged. The entire alveolus can be visually inspected ensuring that all tooth and bone fragments have been removed prior to closure. This procedure is more tedious and time consuming than oral extraction or repulsion. Aftercare is relatively simple and straightforward and found to be relatively free of complications, provided the facial nerves are protected during surgery.[38] Lane describes a modification of a horizontal buccotomy to a vertical incision in the extraction of the fourth and fifth lower cheek teeth.[38]

## RETROGRADE APPROACH TO TOOTH REMOVAL BY REPULSION

The technique for trephining to open the frontal and maxillary sinuses was developed by Lafosse in 1749 as a means of treating nasal diseases caused by glanders or dental disease.[1] This technique was later adapted to approach the apex of the cheek teeth outside of the sinus cavities.[6,26]

Repulsion of teeth is preferred when oral extraction is difficult and impractical. The operation should be performed under general anesthesia with the airway protected using a cuffed endotracheal tube and the mouth held open with an oral speculum. Repulsion involves making a window in the bone to gain access to the apex of the tooth and the use of a dental punch and mallet to drive the tooth from its socket. The principal difficulties of this procedure are gaining access to the base of the tooth without producing excessive damage to the supporting bone and driving the tooth from its socket without fracturing the jaw, splintering the tooth or causing excessive damage to the alveoli of adjacent teeth. The surgeon should elevate the gingiva and attempt to loosen the tooth with spreaders and extraction forceps prior to repelling the tooth. Use of these techniques minimizes the risks of alveolar bone complications.

Repelling is confined to the upper or lower cheek teeth. The horse should be placed on appropriate antibiotics and non-steroidal anti-inflammatory drugs preoperatively and for 5 to 7 days postoperatively. Postoperative care may be required for a few days to several weeks depending on how soon the infection is overcome, involvement of adjacent tissue and how rapidly healthy granulation tissue fills the vacated alveolus.

### Repulsion of the lower cheek teeth

The trephine openings for repulsion of the lower cheek teeth are made on the lateral ventral border of the mandible (Fig. 15.24). Each tooth requires the trephine location to be in a different position. The opening for repelling the first cheek tooth should be made directly ventral to the table surface of the tooth. For the second

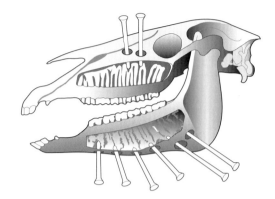

**Figure 15.24.** Proper position of the dental punch for repulsion of the cheek teeth (from Merillat, 1906).[6]

through to the fifth cheek teeth of horses less than 9 years old, the opening is made ventral to the caudal border of the tooth. In horses between 9 and 12 years old, the opening is aligned more closely with the center of the table surface. In horses 12 years of age and older, the opening should be ventral to the center of the table surface.

The trephined opening for the fourth and fifth lower cheek teeth may be near the external maxillary artery and vein and the parotid duct. These should be carefully exposed, freed and retracted from the surgical field.

After surgical preparation of the area, an X-shaped or curved skin incision is made over the site of trephine placement. The center of the incision should mark the center of the opening. The skin flaps are reflected and retracted away from the surgical field. Subcutaneous tissues are dissected and the periosteum incised and carefully elevated from the bone. An alternative approach is to make a full thickness circular incision and discard the tissue leaving the trephine hole to heal by second intention. The center punch of the trephine is set in the center of the field. The instrument is rotated back and forth in an arc until the blades make contact with the bone. At this point the central punch is retracted to prevent damage of highly vascular or sensitive deeper tissues. The instrument is rotated back and forth until the blades cut through the bone. The disk of bone usually remains in the trephine when the instrument is

removed, but in some cases the disk must be freed from underlying attachments with a bone gouge or chisel and forceps. After the trephine opening has been made the base of the affected tooth is carefully located. An intraoperative radiograph will aid in proper punch placement and angulation. An equine dental punch is placed on the base of the tooth and a trustworthy assistant strikes the end of the punch with an orthopedic mallet (Fig. 15.25). If there is insufficient room to do this, the opening should be enlarged with rongeurs or a bone chisel. The accuracy of the punch seating can be determined by palpation of impact with a finger on the crown of the affected tooth. If the punch is properly placed mallet blows have a characteristic ring and rebound not present when the punch penetrates soft tissues. If the tooth has been loosened prior to surgery, it can be repelled with several blows from the mallet.

After the tooth is repelled, examine the base carefully to determine if it is complete. Any dental fragments remaining in the alveolus should be removed with a curette and forceps. Great care must be taken to remove all fragments of the tooth and nodules of cement from the alveolar cavity. Thorough curettage and postoperative radiographs to check the alveolus are

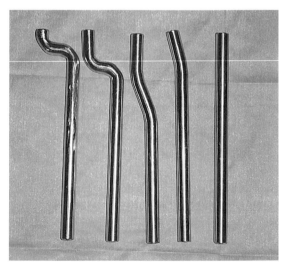

**Figure 15.25.** Full set of equine dental punches. These instruments are fashioned from 8–12 mm diameter stainless steel rods that are 20–25 cm long.

essential. After the socket has been cleansed it should be protected with gauze or a protective patch or plug. The periosteum and skin flaps should be opposed over the incision. If a packing is tied a small central portion of the skin flap should be removed to allow passage of the tie.

Removal of the sixth lower cheek tooth presents several special problems.[39] The tooth root ends approximately midway between the table surface of the tooth and the greatest curvature of the ramus of the mandible. This necessitates trephining on the lateral side of the mandible rather than on the lateral ventral surface. The trephine point underlies the thick and expansive masseter muscle which creates considerable difficulty in exposing the operative site properly. Finally, the curvature of this tooth is greater than that of any other and requires careful attention during repulsion since the line of force established by the mallet and punch must be at an angle rather than a straight line.

A liberal incision is made through the skin and parallel to the fibers of the masseter muscle. The incision should end 4 to 5 cm from the ventral border of the mandible. Care should be taken to avoid damage to the branches of the facial nerve and maxillary artery. The center of this incision should lie midway between the table surface of the tooth and the greatest curvature of the mandible. The muscle fibers are bluntly divided and separated from the bone. A retractor is inserted to separate the musculature and provide exposure to the site.

An alternative approach to the sixth lower cheek tooth is to reflect the body of the masseter muscle away from the bony mandible. This technique involves making a curved incision about 2 cm dorsal lateral to the most ventral aspect of the mandible. The incision begins caudal to the parotid salivary duct and follows the curve of the mandible 12 to 18 cm to the level of the mesenteric artery and vein. The masseter muscle is incised just dorsal to its facial attachment to the ventral mandible. A wide periosteal elevator is used to separate the muscle from the mandible. Careful dissection close to the bone will avoid the large venous plexus in the body of the masseter muscle. This muscle is retracted dorsally to gain access to the lateral aspect of the mandible. The most ventral part of the tooth bed is located by finding the bulging bony prominence of the root and the opening created. A trephine or osteotome can be used to remove a plate of bone at the base of the tooth. Intraoperative radiographs will confirm proper osteotomy placement. A punch with a double bend in its distal end makes it easier to approach this tooth root.[9] The tooth should be repelled along a line parallel to the long axis of the curved tooth crown (Fig. 15.26a–c). The entire tooth can rarely be repelled into the mouth in one piece since the upper sixth tooth is so close. Therefore, the lower tooth must be shortened with a molar cutter or wire saw to complete the extraction.

Postoperative radiographs may reveal remaining alveolar fragments after the socket has been searched. These fragments should be removed prior to irrigating the alveolar socket with antibiotic solution. The defect should be packed or plugged to prevent contamination with food. The incision is closed in layers and should heal by primary intention.

## Repulsion of the upper cheek teeth

It is essential to position the trephine opening properly to avoid damage to the nasolacrimal duct and the lacrimal canal, which run from the medial canthus of the eye rostroventral to the floor of the nasal cavity near the external nares. A base line constructed from the medial canthus of the eye through the infraorbital foramen and extending rostral to the nares marks the location of the nasolacrimal duct (Fig. 15.27). Trephine openings should be made below this line. Due to the length of the teeth in young horses, the trephine opening must be kept as close to the line as possible. In older animals it may be made some distance below the line to compensate for shortening of tooth length and sharpening of facial contours.

For the first and second cheek teeth, a line is drawn vertically through the center of the tooth and the opening is made along this line and just ventral to the baseline. For the third through to the fifth cheek teeth, the opening is made ventral to the base line along a line passing

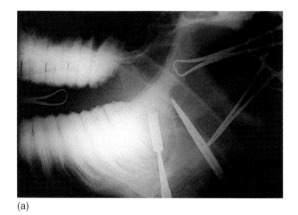

(a)

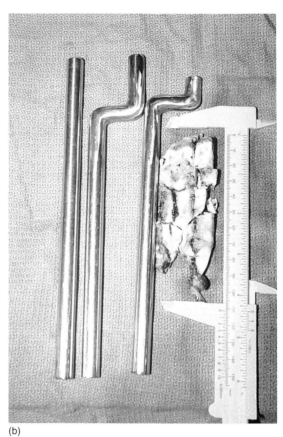

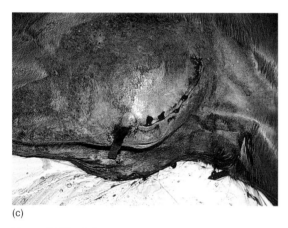

(c)

(b)

**Figure 15.26.** (a) Intraoperative radiographs are important to confirm proper punch placement when repelling teeth. The last lower molar requires the punch to be lined up parallel to the long axis of the tooth crown. (b) Repelled lower last molar showing the punches used to remove the tooth. The fractured tooth crown is typical of a tooth removed by repulsion. This makes it important to reconstruct the tooth after removal and make sure all fragments are accounted for. This will help assure that the alveolus is left free of tooth fragments postoperatively. (c) The curved incision over the caudal cheek teeth is closed in layers. A drain should be placed under the masseter muscle and brought out through a separate stab incision.

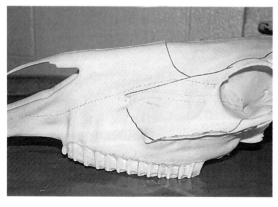

**Figure 15.27.** Equine skull demonstrating landmarks for maxillary sinuses, infraorbital foramen, and nasomaxillary duct.

dorsal parallel to the caudal border of the tooth. For the sixth cheek tooth the opening is made over the frontal maxillary opening and a curved punch used to contact the roots of the tooth. It is fortunate that this tooth seldom needs to be repelled, because it is not easily accessible particularly in young animals in which the base of the tooth lies under the floor of the orbit. As a horse becomes older, the teeth become progressively easier to reach via trephine openings since the gradual eruption of the teeth leaves more space between the baseline and the trephined opening.[33] It is important that this tooth be repelled with the punch in line with the long, slightly backward curved, dental crown.

Maxillary cheek teeth which have their roots within the paranasal sinus system may be removed by the trephine hole technique described above, but this will not allow the management of co-existing secondary dental sinusitis (Fig. 15.28a–d). When there is secondary dental sinusitis, an osteoblastic flap technique may be used.[40] Secondary dental sinusitis is recognized on lateral medial radiographs and the diagnosis confirmed visually by trephining the caudal maxillary sinus (caudal to the ventral rim of the orbit and adjacent facial crest) prior to surgery (sinocentesis). This trephine hole may be useful for sinus lavage postoperatively.

With the horse under general anesthesia and in lateral recumbency with the affected arcade positioned dorsally, the skin overlying the maxillary bone is prepared for surgery. A skin flap is created by incising the skin, subcutis and periosteum around the rostral, ventral and caudal borders of the rostral and caudal maxillary sinuses; to ensure an adequate blood supply to the wound margin during healing, the attached base of the skin flap should be twice the length of its depth. The periosteum is elevated from the underlying maxillary bone and the skin and periosteum are reflected dorsally. A rectangular section of maxillary bone is then marked out 5 to 10 mm inside the margin of the skin flap and using an osteotome and mallet, the bone section is cut and pried away from the underlying sinus lining. The osteotome may need to be run under

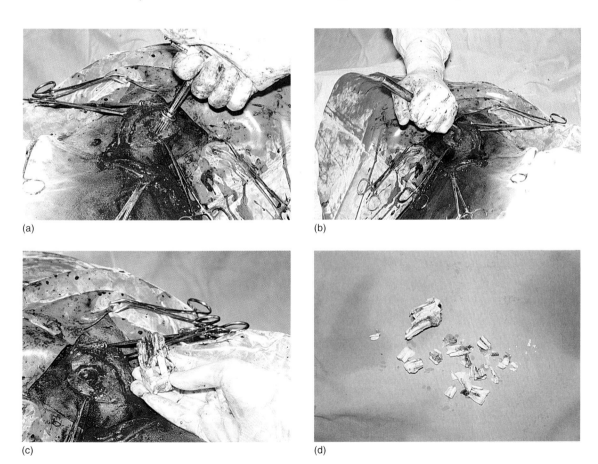

(a)

(b)

(c)

(d)

**Figure 15.28.** (a) Trephine with $\frac{3}{4}$ inch diameter blade being used to open a hole into the rostral maxillary sinus over the root of the first upper molar. (b) Diagram showing proper position (A) of the punch and (B) improper position for repulsion of the first upper molar (from Merillat, 1906).[6] (c) Tooth after removal by repulsion. The roots have been destroyed as has most of the reserve crown. (d) The large crown portion and the crown and root fragments that were removed from the dental socket after repulsion of upper M1.

the bone flap to cut septal attachments before the flap can be mobilized. Care should be taken when cutting the bone flap not to transect the estimated line of the nasolacrimal duct.

It is possible to expose the maxillary sinus by sectioning three sides of the rectangle of maxillary bone and fracturing it along its long dorsal side, allowing replacement at the end of the procedure. This technique requires keeping the soft tissues moist and the periosteum attached to the bone flap (Fig. 15.29). Maintaining a good blood supply prevents postoperative bone sequestra formation.[41]

Once the maxillary sinus has been exposed, the affected cheek tooth is identified and re-pelled as described earlier, again ensuring that all affected tissue and devitalized alveolar bone is completely removed. Likewise the alveolar socket is plugged to prevent contamination of the sinus with ingesta. It is imperative that the oral plug is accurately positioned and remains in situ long enough to prevent contamination of the maxillary sinus with ingesta (i.e. the development of an oroantral fistula).[42]

In cases where there are minimal inflammatory changes to the lining of the maxillary sinus, the sinus is vigorously lavaged and a free flow of irrigation fluid through the normal drainage system (nasomaxillary ostium) to the nasal passages and nares is confirmed. The skin flap is then closed and a postoperative irrigation sys-

tem is placed into the sinus at the previously trephined site, or into the frontal sinus medial to the orbit. Where secondary dental sinusitis is long standing and there are marked inflammatory changes in the sinus, drainage from the sinus will be inadequate or completely obstructed. A fistula must then be created in the ventral turbinate, as ventrally as possible on the floor of the turbinate portion of the maxillary sinus (ventral conchae), to re-establish adequate sinus drainage.

## DRAINAGE OF PARANASAL SINUSES

In certain cases it is necessary to provide drainage to the sinus or perform surgical debridement of the sinus in addition to removing teeth. In chronic sinusitis, debridement of pyogenic membrane from the sinus or removal of soft tissue masses may be necessary. In such cases, the alternative to selective trephination with subsequent enlargement of the opening is to use a bone flap that will allow surgical exposure of both the cranial and caudal compartments of the maxillary sinus simultaneously. A U-shaped incision is made through the bone and the flap is elevated. The flap is left attached at the ventral border. As with trephine holes, careful attention to anatomy is necessary in addition to associated tooth position depending on age.

An effective way to enhance drainage of the cranial maxillary sinus into the nasal cavity is to pass a large, curved blunt instrument (mare urinary catheter) medially over the infraorbital canal and force it gently through the ventral turbinate into the ventral meatus (Fig. 15.30).[43] Setons or drains may be passed into the nasal cavity and exit at the nostril. These may be used to enhance drainage and delay closure of the fenestration site. As mentioned previously, the presence of pyogenic membrane, soft tissue masses (cysts and tumors) and foreign material requires augmentative debridement.[40] Irrigation of the sinus with sterile saline solution containing 2 per cent povidone iodine or 1:1000 potassium permanganate is performed regularly until the problem is considered resolved.[44] Exercise and feeding from the floor will assist in promoting drainage.

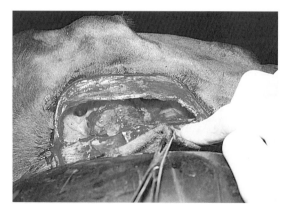

**Figure 15.29.** A frontal sinus being approached through a bone flap technique. This approach gives good exposure to the sinus cavities and is recommended for approaching the root of the last upper molar for repulsion.

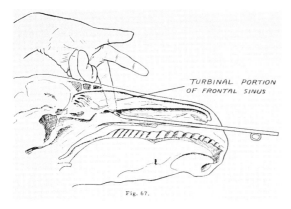

TURBINAL PORTION
OF FRONTAL SINUS

Fig. 67.

**Figure 15.30.** Proper passage of a mare urinary catheter to establish ventral drainage in the maxillary sinus. (from Wheat, 1973, with permission of the editor of the *Proceedings of the 19th Annual Meeting of the American Association of Equine Practitioners).*[43]

When there is involvement of the frontal sinus or caudal compartment of the maxillary sinus, dependent drainage may occur into the cranial maxillary sinus, but trephine openings may need to be made over these specific locations. The conchal portion of the frontal sinus, or conchofrontal sinus (turbinate extension of the frontal sinus), may present a special drainage problem because it is a rostrally placed blind compartment.[45] To drain this area a hole is made 3 cm cranial to a line drawn between the medial canthus of the eyes and off the midline. This will provide access to the turbinate extension of the frontal sinus. A mare urinary catheter is introduced up the nasal passage and pushed through the cranial border of the dorsal nasal concha. Setons or drains can be placed through the hole. Having created a fistula from the nasal passages into the ventral turbinate, further hemorrhage is controlled by packing roll gauze or a sock and gauze bandage tightly into the sinus to produce local compression, and leading the open end out to the nares. The sock and bandage pack is constructed from a length of stockinette bandage (twice the length of the horse's head), folded in on itself to create a sock. Two or three lengths of 2 or 3 inch ribbon gauze are tied end to end and packed into the base of the sock with the free end exiting to the nares. A mare urinary catheter placed retrogradely from

the nares is useful in pulling the sock and bandage pack through to the nares. The skin/periosteal flap is then routinely closed over the packing using a single layer, vertical mattress suture pattern. A postoperative lavage system, consisting of a Foley balloon catheter, is positioned within the sinus and attached to the lateral side of the horse's head leading away from the orbit.

The placement of a nasotracheal tube is mandatory during the horse's recovery from general anesthesia. The combination of the sock and bandage pack obliterating the nostril of the affected side and the prolonged lateral recumbency resulting in vascular engorgement of the mucosa of the dependent nasal passages, may potentially lead to the obstruction of the nasal airway during inspiration and hence, severely compromise the animal during recovery. In view of this some surgeons find it advantageous to perform sinus exploration and drainage on the standing sedated horse.[46]

The inner ribbon gauze of the sinus packing is gradually pulled out over the first 72 postoperative hours and finally the stockinette sock itself is pulled through the nares. Thereafter, the sinus is lavaged twice daily ensuring a free flow to the nares. The flushing is continued until the lavage solution exiting the nares is clear (i.e. for about 7 to 10 days). The Foley catheter is then deflated and removed and the ingress trephine hole is allowed to granulate.

## CONCLUSION

Horses presented for tooth removal should first and foremost have a complete dental examination. Presurgical examination procedures will depend on the horse's age and general health and the requirements of the anesthesiologist. Radiographic evaluation of the head is usually indicated and is the only way to visualize the reserve crowns, roots and support structures of the involved tooth. Radiographs also help with planning the approach to the tooth and can reduce the risk of complications. Exodontia should not be performed unless it has been determined beyond doubt which tooth or teeth are problematic and all methods of corrective, medical, periodontic or endodontic therapy have been exhausted to arrest the disease process and preserve the tooth.

## COMPLICATIONS OF TOOTH REMOVAL

The removal of a tooth or a number of teeth from a horse should not be approached casually. Reports on the incidence of complications that accompany cheek tooth removal range from a low level of 4 per cent for oral extraction to as high as 47 per cent for repulsion of maxillary cheek teeth.[28,47] Other studies have shown a 22 to 40 per cent rate of complications from traditional tooth repulsion.[37,42,48] Complications can be divided into categories beginning with problems associated with restraint, general anesthesia, and long-term hospital care. Problems associated with the extraction itself include hemorrhage, removal of the wrong tooth, damage to structures adjacent to the tooth being removed (i.e. palatine artery, sinuses, alveolar bone, jaw, adjacent teeth, nasolacrimal duct, parotid salivary duct and facial nerve).

Complications associated with wound healing can include wound dehiscence or persistent draining due to fistula formation, resulting from incomplete tooth removal, bone sequestrum, infected membrane socket, packing breakdown, mucous membrane healing prior to wound granulation or a foreign body in wound. Long-term complications can be associated with a misdiagnosis of the initial problem that can result in removal of a wrong or inappropriate tooth, leaving behind a tumor, infected sinus with inspissated pus or diseased tooth. Additionally, long-term consequences can occur with abnormal wear of opposing teeth and mesial drift of adjacent teeth that, over time, can lead to periodontal pockets and further dental disease.

Careful and complete examination of the equine patient will allow an accurate diagnosis of the dental problem and any associated medical conditions that could possibly cause problems during restraint and anesthesia. Surgery should be planned with facilities and equipment adequate to support the patient. Prolonged

periods of keeping the mouth open with a speculum or rough use of a speculum can also lead to postoperative pain and damage to muscles or to the temporomandibular joint. Special considerations need to be given to upper airway maintenance and lower airway protection from oral fluids and debris. Nasotracheal intubation or a tracheotomy tube may be necessary. Reports in the literature quote the average hospital stay after tooth repulsion to be 2 to 61 days (median 22 days) for maxillary teeth and 3 to 35 days (median 8 days) following mandibular tooth repulsion.[47] Every effort should be made to minimize the patient's postoperative stay thus reducing the chance of acquiring a nosocomial infection and shortening the ultimate recovery phase.

During the surgical procedure, hemorrhage is a consideration from the very nature of the surgery. The nasal turbinates, oral mucosa and sinuses are very vascular. It has been recommended that packing the nasal passages or sinuses is the most important factor in preventing postoperative blood loss. Infusion of balanced electrolyte solutions, hypertonic saline solutions and administration of dobutamine may be needed to maintain adequate blood pressure after severe blood loss. The decision to perform a whole blood transfusion should be made on the basis of mucous membrane color, capillary refill time, oxygen saturation, packed cell volume hemoglobin concentration and arterial blood pressure.[49]

Careful surgical planning and review of anatomy can reduce the chance of damaging structures that should be protected during surgery. The parotid salivary duct, palatine artery, nasolacrimal duct and facial nerves are structures to be considered when surgery is anticipated.

Judicious use of intraoperative radiographs or fluoroscopy are indicated to avoid operative problems such as removal of the wrong tooth or damage to structures adjacent to the tooth being removed (see Fig. 11.21). These would include the palatine artery, mesial or distal alveolar bone and adjacent teeth. Additional radiographs taken after tooth removal are useful in confirming that the proper tooth was removed and the alveolus is clear of unattached pieces of bone, slivers of crown enamel or root fragments (see Fig. 11.12).[50]

Many factors can contribute to delayed healing of the dental socket. In the normal course the vacant alveolus fills with a sterile hematoma. This blood clot, protected from oral contamination, is the framework for a vascularized bed of granulation tissue that migrates inward from the outside margins of the wound, filling the void left by the removal dental crown and roots. The mucosa of the oral cavity, paranasal sinus, nasal passage or skin adjacent to the wound migrates over the bed of granulation tissue and, along with wound contraction, covers the alveolus with a layer of epithelium to complete socket healing. Many factors can delay or completely interrupt this healing process, causing long-term problems for the horse, and in some cases further corrective surgery.

Persistent sinus formation is a common complaint following tooth removal.[34] A sinus is a tubular ulcer that refuses to heal owing to the presence of a foreign body or dead tissue. A draining sinus is lined by granulation tissue and will heal rapidly once the offending material is removed. Sources of sinus formation can be pieces of avascular bone, dental fragments, dental packing materials, feed or debris from the oral cavity, avascular or infected nodules of cementum or any foreign body in the depth of the healing wound. Characteristically, a sinus will discharge purulent material then appear to heal. However the infection or irritation persists and the sinus tract reforms periodically. Transient response is often seen following systemic antibiotic therapy.

The successful treatment of a sinus tract involves removing the cause of the irritation to allow the tract to heal spontaneously. The source of the sinus should be identified with plain and/or contrast radiographs and a complete examination of the involved area should be performed (Fig. 15.31). Generally, it can be determined where the source of the sinus is likely to be and this area should be approached surgically via the most suitable route. Placement of drainage tubes or antibiotic impregnated

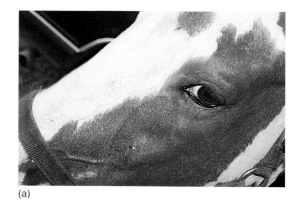
(a)

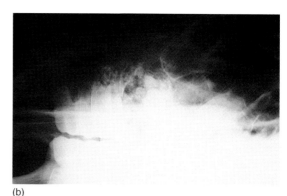
(b)

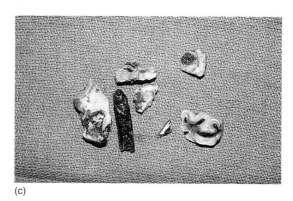
(c)

**Figure 15.31.** (a) A 20-year-old paint gelding with an orocutaneous fistula that had been draining for 2 years. An upper left third cheek tooth (208) had been removed by repulsion and the trephine hole had healed, only to break open and begin draining 6 months after surgery. Repeated bouts of systemic antibiotic therapy and fistula irrigation failed to resolve the problem. (b) A radiograph of the head area revealed a dental socket with radiopaque objects in it. The root of the left upper fourth cheek tooth (209) appears to be fragmented. (c) Dental fragments removed from the alveolus of 208 and a diseased 209. The dental sockets were surgically cleansed and debrided. The mucosal lining of the fistula was removed with a curette. The sockets were covered with a methylmethacrylate patch secured to 207 rostral and 210 caudal. The wound healed without difficulty.

beads of methylmethacrylate and protection of the surgical area from oral contamination can speed healing. Plugging the dental socket with bone cement has been shown to be superior in protecting the alveolus.[34]

A fistula is a similar non-healing wound connecting skin with a mucosal surface or one mucosal surface to another. In a fistula, the tract can be lined with either granulation tissue, scar tissue or epithelium that has grown along it from either or both ends. Dental fistulae can form connecting the oral mucosa to the skin (orocutaneous), to the paranasal sinus (oroantral) or to the nasal mucosa (oronasal). The treatment of fistulae is usually complex and detailed anatomical reconstruction may be required. The tube lining a fistula is covered by epithelium and this must be completely removed to allow the defect to fill with granulation tissue. Fistulae have been known to form over the paranasal sinuses after they have been opened by trephination or a sinus flap. Fistulae between the nasal passages and paranasal sinuses are not usually a concern and can be useful in some situations to allow better ventral drainage of the paranasal sinuses.

Detailed descriptions for management of surgical and post surgical complications can be found in the literature.[34,42,50,51] The objective to exodontia should be to carefully plan and execute the extraction and protect the dental socket, thereby minimizing complications.

## ACKNOWLEDGEMENTS

Dave Becker, Central Kentucky Equine Practitioner. For referrel of the case for Figure 15.1.

Jeff Greer, Waddy, Kentucky. For referrel of the case used for Figure 15.10.

Peter Emily, DDS Colorado, For collection of the skull and models used in Figures 15.23 a–j.

## REFERENCES

1. Harvey CE (1994) The history of veterinary dentistry part one: from the earliest record to the end of the 18th century. *Journal of Veterinary Dentistry*, 11(4), 135–139.
2. Kertesz P (1993) *Colour Atlas of Veterinary Dentistry and Oral Surgery*. Wolf Med Pub Co, London.
3. Blunderville T (1566) *The fower chiefyst offices belonging to horsemanshippe*. London.
4. Markham G (1723) *Markham's masterpiece*, G Conyers, London.
5. Bartlett J (1782) *The gentleman's farriery*. London.
6. Merillat LA (1906) Equine dentistry and diseases of the mouth. *Veterinary Surgery, Vol. 1*, Alex Eber, Chicago, Chap. – *Tooth Removal*.
7. Hofmeyr CFB (1974) The digestive system. In: *Textbook of Large Animal Surgery*, ed. EW Oehme and JE Prier, William and Wilkins, Baltimore.
8. Frank ER (1964) *Veterinary Surgery* (7th edn). Burgess Publishing, Minneapolis.
9. Cook WR (1965/1966) Dental surgery in the horse. *British Equine Veterinary Association Bulletin*.
10. Baker GJ (1972) Surgery of the head and neck. In: *Equine Medicine and Surgery* (2nd edn), ed. RA Manesmann and ES Mcallister, American Veterinary Publications, Wheaton, IL, pp. 752–791.
11. Orsini PG (1992) Oral cavity. In: *Equine Surgery*, ed. JA Auer, WB Saunders, Philadelphia, pp. 296–305.
12. Pascoe J (1991) Complications of dental surgery. *Proceedings of the 37th Annual Meeting of the American Association of Equine Practitioners*, 37, 141.
13. Prichard MA, Hackett RP and Erb HN (1989) Tooth repulsion in horses: complications and long-term outcome. *Proceedings of the 35th Annual Meeting of the American Association of Equine Practitioners*, 35, 331.
14. Conner HD *et al.* (1967) Bacteremias following periodontal scaling in patients with healthy appearing gingiva. *Journal of Periodontology*, 38: 466–471.
15. Black AP *et al.* (1980) Bacteremia during ultrasonic teeth cleaning and extraction in the dog. *Journal of American Animal Hospital Association*, 1980, 16: 611–616.
16. Hamlin RL (1991) A theory for the genesis of certain chronic degenerative diseases of aged dogs. *Veterinary Scope*, 1(1), 6–10.
17. McIlwraith CW (1984) Equine digestive system. In: *The Practice of Large Animal Surgery*, ed. PB Jennings, WB Saunders, pp.554–664.
18. Garcia F, Sanroman and Lioneno MP (1990) Endodonics in the horse: an experimental study. *Journal of Veterinary Medicine*.
19. Pascoe RR (1980) Surgical Removal of all Incisors and Canine Teeth from a mature Thoroughbred Stallion. *Australian Veterinary Practitioner*, (10) 4, 253–251.
20. Sisson S and Grossman JD (1965) Digestive system of the horse. In: *The Anatomy of Domestic Animals* (4th edn), ed. R Getty, WB Saunders, Philadelphia, p. 387.
21. Nickel R, Schummer A and Seiferle E (1979) *The Viscera of Domestic Animals* (2nd edn). Paul Parey, Berlin and Hamburg.
22. Grove TK (1991) Extractions and simple oral surgery in equines. *Proceedings of the Eastern States Veterinary Conference*, vol. 5, 337.

23. Colyer JF (1990) *Variations and Diseases of the Teeth of Animals* (revised edn), Cambridge University Press, Cambridge.

24. Mair T, Love S, Schumacher J and Watson E (1998) *Equine Medicine, Surgery and Reproduction.* WB Saunders, Philadelphia, p. 106.

25. Easley J (1991) Recognition and management of the diseased equine tooth. *Proceedings of the 37th Annual Meeting of the American Association of Equine Practitioners*, 37, 129–139.

26. Guard WF (1951) *Surgical Principles and Techniques.* Columbus, OH, pp. 78–89.

27. Tremaine WH (1997) Oral extraction of equine cheek teeth: a Victorian technique revisited. *Proceedings of the 5th World Veterinary Dental Congress,* Birmingham, 139–141.

28. Easley KJ (1997) Cheek tooth extraction: an old technique revisited. *Large Animal Practice*, 18(1), 22–24.

29. Easley KJ (1998) Dental care and instrumentation. In: *Veterinary Clinics of North America Equine Practice,* WB Saunders, Philadelphia, August 1998.

30. O'Conner JJ (1942) *Dollar's Veterinary Surgery* (2nd edn). Baillère, Tindall and Cox, London, pp. 250–261.

31. Fischer DJ and Easley KJ (1993) Equine dentistry: proper restraint. *Large Animal Veterinarian*, 49(9), 14–22.

32. Easley KJ and Fischer DJ (1993) Equine dentistry regional anesthesia. *Large Animal Veterinarian*, 48(9), 14–25.

33. Baker GJ (1991) Diseases of the teeth. In: *Equine Medicine and Surgery* (4th edn), vol 1, *American Veterinary Publications*, Goleta, CA, pp. 551–570.

34. Dixon PM (1997) Post-extraction oro-maxillary (antral) fistula: is a bone cement prosthesis the solution? *Proceedings of the 5th World Veterinary Dental Congress,* Birmingham, 147–150.

35. Williams WL (1906) Surgical and Obstetrical Operations, 2nd ed., Published by the author, Uthica, N.Y., 1–16.

36. Evans LH, Tate LP and LaDow CS (1981) Extraction of the equine 4th upper premolar and 1st and 2nd upper molars through a lateral buccotomy. *Proceedings of the 27th Annual Meeting of the American Association of Equine Practitioners*, 27, p. 249.

37. Lane JF and Kertesz P (1993) Equine dental surgery. In: *A Colour Atlas of Veterinary Dentistry on Oral Surgery*, ed. P Kertesz, Wolf, London, pp. 35–50.

38. Lane GJ (1997) Equine dental extraction – repulsion vs buccotomy: techniques and results. *Proceedings of the 5th World Veterinary Dental Congress,* Birmingham, 135–138.

39. McIllwraith CW and Turner SA (1987) *Equine Surgery: Advanced Techniques.* Lea and Febiger, Philadelphia, pp. 260–263.

40. Howarth S (1995) Equine dental surgery. *Journal of Veterinary Postgraduate Clinical Study 'In Practice'*, 17, 178–188.

41. Schumacher J and Honnas CM (1993) Dental surgery. In *Veterinary Clinics of North America Equine Practice*, 9(1), 133–152.

42. Orsini PG, Ross MW and Hamir AN (1992) Levator nasolabilis muscle transposition for prevention of oro-sinus fistulation following tooth extraction in the horse. *Veterinary Surgery*, 21(2), 150–156.

43. Wheat JD (1973) Sinus drainage and tooth repulsion in the horse. *Proceedings of the 19th Annual Meeting of the American Association of Equine Practitioners*, 171.

44. Schneider JE (1974) The respiratory system. In: *Textbook of Large Animal Surgery*, eds FW Oehme and JE Prier, William and Wilkins, Baltimore.

45. Trotter GW (1993) Paranasal sinus. In: *Veterinary Clinics of North America Equine Practice*, 9(1), 153–169.

46. Scrutchfield WL, Schumacher J, Walker M and Crabill M (1994) Removal of an osteoma from the paranasal sinuses of a standing horse. *Equine Practice*, 16, 24–28.

47. Prichard MA, Hackett RP and Erb HN (1992) Long-term outcome of tooth repulsion in horses, a retrospective study of 61 cases. *Veterinary Surgery*, 21(2), 145–149.

48. Baker GJ (1979) Dental diseases in horses. *Journal of Veterinary Postgraduate Clinical Study 'In Practice'*, November 1979, 19–26.

49. Trimm CM, Eaton SA, Pharm B and Parks AH (1997) Severe nasal hemorrhage in an anesthetized horse. *JAVMA*, 210, 1324–1327.

50. Baker GJ (1982) Dental disorders in the horse. *The Compendium on Cont Ed*, 4(12), 5507–5514.

51. Leitch M (1997) *Complication of dental surgery and postoperative management. Handout notes from Int Equine Dental Tech Annual Meeting*, Cochranville, PA, September.

# 16

# ENDODONTIC THERAPY

Gordon J Baker, BVSc, PhD., MRCVS, Diplomate ACVS, University of Illinois, College of Veterinary Medicine, Urbana, IL 61802

## INTRODUCTION

Endodontics is that branch of dentistry that covers the diagnosis, management and prophylaxis of diseases of the dental pulp and periapical tissues.[1] As early as 1884, it was commented that 'A few moments consideration of the original cause of trouble at the apex of roots will enable us to realize what is required to be accomplished in the way of successful treatment. If the original cause is admitted to be irritation from decomposing pulp, its removal will, in most cases, affect a cure.'[2]

In man, at least, dental caries and dental trauma are the most common causes of acute pulpitis. The etiopathogenesis of pulpitis in the horse is less well documented, but it is seen that trauma, impaction, periodontal disease and caries of cementum may all be involved.[3] Prior to 1900, many surgical techniques were developed that did, in many cases, successfully drain and resolve periapical abscesses and preserve the teeth.[4]

Many of the principles of endodontic therapy used in man can be applied to the horse and in recent years, clinical experience and case results have shown success in preserving teeth.[5,6] As in man, the re-implantation of teeth – particularly incisors – is frequently successful in that the teeth and associated permanent tooth germs have survived. It is not uncommon, however, for maleruptions to follow such events. In 1959 it was suggested that some cases of 'alveolar periostitis' in young horses could be managed by apicoectomy (root end resection) and drain-age of root abscesses.[7] More recently, mixed results have been reported from pulp ablation and root canal therapy in horses. The indications are that the results are better in mandibular teeth than maxillary teeth.[5] In an experimental study of a coronal access (through erupted crown) to the pulp chamber of normal incisor teeth in the horse, it was shown that when 44 incisor teeth of 8 horses aged from 6 to 11 years of age were treated, there were no surgical complications and the teeth continued to erupt and to wear over an 18-month period.[8]

In this chapter, the principles of endodontic therapy will be described together with important guidelines for the choice of care and the management of complications and sequelae.

## MANAGEMENT OF ACUTE PULP EXPOSURE

Accidental fractures of the teeth may expose the pulp. In some instances this may occur during dental work when incisor bites (e.g. parrot-mouthed horses) or major arcade irregularities and overgrown teeth are cut. Under such circumstances the clinicians should be prepared to offer first aid that is directed at minimizing the degree of pulp necrosis and complications. It has frequently been claimed that pulp exposure under such conditions does not require treatment as the natural defense mechanisms of reparative dentin are adequate and no complications result. In fact, in some species it is routine, as a management technique, to cut particular teeth, for example the canines of piglets and fighting teeth (canines) of new world camelids (llamas). This apparent conflict in complication detection is possibly due largely to lack of observation. If cases in which the pulp has been exposed are followed up, it will be found that at least 25% of them develop apical swellings that are painful to pressure and which may form root abscessations. In young animals, when deciduous teeth are involved, these swellings are often missed and many complications resolve when the permanent teeth erupt.

When the crown is fractured and the pulp exposed, it should be either capped or the pulp removed by a pulpotomy procedure. Many materials have been used as pulp-capping agents. Most of these supplement the most widely used material, calcium hydroxide. The supplementation consists of the use of enzymes, antiseptics, antibiotics and anti-inflammatory agents.[9,10] Pulp capping is the covering of exposed pulp with a medicated dressing in an attempt to preserve the pulp's vitality. Pulpotomy is the removal of the coronal portion of the pulp and covering of the remaining pulp to inhibit periapical disease and preserve the vitality of the radicular (tooth root) pulp tissues.

Calcium hydroxide has been the material of choice since the 1930s.[11] Prior to that time, pulp therapy had consisted of the application of arsenic and other fixative agents that devitalized the exposed pulp. The advantages of calcium hydroxide are its initial devitalization of contact pulp and contiguous tissues, followed by the formation of a dentin bridge (reparative dentin) at the junction of the necrotic and vital tissues. The exact mechanism of this process is not clearly understood, however, when other compounds of similar alkalinity (pH 11) are used, an extremely unhealthy liquefactive necrosis takes place. Consequently calcium hydroxide (e.g. Pulpdent, Henry Schein Inc. 5, Harbor Park Drive, Port Washington, New York 11050) has remained the material of choice.

## TECHNIQUE FOR TOOTH CAPPING

The extent and duration of pulp exposure is evaluated and documented. If necessary, crown fragments from the damaged tooth are removed and prepared. Depending on the site of the tooth this may be carried out under sedation and peripheral nerve blocks. Some cases will require general anesthesia to facilitate the procedure. It is important that damaged pulp tissue be removed. The use of an operative loupe (for magnification) and spoon excavator allow the surgeon to cut down to the vital pulp. Any hemorrhage must be controlled before the pulp cap material (calcium hydroxide) is applied. This may be achieved by epinephrine mixed with saline washes and by pressure packing. The use of vacuum and air drying achieves the ideal operative site. Calcium hydroxide is mixed according to the manufacturer's instructions and used to cover the exposed pulp.

Care is then taken, once the material has set up, to modify the occlusal contact made by the treated tooth so that occlusion is prevented for 3 months or more. In this manner the reparative dental bridge is completely formed before attrition from dental wear begins. In the horse, provided occlusal contact is avoided, then additional restorative covers are not needed over the calcium hydroxide.

Follow-up care requires that the tooth apex be monitored for periapical swellings and gingival ulceration and bone erosion (radiographic check-ups may be indicated). If complications arise it may be necessary to either complete a pulpectomy or extract the tooth.

Pulpectomy may also be used when there is chronic coronal pulp exposure. In such cases, the pulp chamber is opened from the crown or from the fracture site. The pulp chamber is cleaned out and prepared for filling (see root end resection pp. 251–254).

## SURGICAL ENDODONTICS

In clinical practice most cases of pulpitis are not presented in the acute stage of the disease. The diagnosis of pulp infection is based on clinical findings and radiographic analysis. The selection of endodontic therapy versus tooth extraction in the management of equine dental disease is based upon the summation of the following observations: (a) the absence of other significant disease, (b) the localization of the periradicular disease process, (c) the availability of equipment and operative expertise and (d) client compliance and economic factors.

It is particularly important that the clinician evaluates if there are local factors indicating complications. Mandibular fistulae should be probed and pressure flushed to ensure there is no periodontal leakage. If there is active periodontal leakage or accompanying periradicular pathology, for example maxillary sinus empyema, this may inhibit the use of root end resection, endodontic therapy and tooth preservation. In young horses (4 to 6 years old), there may not be adequate maturation of the tooth roots to enable root filling to be achieved. There are only a few anecdotal stories of successful endodontic therapy in young horses. The technique of apexification, to promote root closure, is an important precursor of endodontic therapy. Apexification (surgical exposure, drainage of periradicular disease and application of calcium hydroxide), however, requires more than one general anesthetic and consequently may not be acceptable to the client. During interactions between clinician and client the potential of failure of endodontic techniques and ultimate extraction of the diseased tooth must be discussed. The client's compliance may be achieved if it is explained that endodontic success will avoid all the complications of tooth extraction, and if it fails then at least every effort has been made to save the tooth. The economics may then be weighed by both the veterinarian and the owner to allow a management plan to be agreed upon.

## TECHNIQUE FOR ROOT END RESECTION

The terms surgical endodontics, apicoectomy and root end resection are synonymous. In this account the term root end resection will be used. As has been described, it is commonly seen that the indications for endodontic therapy in the horse are the clinical signs associated with periradicular disease, swellings, drainage and radiological evidence of apical haloes (or bone lysis). A final check for conditions suitable for endodontic surgery are carried out under general anesthesia and include testing for periodontal leakage into and from the oral cavity as well as crown impactions. The relief, by interproximal grinding, of occlusal impaction should be carried out as the first procedure in the endodontic treatment surgery.

## EQUIPMENT

In addition to the equipment and facilities for general anesthesia with monitoring, general surgical instruments and the use of intra-operative radiology, the following are required for root end resection and endodontic therapy:

1. suction
2. electrical hemostasis (diathermy)
3. bone trephines and rongeurs (angled and straight)
4. low and high speed drills with 10:1 reduction hand piece
5. diamond discs and abrasive burrs
6. short and long inverted cone burrs
7. lentula spiral
8. endodontic files and broaches
9. endodontic spoon excavator
10. periodontal probes and explorer
11. 2 per cent hypochlorite solution
12. paper points
13. zinc oxide powder and eugenol
14. glass mixing slab, syringes
15. plastic instruments and spatula
16. gutta-percha (warm gutta-percha delivery system is ideal, e.g. Obtura II system)
17. endodontic spreaders
18. amalgam, mixer and carrier
19. as an alternative to amalgam is Super EBA with Alumina (Bosworth Co., Skokie, IL).

Equipment required for hemostatic support:

1. diathermy
2. suction
3. saline with 8 per cent epinephrine
4. retraction cord (SilTrax, Pascal Co. Inc. 2929 N.E. Northrup Way, Bellevue, WA 98004).

## SURGICAL TECHNIQUE

Successful endodontic therapy in the horse, defined as the resolution of periradicular disease, and the retention and continued eruption of the diseased tooth, is dependent upon the application of good endodontic technique.

### Access

After completing the oral examination, correction or relief of impactions and final radiographic analysis, drape off the surgical site after routine clipping, shaving and skin sterilization. Approach through a cruciate skin incision with retraction of the periosteum along the incision lines. The precise site is tooth dependent, it is easier to complete the root canal procedure on 107, 108, 207 or 208 if the horse is positioned on its back. Maxillary teeth are approached from a dorsolateral site. Bone over the disease root is removed by using a combination of a trephine, rongeurs and a Hall air drill. Complete exposure of the site is essential to afford complete excision of all periradicular disease. This is relatively easy in mandibular teeth but more difficult in maxillary teeth. In some cases of maxillary tooth disease associated with sinus empyema this may prove to be impossible and it may mean that the endodontic therapy treatment option is abandoned at this stage and the tooth is repelled.

After suitable exposure, the root end is divided using either a diamond disc attached to the dental drill and reduction hand piece or it may be cut off with a conical abrasive burr. The object is to produce an angled cut which is shorter to the outside on a 15 to 20 degree plane.

### Sterilization

It has been documented that inadequate sterilization of the diseased pulp chamber is the cause of long-term complications and failure of endodontics. Sterilization is achieved by the physical removal of all of the non-vital, necrotic pulp tissue, and this is done by shaving away portions of the dentinal walls with a file. Thorough and high-volume irrigation of the cavities with sterile saline and 2.5 per cent sodium hypochlorite solution is essential in this procedure. The complexity of the shape of the pulp chambers of the horse, however, makes endodontic curettage, (filing etc.) particularly difficult and it means that complete cleansing of the pulp chamber is almost impossible. However, if carried out thoroughly with complete sealing and obturation, success is still achieved. This may be explained using the 'Dom Perignon' analogy, that is if you place a perfect cork in the bottle, the result inside the bottle is champagne not vinegar. Hence, the key to success is in sealing, obturation and root end closure.

## OBTURATION

Obturation is the process of complete filling of the exposed pulp chamber. The objectives are first to eliminate all avenues of leakage from the oral cavity or the periradicular tissues into the root canal system. Second, effective obturation should seal within the system any irritants that cannot be fully removed during canal cleaning and shaping. This recognizes that microbial irritants (micro-organisms, toxins and inflammatory products from pulp residues) are the prime cause of pulpal disease and its subsequent extension in periradicular disease.[12] The American Association of Endodontists has defined obturation as the three-dimensional filling of the entire root canal system as close to the cementodentinal junction as possible. Biologically compatible root canal sealers are used in conjunction with the core filling material to establish an adequate seal.[13]

A plethora of materials have been used over the past 150 years for root canal filling in man and historically, gutta-percha has been the material of choice. Despite its relative lack of rigidity and adhesiveness and its ease of displacement under pressure, it is still the ideal material for use in retrograde filling, after root end resection, as done in the horse.

The characteristics of the ideal root canal filling, as modified after Grossman *et al.*[14] by Wiggs and Lobprise[15] are that it is

1   easily manipulated and placed, allowing adequate working time prior to setting up

2  dimensionally stable, there is no shrinkage or expansion after compaction

3  conformable and adaptable to the various shapes and contours of the canal, while sealing it apically (coronally in retrograde filling) and laterally

4  non-irritating to periapical tissue (this is not significant in the horse where retrograde filling is the rule)

5  non-porous, impervious to moisture

6  unaffected and insoluble in tissue fluids; incapable of corroding or oxidizing

7  bacteriostatic

8  non-staining to dental or peridental structures (this is not significant in the horse where retrograde filling is the rule)

9  sterile or easily and quickly sterilized for immediate use

10  removable without difficulty

11  biologically unharmful

12  radiopaque.

In practice, the combination of gutta-percha and a mixture of zinc oxide and eugenol affects the best material. After exposure and preparation/sterilization, it is key for the endodontist to be able to work in a dry surgical field. The root canal and pulp chamber is dried with paper points and warm air and the periradicular area is packed off to control osseous bleeding. The surgical assistant should have the primary responsibility of ensuring the integrity of the working area using suction and packing. The zinc oxide and eugenol mixture is mixed on the glass slab so that it will form a thick viscus mixture that can be injected by syringe through an 18 guage catheter. The pulp chamber is then lined with this material and filled with gutta-percha. This process is made easier using the entrance heating systems for intracanal softening of gutta-percha before compaction (such as the Obtura II system, Obtura Corp, Fenton, MO).[13] Canal and chamber obturation may be checked using lateral and oblique radiographs.

## APICAL SEALS

As the root canal filler sets up, the clinician uses either the short or the long inverted cone burr to construct an apical inlay cut to hold the apical sealer. The size of this apex after root end resection may well be quite large and require multiple mixes of standard amalgam to fill. This introduces the potential for an incongruity of amalgam sealer and subsequent failure of the seal. For this reason, although more expensive, other seals may be used such as glass ionomers or Super EBA.

Having completed the procedure, the apex is packed with a surgical dressing and the surgical site closed leaving drainage access.

Postoperative care includes analgesic and anti-inflammatory drugs (Phenylbutazone) and antibiotics. The surgical site is checked daily and the wound pack removed after 3 to 4 days. Special diets are usually not needed in the care of horses after endodontic therapy (see Figures 16.1–16.10 for endodontic technique)

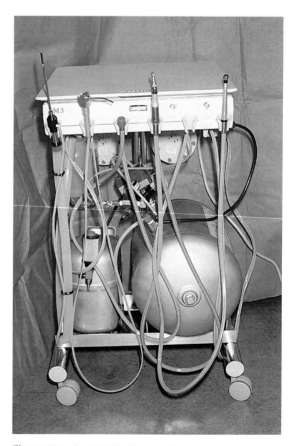

**Figure 16.1.** Dental drill with reduction gear handpiece.

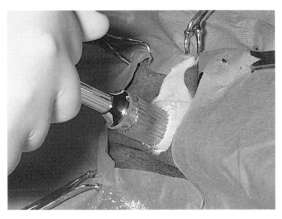

Figure 16.2.

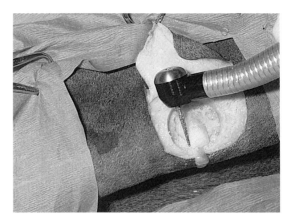

Figure 16.3.

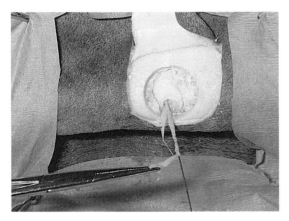

Figure 16.4.

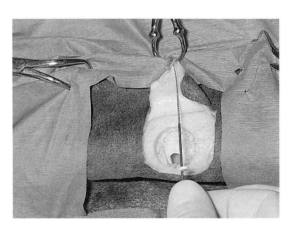

Figure 16.5.

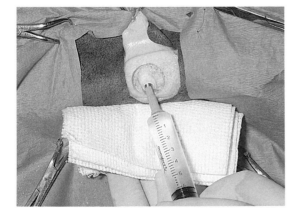

Figure 16.6.

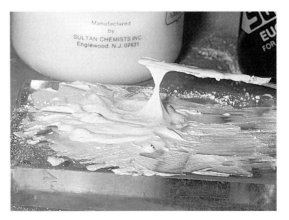

Figure 16.7.

**Figures 16.2–16.10.** Endodontic technique: documented in anatomical preparations.

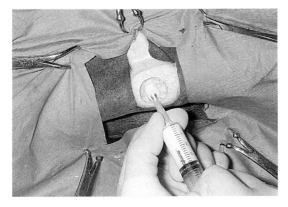

**Figure 16.8.**

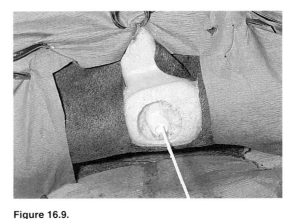

**Figure 16.9.**

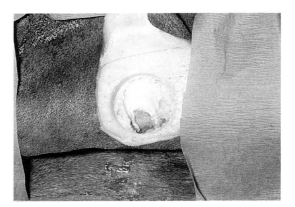

**Figure 16.10.**

## RESULTS OF ENDODONTIC THERAPY IN THE HORSE

The literature contains a number of descriptions of the use of endodontic techniques but there are no detailed accounts of long-term follow up of the results and complications. It has been shown in experimental studies of endodontic therapy in the normal incisor teeth of horses that in 44 teeth that were treated and followed over an 18-month period, there continued to be normal eruption and wear. In personal communications with numerous veterinarians in the USA, Canada, Europe and Australia, the author estimates that with careful case selection up to 80 per cent success may be achieved. It appears that experience with endodontic technique and care in case selection, particularly in the maturity of the teeth affected, are the key factors to success.[16]

The following is an analysis of some 42 endodontic therapies carried out at the University of Illinois over the past 12 years. There were thirty-eight horses, four of which had two separate teeth treated, either 306 and 307 or 406 and 407. Of the forty-two treatments, only two were in horses under 3 years of age, and only nine involved maxillary teeth. No success was achieved in five maxillary teeth in association with sinus empyema on initial therapies, in four of these cases the teeth were subsequently extracted and the other one had two follow-up periradicular drainage procedures with an eventual successful outcome. Four horses with periradicular disease associated with 108 or 208 had successful outcomes (Figs 16.11–16.14). The 33 other teeth were all rostral mandibular teeth. There were seven distal root 307s, five distal root 407s, nine mesial root 308s and four mesial root

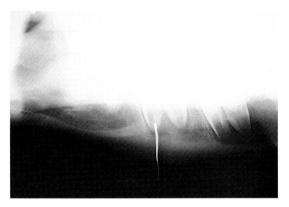

**Figure 16.11.** Mandibular dental fistula rostral root 307.

**Figure 16.12.** Probe along dental track.

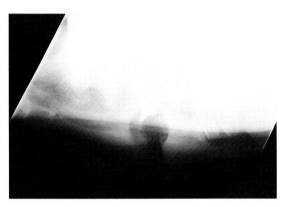

**Figure 16.13.** 1 month post root end resection.

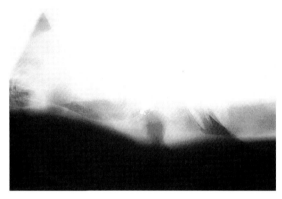

**Figure 16.14.** 6 months post root end resection.

408s, two each distal root 308 and 408 and two and one proximal root 309 and 409 respectively. Of the mandibular teeth, the mean duration of clinical signs was 6 months (range 2 to 14 months). Of the 33 mandibular endodontic treatments with follow ups of 8 months and more, only three teeth required further surgery. Of these three, one tooth was preserved and two were extracted. The overall success rate as defined by absence of complications and preservation of the tooth was 32 out of 38 horses (84 per cent).

## SUMMARY

Endodontic therapy, tooth preservation rather than extraction, is a viable technique for use in selected dental disease cases in horses. The keys to success are clear and effective client education leading to compliance, concentration on thorough techniques and adherence to proven endodontic practices.

### REFERENCES

1. Jensen JR and Serene TP (1984) *Fundamentals of Clinical Endodontics.* Kendall Hunt, Dubuque, Iowa, pp. 1–5.
2. Whitehouse W (1884) Dental Decay. *British Dental Journal*, 27, 238–240.
3. Baker GJ (1985) Oral examination and diagnosis: management of oral diseases. In: *Veterinary Dentistry* (1st edn), ed. CE Harvey, WB Saunders, Philadelphia, pp. 217–234.
4. Weinberger BW (1948) *Introduction to the History of Dentistry*, CV Mosby, St Louis, p. 205.
5. Baker GJ and Kirkland DK (1992) Endodontic therapy in the horse. *Proceedings of the 38th Annual Meeting of the American Association of Equine Practitioners*, 329–335.

6. Dixon PM (1997) Dental extraction and endodontic techniques in horses. *Compendium on Continuing Education for the Practicing Veterinarian*, 19, 628–638.

7. Eisenmenger F (1959) Surgical treatment of alveolar periostitis in young horses. *Wienna Tierarzle Mochenschrift*, 46, 51–70.

8. Garcia F, Sanroman and Llonens MP (1990) Endodontics in the horse: an experimental study. *Journal of Veterinary Medicine*, 37, 205–214.

9. Cvek M (1981) Endodontic treatment of traumatized teeth. In: *Traumatic Injuries of the Teeth* (2nd edn), ed. JO Andreasen, WB Saunders, Philadelphia, pp. 318–349.

10. Seltzer S and Bender IB (1990) Pulp capping and pulpotomy. In: *The Dental Pulp Biologic Considerations in Dental Procedures* (3rd edn), eds S Seltzer and IB Bender, Ishiyaku EuroAmerica, St Louis, pp. 215–249.

11. Hermann BW (1930) Dentinobliteran der Wurzelkanale nach der Behandlung mit Kalzium. *Zahertzl Rund*, 39, 888.

12. Naidorf IJ (1974) Clinical microbiology in endodontics. *Dental Clinics of North America*, 18, 329.

13. Gutmann JL and Witherspoon DE (1998) Obturation of the cleaned and shaped root canal system. In: *Pathways of the Pulp* (7th edn), eds H Cohen and RC Burne, CV Mosby, St Louis, pp. 258–361.

14. Grossman LI, Obiet S and Del Rio C (1988) *Endodontics* (11th edn), Lea and Febiger, Philadelphia, pp. 226–245.

15. Wiggs RB and Lobprise H (1997) Basic endodontic therapy. In: *Veterinary Dentistry Principles and Practice*, eds RB Wiggs and H Lobprise, Lippincott-Raven, Philadelphia, pp. 280–328.

16. Emily P, Orsini P, Lobprise HB and Wiggs RB (1997) Oral and dental disease in large animals. In: *Veterinary Dentistry Principles and Practice*, eds RB Wiggs and H Lobprise, Lippincott-Raven, Philadelphia, pp. 559–579.

# MANDIBULAR AND MAXILLARY FRACTURE OSTEOSYNTHESIS

MR Crabill, DVM, Diplomate ACVS, ABVP; CM Honnas, DVM, Diplomate ACVS; Las Colinas Veterinary Clinic, Equine Medical and Surgical Centre, Irving, Texas 75039

## ANATOMY

The equine mandible is composed of two halves that are mirror images of one another. Each hemimandible contains a horizontally oriented body and a vertically oriented ramus. The body is composed of two parts. Rostrally the incisive portion contains the incisor teeth and caudally the molar portion contains the premolar and molar teeth. The interdental space lies between the third incisor tooth and the second premolar tooth. The vertical ramus contains the coronoid and condylar processes at its dorsal aspect (Fig. 17.1). The condylar process comprises the mandibular portion of each temporomandibular joint and articulates with the squamous portion of the temporal bone via an interposing articular

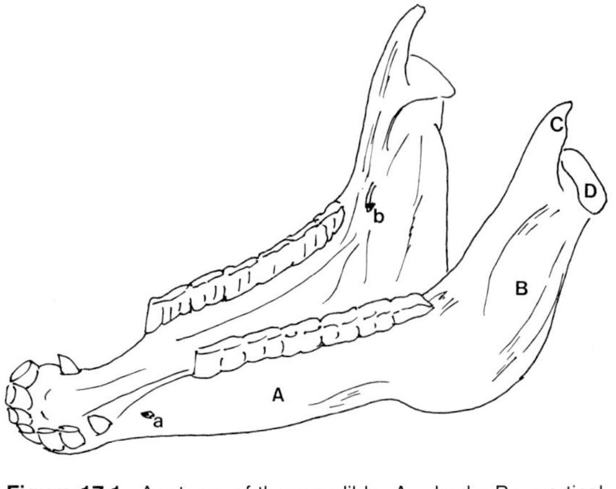

**Figure 17.1.** Anatomy of the mandible. A – body; B – vertical ramus; C – coronoid process; D – condylar process; a – mental foramen; b – mandibular foraminae.

disc. Fusion of the two halves of the mandible occurs along the mandibular symphysis at 2 to 3 months of age.

The mandibular alveolar nerves enter the mandibular foraminae on the medial aspect of each vertical ramus. The mandibular alveolar nerves course through their respective mandibular canals, ventral to the mandibular cheek teeth, innervating the teeth and gingiva.[2] Each mandibular alveolar nerve is accompanied by a mandibular alveolar artery. The mandibular alveolar nerves bifurcate giving rise to the mental nerves which emerge from the mental foraminae, and the inferior alveolar nerves which course rostrally in the incisive portion of the mandible and innervate the canine and incisor teeth and gingiva.[3]

Overlying the lateral aspects of the mandible, the facial artery, facial vein and parotid salivary duct course from medial to lateral across the ventral surface of the bodies of the mandible and turn to course dorsally over the lateral aspects of the mandible along the rostral margin of the masseter muscles. The facial nerve courses rostrally across the lateral aspects of the face, approximately at the level of the cheek teeth. Ventral to the eye the facial nerve divides to supply motor innervation to the ipsilateral upper and lower lips.

Related anatomy of surgical concern on the ventral aspect of the mandible includes the mandibular lymphocenter and the facial artery, facial vein and parotid salivary duct. These structures course rostrally along the medial

259

aspect of each hemimandible before turning to run lateral and dorsal at the rostroventral margin of the masseter muscles.

The mandible changes in shape as the mandibular teeth erupt. The incisive and molar portions of the body of the mandible are thicker in the young horse and thin progressively as reserve crown is reduced as the teeth erupt.[1]

## FRACTURES OF THE MANDIBLE

The mandible is the most commonly fractured bone of the horse.[4] The inquisitive nature of the horse and the use of the lips and nose to gather information about the environment predispose the horse to mandibular trauma. The rostral mandible is not protected by large amounts of soft tissue, rendering the bone more susceptible to trauma. Fractures of the mandible occur after being kicked, after hitting the mandible on solid objects or, in cases of rostral mandibular fractures, catching the mandibular incisors on stationary objects and pulling back.[4-6]

Fractures of the mandible may be categorized by anatomic location[7] including the incisive portion of the body, the interdental space, the molar portion of the body and the vertical ramus including the temporomandibular joint and coronoid process. Fractures of the mandible rostral to the cheek teeth are most commonly encountered, while fractures of the ramus are rare.[5,8]

Clinical signs exhibited by affected horses vary with the site of mandibular fracture.[5] Oral pain is manifested by difficulty or unwillingness to eat. Ptyalism, halitosis and incisor malalignment are the most common clinical signs (Fig. 17.2).[4,9] Fracture of the incisive portion of the mandible may be overlooked due to lack of overt external signs (Fig. 17.3).[10] The majority of rostral mandibular fractures result in avulsion of teeth and contain feed and debris accompanied by a foul odor. Fractures of the interdental space are commonly bilateral and result in instability of the rostral mandible that is readily palpable. Hemorrhage from the oral cavity may be present. Clinical signs of facial swelling, soft tissue trauma, ptyalism, dysphagia and malalignment of teeth should prompt

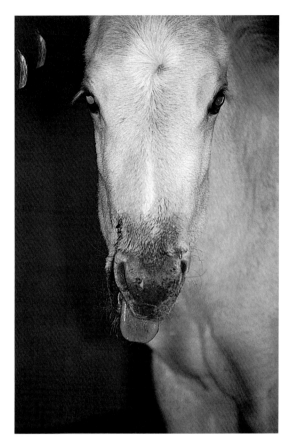

**Figure 17.2.** Appearance of a foal that has sustained a fracture of the mandible through the interdental space of each hemimandible. Because of ventral deviation of the rostral mandible resulting in inability to occlude the incisors, the tongue continually protrudes out the mouth. Neurologic function of the tongue is normal.

an investigation for the presence of a caudal mandibular fracture.[7] Horses with disease of the temporomandibular joints may exhibit external swelling, pain upon palpation of the temporomandibular joint, unwillingness to open the mouth, crepitation, rostral or caudal displacement of the mandible, malocclusion of the caudal cheek teeth preventing apposition of the incisors and crossbite conformation of the incisors.[9-12] Oral examination should always be performed and will enable diagnosis of rostral mandible and interdental space fractures (Fig. 17.3). Mucosal laceration, broken, loose or displaced teeth and malocclusion are oral signs indicating that a mandibular fracture should be suspected. Although temporomandibular joint

ity or unwillingness to eat or drink. Fixation of mandibular fractures can be delayed with little impediment to healing so as to allow stabilization of the horse with fluids. Administration of antimicrobials, non-steroidal anti-inflammatory drugs, and tetanus prophylaxis are indicated. Penicillin is a suitable antimicrobial for most fractures. Broader spectrum antimicrobials are indicated when internal fixation is used.

Following sedation and local or general anesthesia, fracture therapy begins with cleansing and debridement of the fracture line. Feed, blood clots and bone fragments are removed from the fracture and a dilute antiseptic solution (0.1 per cent povidone iodine, 0.05 per cent chlorhexidine) is used to thoroughly lavage the wound. Alignment of the incisor occlusal surfaces is used as a guide during reduction of the fracture. Alignment of the fracture may be maintained by an assistant during surgical fixation or by wiring the incisors of the incisive bone and the mandible together.[5] Lacerations and tears of the gingival mucosa may be sutured using polypropylene or polydioxanone in a simple continuous or continuous horizontal mattress pattern, or allowed to heal by second intention.

Fractures involving alveoli can result in infectious periodontitis and pulpitis necessitating removal of the tooth. The decision to remove affected teeth should be deferred until the fracture has healed.[5] Premolar and molar teeth may lend stability to the mandible during healing as compared to an empty alveolus. Detached and broken teeth are candidates for removal.[4] Loose incisors may be wired in place and can be used to bolster repairs in some cases.[10] Exposed permanent teeth that are unerupted should be left in place and manipulated as little as possible. If viability of a tooth is in question, it may be left in place and removed, if necessary, after bony healing has occurred.[4]

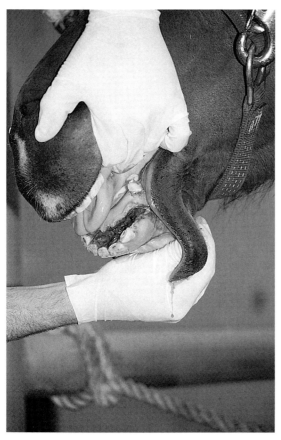

**Figure 17.3.** Fracture of the incisive portion of the mandible. The horse looked normal on clinical presentation and had no externally obvious clinical signs that a fracture had occurred.

injuries are uncommon, palpation of the joints is advisable.

Radiography is indicated for fractures caudal to the incisor teeth. Radiography of rostral fractures involving only the incisors may not be indicated in every case based on findings of a physical examination. Lateral, dorsoventral and oblique views allow fracture definition and comparison to the contralateral portion of the mandible. Intra-oral placement of radiographic cassettes will allow better definition of rostral mandibular fractures. Improved definition of the condyle and coronoid process of the ramus is obtained by taking a lateral projection with the mouth held open with a speculum.[10,11]

The overall general health of the horse and cardiovascular status should be assessed, especially in horses with fractures that cause inabil-

## FRACTURES INVOLVING THE INCISIVE PORTION OF THE MANDIBLE OR MAXILLA

Fractures of the rostral incisive portion of the mandible are common and are amenable to fixation in most settings. Evaluation and fixation of these fractures may be completed in the standing sedated horse. Anesthesia of the mandibular alveolar nerves at either the mandibular alveolar foramina or the mental foramina will facilitate debridement and fixation of these fractures in the standing horse.

Oral examination reveals the extent of the fracture and teeth involved. 'Corner fractures', running from midline near the first or second incisor to the area of the ipsilateral third incisor are common. Radiographs can be used to define fractures of the incisive portion of the mandible but are often not necessary in most cases.

Appropriate attention to debridement of the fracture line will facilitate reduction of the fracture.[13] Wire fixation is widely used to stabilize rostral mandibular fractures involving the incisors. Wire fixation carries the advantage of providing a stable fixation along the tension surface of the mandible and is an uncomplicated method. A minimum of one wire is used on each side of the fracture with overlapping of the wires.[13] Exact placement of wires is dependent on the configuration of the fracture. Holes are placed between the incisive teeth at the gingival margin using a Steinman pin or 3.2 mm drill bit. Cannulation of the holes with a 14 gage needle facilitates placement of the wire between teeth (Fig. 17.4). Fourteen gage needles may be used in young horses without prior drilling of holes. The occlusive surfaces of the incisors are aligned to attain proper fracture reduction.[5] Stainless-steel wire, 1.2 mm or larger, is placed through the holes, twisted together on the labial surface of the mandible and bent down into the gingiva. Fencing pliers are useful for tightening the wires. Wires should be pulled away from the gingiva as they are twisted together to avoid breakage during the tightening process. Notches may be cut into the caudal margin of the third incisor teeth or canine teeth to allow the wire to be anchored around these structures. Holes may be drilled through the mandible in the interdental space, permitting wire placement from the incisors in a caudal direction (Fig. 17.5).[5] Suturing mucosal lacerations prevents continued gross contamination of the fracture site but is not necessary in most cases.

Fractures of the rostral mandible involving the incisors can propagate caudally into the

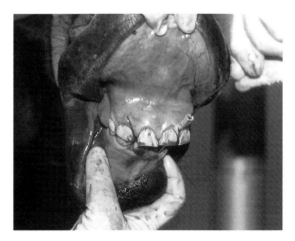

**Figure 17.4.** Cannulation of pre-drilled holes with a 14 gage needle, facilitates wire placement when repairing rostral maxillary or mandibular fractures.

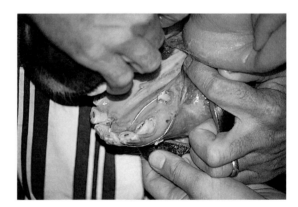

**Figure 17.5.** Repair of the corner fracture in Figure 17.3 was accomplished with wire placed on either side of the fracture. This photograph was taken 6 weeks postoperatively when the horse presented for removal of wire implants. Healing was uncomplicated with a good cosmetic result.

interdental space creating large bone fragments. A combination of wire fixation and pins or cortical bone screws is indicated in these instances to provide stability that cannot be obtained with wire fixation alone.[9,14] Following preparation of the fracture, reduction is achieved and may be maintained with reduction forceps during implant placement. Pins or cortical bone screws placed in lag fashion are placed strategically to provide compression across the fracture line. Stab incisions are made in the gingiva and a drill guide is used to protect surrounding soft tissues. Implants should be placed so as to avoid tooth roots. The size and configuration of the fragments will dictate the number of implants used. Concurrent wire fixation is used as needed to counter rotational instability.[14] Implants are removed 8 weeks after fixation.

After fixation of rostral mandibular incisive fractures the horse may be fed hay and grain. Hay should be pulled apart so the horse does not have to prehend with the repaired teeth. Grazing grass or eating other feeds requiring cutting with the incisors is prohibited until the fracture has healed. Daily examination of the wires is indicated to identify loose or broken wires. The mouth may be rinsed with water to remove feed material trapped in wires or to lavage open wounds. Wires are removed from the oral cavity 4 to 8 weeks postoperatively. The prognosis for healing of these fractures is good to excellent. Ultimate cosmetics of the dentition is dependent on the damage that has occurred to the teeth and permanent tooth buds during the original injury.

## FRACTURES OF THE INTERDENTAL SPACE

Fractures through the interdental space commonly involve the left and right sides of the mandible, causing instability of the rostral aspect of the mandible.[7] Fractures of the maxillary interdental space can also occur but are not as commonly encountered (Fig. 17.6). A full radiographic series, including dorsoventral, lateral and oblique views, is indicated to delineate the fracture and identify involvement of adjacent teeth and the presence of osseous fragments. Fractures of the mandibular interdental space are most often transverse or short oblique in configuration with minimal comminution.[10]

Fixation of fractures involving the interdental space is performed under general anesthesia. Intravenous anesthesia or nasotracheal intubation increases space for the surgeon to work in the oral cavity and is recommended in most cases. Dorsal recumbency is recommended as it permits the surgeon to access both sides of the mandible. Methods of fixation of fractures of the interdental space include tension-band wiring, oral acrylic splints, U-bars, external fixators and bone plating.[4–7,10]

Fractures of the interdental space that are not significantly displaced and have sufficient interdigitation at the fracture line limiting movement, may be repaired using tension-band wiring.[5–7,10] The tension surface of the mandible lies along the dorsal border (oral surface) allowing tension-band wiring to be successful when minimal displacement is present.

Following anesthesia of the patient and preparation of the oral cavity and left and right external cheek surfaces for surgery, holes are drilled between all mandibular incisors as described above. Stab incisions are made bilaterally through the cheek over the space between the second and third mandibular premolar teeth. Hemorrhage is minimized by incising through the skin and using blunt dissection to separate underlying soft tissues.[7] The buccal mucosa is incised and the drill bit is positioned between the second and third premolars just ventral to the gingival margin.[5] Soft tissues are protected during drilling by use of a drill guide. Wire is threaded through the holes between the premolar teeth and directed rostrally to be laced through holes previously made between the incisors. Differing patterns for wire placement may be used incorporating one or two wires.[5–7] The wire spanning the interdental space is twisted together to increase compression at the fracture line.[6,7] The stab incisions through the cheeks are left to heal by second intention or closed with a single suture. The wires are removed 6 to 8 weeks after fixation.

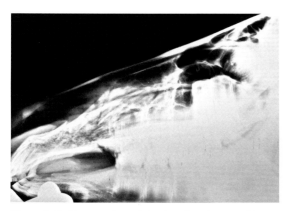

**Figure 17.6.** Fracture through the interdental space of the maxilla in a young horse. These fractures are not as common as fractures through the same location in the mandible.

Intra-oral acrylic splints provide stable fixation of interdental space fractures and are technically easy to use.[7,10,15] Following anesthesia and preparation of the oral cavity and cheeks, multiple 1.2 mm wire loops are placed through holes drilled into both sides of the mandible rostral and caudal to the fracture line. Loops of wire are formed to extend into the mouth past the lingual aspect of the mandible. The wire ends are left on the buccal or labial aspect of the mandible. Wire loops may also be placed around the second premolar teeth to provide anchorage at sites caudally.[7] Holes for these wires are placed as described above for tension-band wiring. Polymethylmethacrylate or cold-curing acrylic is mixed and molded to fit the oral surface of the mandible and incorporate the wire loops. A thickness of 6 to 8 mm is sufficient for most splints; the acrylic may be thickened at sites of wire incorporation to reduce fatigue and breakage of the splint.[10,13] The acrylic splint should be molded along the horizontal bodies of the mandible and the premolars, leaving room for the tongue. After the acrylic has hardened the free wire ends are twisted together and bent down into the gingiva.

Intra-oral acrylic splints require minimal surgical invasion of the mandible, avoid the risk of damage to tooth buds or roots and provide fixation along the tension side of the fracture.[9] Acrylic splinting can be used successfully in foals that have not erupted incisors suitable for placement of wires.[15] When molding the splint, care should be taken to avoid the presence of sharp points or edges. The oral cavity should be flushed daily and the splint inspected for breakage. The splint is removed 6 to 8 weeks after surgery and can often be removed with the patient sedated and standing.

Intra-oral placement of U-bars with fixation around the teeth using wire has been described to treat fractures of the interdental space.[4,5,16,17] Aluminum rod, 6.3 to 9.5 mm is contoured to fit around the labial and buccal aspect of the mandibular incisors and second and third premolar teeth, respectively. Holes are drilled into the bar corresponding with the sites between the rostral second and third cheek teeth and incisor teeth. The rod may be flattened to make drilling

through the bar easier. Holes are drilled between the mandibular premolar teeth and the incisors as previously described. Stab incisions in the cheeks are necessary to access the sites between the premolar teeth. If accessible, the fracture site is debrided, lavaged and reduced. The formed rod is placed in the oral cavity around the mandibular teeth and the holes in the bar are aligned with holes between the teeth. Wire (1.2 mm) is placed through the bar, around an adjacent premolar or incisor tooth, and then back through the bar. Wire ends are twisted together on the buccal and labial aspect of the teeth and bent down into the gingiva to prevent laceration.

Placement of wire through holes in the bar and between teeth is difficult due to lack of visualization and limited working space. As an alternative, fixation of the U-bar to the teeth has been performed (Honnas, unpublished data, 1997) (Fig. 17.7). The bar is contoured prior to surgery as described previously and 5.0 mm holes are drilled in the bar at sites corresponding to the rostral 2 premolar teeth. Stab incisions are made in the cheeks over the premolar teeth and the bar is positioned following reduction of the fracture. Holes are drilled into the premolar teeth with a 3.2 mm drill bit and are tapped to accept a 4.5 mm cortical bone screw. Wire is used to attach the rostral portion of the bar to the mandible as previously discussed. The U-bar is removed 6 to 8 weeks after surgery.

U-bars allow fixation of mandibular fractures with minimal surgical invasion and places the fixation on the tension side of the fracture.[9] Long-term outcome of the effects to premolar teeth that have been utilized for screw fixation of the U-bar has not been reported. Immediate results using this fixation have been good and resultant dental disease has not been a problem (Honnas, personal observation).

Type II Kirschner-Ehmer frames, with intramedullary pins placed completely across the mandible rostral and caudal to the fracture line, can be successfully used to stabilize interdental space fractures.[4,5,7,10] Stab incisions are made into the skin overlying the mandible and pilot holes are drilled across the mandible. Radiographic guidance is used to avoid damaging teeth. Protection of soft tissues during drilling

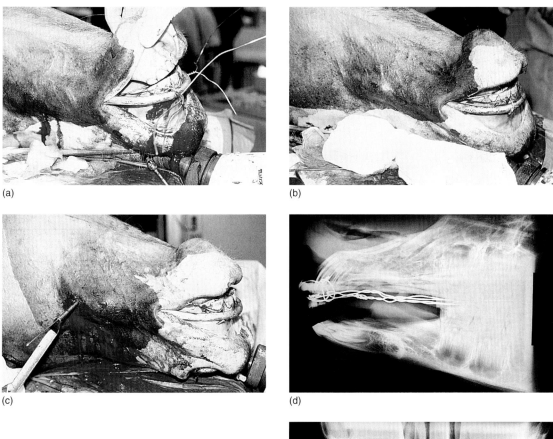

(a)

(b)

(c)

(d)

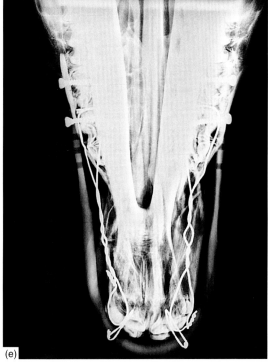

**Figure 17.7.** Stabilization of the maxillary fracture in Figure 17.6 with a U-bar that has been attached to the rostral premolars with cortical bone screws. With the horse in dorsal recumbency and nasally intubated, the U-bar is contoured to fit around the labial and buccal surfaces of the incisors and rostral premolars. (a) Holes are drilled between the incisors and wire threaded between the teeth and around the bar. (b) The wires are twisted around the rostral portion of the U-bar to anchor the appliance. (c) Stab incisions are made through the cheeks, the fracture is reduced and the incisors aligned prior to drilling 3.2 mm holes through the second and third premolars on each side of the maxilla. The holes in the teeth are tapped and a 4.5 mm screw inserted to attach the U-bar to the premolars. (d) and (e) Tension-band wiring spanning the interdental space was also employed to supplement fixation in this case.

(e)

and pin placement decreases the incidence of pin tract infection. Pins ranging in size from 3.1 to 6.3 mm diameter are used depending on the size of the horse. Use of two pins on either side of the fracture is recommended when possible.[5,10,11] Pins should be placed in a straight line to allow connection to the side bar. Pins are cut approximately 4 cm from the skin surface. Clamps and metal rods or acrylics are used as side bars to connect pins placed through the mandible (Fig. 17.8). The fixator should be bandaged to reduce the risk of the horse catching the side bars on objects in the environment. Side bars made of acrylic may be molded to decrease entanglement of the external fixator with objects in the environment.[11] Approximately 6 weeks will be needed to allow sufficient healing of the mandible fracture. Following removal of the external fixator, pin tracts are lavaged daily until healed.

Advantages of a Kirschner-Ehmer frame include the ability to obtain purchase into rostral fragments of the mandible when limited space for plate fixation is present, relative ease of application compared to plating, decreased amount of tissue dissection needed for placement, lower risk of disseminating infection, patient acceptance and decreased risk of damage to teeth, especially in younger horses.[5,7,11,13]

Bone plating can provide a successful repair of fractures of the interdental space and mandibular body and is recommended in adult horses when increased stability is needed.[10,13] Bone platings discussed below under caudal mandibular fractures.

Rarely, fractures of the rostral mandible, involving either the incisive area or interdental space, are accompanied by severe damage to the bone and overlying soft tissues resulting in a poor prognosis for healing and survival of the tissues of the rostral mandible. Rostral mandibulectomy can be used in these cases and is performed by excising the rostral fragments, debriding the area of the fracture and soft tissues, and apposing mucosa over the mandibular stump when possible. Rostral mandibulectomy has been reported for the treatment of rostral mandibular tumors.[18] The ability of the horse to eat hay and grain is not inhibited and the cosmetic results are good in most cases.

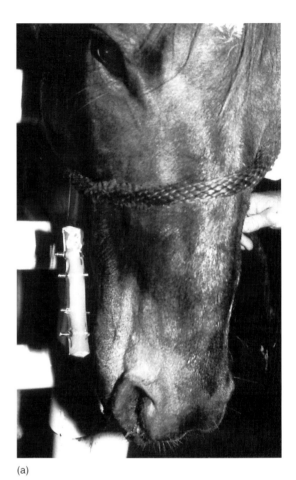

(a)

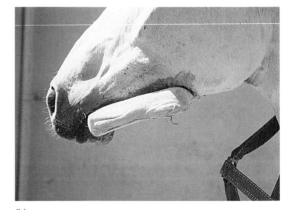

(b)

**Figure 17.8.** A Kirschner-Ehmer frame was utilized in this horse to stabilize a fracture through the mandibular interdental space. (a) Acrylic side bars were used to connect the pins placed through the mandible. (b) Following surgery the side bars should be bandaged to prevent the horse from catching the apparatus on objects in the environment.

## FRACTURES OF THE CAUDAL MANDIBLE

Fracture of the molar portion of the mandibular body and vertical ramus are uncommon.[5] Radiography is used to define involvement of teeth, temporomandibular joints, the hyoid apparatus and comminution and guides the surgeon to applicable treatment options and implant positioning.[13] Fractures of the molar portion of the mandibular body are typically unilateral with minimal displacement and comminution.[7,10] Reported fractures of the vertical ramus include transverse, oblique and degloving fractures of the angle of the mandible.[10,19] Caudal mandibular fractures can be treated using conservative therapy, bone plating or external fixation.[5,7,10,20,21]

Fractures of the caudal region of the body or ramus of the mandible resulting in minimal instability, malocclusion and pain and that permit the horse to eat are candidates for conservative therapy.[9,13] In these cases, the overlying pterygoid and masseter muscles confer stability to the fracture.[19] Anti-inflammatory medications, lavage of the oral cavity and feeding mashes of complete pelleted feeds increase patient comfort and provides nutrition in an easily consumed fashion. Antimicrobial therapy is indicated when the fracture is open to the oral cavity. Care providers should ensure that the horse continues to eat and drink. Radiographic evaluation of the fracture should be performed periodically. Evidence of lack of progression of healing within 6 weeks post-fracture or bony lysis denoting osteomyelitis at the fracture site are indications for internal fixation of the fracture.[9]

Fracture of the caudal angle of the mandible with degloving of the overlying soft tissues has been described.[10] The injury results from placement of the head between fence posts or gratings and then pulling back. Communication of these fractures with the oral cavity or adjacent alveoli is uncommon. Surgical removal of the small fractured segments of the mandible can be performed with minimal functional or cosmetic disturbance.[10] Internal fixation may be indicated for larger fragments.

Indications for fixation of caudal mandibular fractures are instability, malocclusion pre-

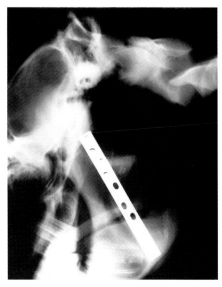

**Figure 17.9.** Comminuted fracture of the vertical ramus of the mandible that was repaired with a dynamic compression plate. The masseter muscle was elevated and reflected dorsally to allow access to the mandible for plate application. The fracture healed without complication.

venting prehension or mastication, pain with unwillingness to eat and bilateral involvement.[5,7,9,10] Internal or external fixation can be used to stabilize caudal mandibular fractures. Bone plating provides a strong bone-implant construct and can be used successfully in unilateral or bilateral body fractures and fractures of the vertical ramus (Fig. 17.9).[19,21] Bone plating is recommended for adult horses in which healing may be delayed.[13] External fixation provides stable fixation of fractures of the mandibular body and carries benefits of decreased surgical dissection and increased latitude in placement of implants.

A ventrolateral approach to the mandible is used for bone plating mandibular fractures. The facial artery, facial vein, parotid salivary duct and mental nerve are identified and preserved during surgical dissection. Elevation of the masseter muscle from the mandible is necessary and is accomplished by transecting the attachments of the muscle at the ventral border of the mandible and reflecting the muscle proximally. The size of plates used ranges from 3.5 to 4.5 mm narrow or broad, depending on fracture configuration and size of the patient. Positioning of the bone plate on the ventrolateral aspect of the mandible is preferred.[10] Alternative plate positions include ventral and ventromedial.[4,10] The plate is contoured and attached to the bone; a minimum of three screws on either side of the fracture is recommended.[11] Teeth roots should be avoided when applying plates.[4,5,10,11] The use of masonry drill bits to drill through teeth roots without causing tooth loss has been reported.[7]

Wilson and co-workers have described a surgical approach to the ramus of the mandible for internal fixation.[19] An incision is made 2 to 3 cm rostral and parallel to the caudal border of the mandible from the zygomatic arch to the point where the facial artery crosses the ventral border of the mandible. The transverse facial artery and vein, facial nerve and auriculotemporal nerve are retracted dorsally and the insertion of the masseter muscle along the caudal mandibular border is sharply incised, allowing subperiosteal elevation of the masseter muscle. Plates used rostrally and caudally on the lateral surface of the ramus provide secure fixation. Care is warranted when tapping and placing screws in the thinner rostral portion of the ramus.[19] Following internal fixation, the masseter fascia and periosteum are closed followed by subcutaneous and skin closure.

Although bone plating provides a very stable construct, extensive surgical dissection is required. Fractures open to the oral cavity can be expected to become infected, necessitating removal of plates after bone healing.[4,11] Bone plating may be a necessity despite the presence of an open fracture when treating unstable fractures in adult horses and when buttress plating is needed in conjunction with corticocancellous bone grafting.[4,10]

External fixators, including type II Kirschner-Ehmer frames previously discussed, can be used in treatment of caudal fractures of the body.[7] Recently, the use of a pinless external fixator has been reported in cattle for fixation of mandibular body fractures.[20] In the place of pins, special bone clamps were used in series along the ventral border on the mandible. The clamps embed into the cortex of the mandible without penetrating the medullary cavity. The clamps were tightened in place using a nut on a central

hinge. An additional short bar ran laterally from the central hinge and enabled all clamps to be connected to a common connecting bar coursing longitudinally along the mandible. Stab incisions followed by blunt dissection of soft tissues were necessary for placement of the clamps into the mandibular body. Fixators were removed 5 to 8 weeks after fixation and stability of the healed mandible allowed immediate return to mastication. Draining tracts around the implants healed with local wound therapy and complications encountered with healing of the mandibular fractures were not attributable to the external fixator.

Prognosis for healing of caudal mandibular fractures is guarded to good.[7,10,11] Complications do occur however, and are generally associated with communication with the oral cavity and involvement of alveoli. When possible aggressive debridement of fracture lines with thorough lavage, closure of oral mucous membranes and antimicrobial use are the best means of prevention of osseous infection and sequestration. Treatment of osseous infection developing postoperatively follows the guide lines of debridement, autogenous cancellous bone grafting when indicated and antimicrobial therapy. Involvement of alveoli with consequential infectious periodontitis and pulpitis will require removal of affected teeth.[5,10,11] Removal of a tooth or destruction of a permanent developing tooth mandates regular dental care to prevent serious malocclusion. Implant associated infection requires removal of plates or pins, debridement of soft tissues, lavage and antimicrobials. Resolution of infection after implant removal often proceeds without further complication.[11]

Failure of fixation is an additional potential complication. Assessment of the initial fixation, degree of stability and presence of infection should be considered in planning further treatment. Use of a more stable means of fixation and concurrently addressing any additional problems such as infection will provide the best prognosis for complete healing. Adjunctive therapy, including autogenous cancellous bone grafting and antimicrobial impregnated beads, may be indicated.

## FRACTURES INVOLVING THE TEMPOROMANDIBULAR JOINT

While fractures involving the temporomandibular joint are rare, they are associated with a higher degree of morbidity.[10,12,22] Radiography, including lateral, oblique and dorsoventral views, is indicated. Lateral projections with the mouth held open with a speculum may give better definition to the temporomandibular region as the condylar and coronoid processes will be subluxated.[10,11]

Internal fixation of fractures involving the temporomandibular joint has not been reported to the authors' knowledge. Conservative therapy or condylectomy are the treatment recommendations that have been published.[12,22] Bilateral mandibular condylar fractures have been reported in a stallion.[12] Treatment of the horse in that report included floating the caudal cheek teeth to allow improved prehension and mastication as premature occlusion of the molars prevented occlusion of the incisors.

Condylectomy of the mandible has been advocated for treatment of fractures involving the temporomandibular joint.[22] A 5 cm skin incision is made over the temporomandibular joint, curving caudoventrally. Branches of the auriculopalpebral nerve are retracted ventrally and portions of the parotid gland are retracted caudally. A horizontal incision is made in the lateral mandibular ligament and joint capsule over the meniscomandibular compartment of the temporomandibular joint. A vertical periosteal incision is made in the lateral surface of the condyle and the periosteum is liberally elevated. Condylectomy is performed 2.5 cm ventral to the articular surface of the condyle. The joint capsule, subcutaneous tissues and skin are closed.

Temporomandibular joint fractures carry a guarded prognosis as degenerative joint disease and resultant inhibitions to prehension and mastication render the horse susceptible to weight loss.[12,23] The prognosis after condylectomy to treat degenerative disease of the temporomandibular joint appears to be guarded to good.[23]

## SUMMARY

Because the mandible of the horse is frequently fractured, knowledge of mandibular surgical anatomy and the most common types of mandibular fractures encountered is essential to the equine veterinarian. This chapter reviews pertinent mandibular surgical anatomy, clinical signs and diagnosis of fractures of the mandible and discusses their treatment on an anatomical basis.

Fractures of the mandible are defined by physical and radiographic examination. Use of fixation methods that counter the tensile forces on the dorsal or oral surface of the mandible should provide the best opportunity for successful healing. The prognosis for the majority of mandibular fractures is good when thorough debridement and use of proper bone-implant constructs are employed.

### REFERENCES

1. Hillmann DJ (1975) Equine skull. In: *Sisson and Grossman's The Anatomy of the Domestic Animals* (5th edn), ed. R Getty, WB Saunders, Philadelphia, pp. 335–336.
2. Godinho HP and Getty R (1975) Equine cranial nerves. In: *Sisson and Grossman's The Anatomy of the Domestic Animals* (5th edn), ed. R Getty, WB Saunders, Philadelphia, p. 656.
3. Kainer RA (1993) Clinical anatomy of the equine head. *Veterinary Clinics of North America Equine Practice*, 9(1), 1–23.
4. Sullins KE and Turner AS (1982) Management of fractures of the equine mandible and premaxilla (incisive bone). *Compendium Continuing Education for the Practicing Veterinarian*, 4(11), S480–S489.
5. Meagher DM and Trout DR (1980) Fractures of the mandible and premaxilla in the horse. *Proceedings of the American Association of Equine Practitioners*, 26, 181–192.
6. Monin T (1977) Tension band repair of equine mandibular fractures. *Journal Equine Medicine and Surgery* 1, 325–329.
7. Schneider RK (1990) Mandibular fractures. In: *Current Practice of Equine Surgery*, eds NA White and JN Moore, JB Lippincott, Philadelphia, pp. 589–595.
8. Little CB, Hilbert BJ and McGill CA (1982) A retrospective study of head fractures in 21 horses. *Australian Veterinary Journal*, 62(3), 89–91.
9. Watkins JP (1991) Diseases of the head and neck. In: *Equine Medicine and Surgery* (4th edn), eds PT Colahan, IG Mayhew, AM Merritt and JN Moore, American Veterinary Publications, Goleta, CA, pp. 1461–1464.

10. DeBowes RM (1996) Fractures of the mandible and maxilla. In: *Equine Fracture Repair*, ed. AJ Nixon, WB Saunders, Philadelphia, pp. 323–332.

11. Blackford JT and Blackford LW (1992) Surgical treatment of selected musculoskeletal disorders of the head. In: *Equine Surgery*, ed. JA Auer, WB Saunders, Philadelphia, p. 1075.

12. Hurtig MB, Barber SM and Farrow CS (1984) Temporomandibular joint luxation in a horse. *Journal of the American Veterinary Medical Association*, 185, 78–80.

13. Ragle CA (1993) Head trauma. *Veterinary Clinics of North American Equine Practice*, 9(1), 171–176.

14. DeBowes RM, Cannon JH, Grant BD, *et al.* (1981) Lag screw fixation of rostral mandibular fractures in the horse. *Veterinary Surgery*, 10, 153–158.

15. Colahan PT and Pascoe JR (1983) Stabilization of equine and bovine mandibular and maxillary fractures using an acrylic splint. *Journal of the American Veterinary Medical Association*, 182, 1117.

16. Gabel AA (1969) A method of surgical repair of the fractured mandible in the horse. *Journal of the American Veterinary Medical Association*, 155, 1831–1834.

17. Krahwinkel DJ, Heffernan HJ and Ewbank RL (1969) Surgical repair of fractured maxillae and premaxillae in a horse. *Journal of the American Veterinary Medical Association*, 154, 53–57.

18. Richardson DW, Evans LH and Tulleners EP (1991) Rostral mandibulectomy in five horses. *Journal of the American Veterinary Medical Association*, 199, 1179–1182.

19. Wilson DG, Trent AM and Crawford WH (1990) A surgical approach to the ramus of the mandible in cattle and horses. *Veterinary Surgery*, 19, 191–195.

20. Lischer CJ, Fluri E, Kaser-Hotz B, *et al.* (1997) Pinless external fixation of mandible fractures in cattle. *Veterinary Surgery*, 26, 14–19.

21. Murch KM (1980) Repair of bovine and equine mandibular fractures. *Canadian Veterinary Journal*, 21, 69–73.

22. Barber SM, Doige CE and Humphreys SG (1985) Mandibular condylectomy, technique and results in normal horses. *Veterinary Surgery*, 14, 79–86.

23. Patterson LJ, Shappell KK and Hurtig MB (1989) Mandibular condylectomy in a horse. *Journal of the American Veterinary Medical Association*, 195, 101–102.

# INDEX

Figures and Tables in *italic*

Achondroplasia, *212*
Acrylic splints, 263, 264, *266*
Adamantinoma, 86–8, *86–8*, 92, 165
Aging, 23, 35–45, 133
    different breeds, 39–45, *40–5*
    eruption, 35–6, *35–6*
    examination, 109–10, 117
    incisors, changes in shape, 37–8,
        *37–8*
    occlusal surface changes, 36–7,
        *36–7*
    prophylaxis, 198–9, *199*
    wear, 70–4, *71–4*
    see also Periodontal disease
Alberts molar forceps, 226, 228
Alignment, examination, 105
Alimentary tract, obstruction, 134
Alveolar
    bone, 24–5, 74, 75
    crest, 25
    nerve, 259
    periostitis, 74, *137*, 250
    plate removal, 236–9, *237–9*
    socket, 49
    see also Periodontal disease
Ameloblastic odontoma, 86–8, *86–8*
Ameloblastoma, 86–8, *86–8*, 92, 165
Ameloblasts, *6*, 8, 9, 10, 49, *49*
Amelodentinal junction, 9, *17*
American Paint Horse Association, 116
American Quarter Horse
        Association, 116
Amylase, saliva, 62
Anadontia, 156, *156*
Anaplastic sarcoma, *166*
Anatomy, 3–27
    blood supply, 24
    bones and muscles of prehension
        and mastication, 24–7

canine teeth, 22
cheek teeth, 22–4
embryology, 5–10, *6–10*
evolution, 3–5
incisors, 19–22, *20–1*
nerve supply, 24
nomenclature, 3
structures
    cement, 16–19, *17–18*
    dentin, 13–15, *13–15*
    enamel, 10–13, *11–12*
    occlusal surface, 19
    pulp, 15–16, *15*
Anelodont teeth, 4
Anesthesia
    imaging, 139, 142
    oral examination, 61
    prophylaxis, 203
    tooth removal, 221, 222, 223, 230,
        231, 236, 246
Anisognathism, 23, 30, 32, 209
Anorexia, 129
Antibiotics, 68, 220
Antimicrobials, 69, 261, 267, 268
Apexification, 252
Apical, nomenclature, 3, 4
    delta, 82
    osteitis, 59, 83, 84
    periodontitis, *83*
    seals, 254, *255*
Apicoectomy, 250, 252
Approximal, nomenclature, 3
Arabian horses, 115, 150
    aging, 39–45, *40–2*, *44*
    developmental abnormalities,
        55
    orthodontic, 209–10, 216
Arcade see Dental arcade
Arnold's mouth gag, 112

Arthroscope, 121, 122
Auto-immune disease, 132, *132*

Bacillus Calmette Geurin (BCG), 95
Bacteremia, 75
Bacteria, 62, 228
Ball burrs, 181
Barium sulfate, 61
Basal cell carcinoma, 95
Basket retractor, 119, *120*
Bayer mouth wedge, 111, 174
Beaks
    examination, 109
    floating, 185, 197–8
Behavioral consequences, dental
        disease, 127–9, *128*
Belgian draft horse, aging, 39–45,
        *40–3*
Bell stage, tooth development, 5–8, *6*,
        81
Beveling, 190–1, *192*
Big-head disease, 131
Biomedical orthodontics, 207
Bit
    exondontia, 220
    gnathism, 128–9
    injuries, 116, 128, 204
    oral trauma, 61, 65, 69
    seats, 190–3, *191–3*
'Bite plane', 70
Blade retractor, 119
'Blind wolf teeth', 224
Blister-beetle toxicity, 132
Blood supply, teeth, 7–9, 10, 24
Body condition score, 114, *114–5*,
        123
Bone flap technique, 244, *244*
Bone plating, 263, 266, 267–8, *267*
Bone rongeur, 226

Brachydont compared to hypsodont, 3, 4–5, 13, 14, 15–16
  cheek teeth, 22, 24
  developmental abnormalities, 51
  embryology, 6–7, 10
Brachygnathia see Parrot mouth
Bran disease, 131
Buccal
  nomenclature, 3
  points, 109, 119
  see also Cheek
Buccinator muscle, 30
Buccotomy, 236––, 237–9
Bud stage, tooth development, 5, 6
Bullous pemphigoid, 132, 133
Burgess wolf tooth instrument, 179, 194, 226, 225–6
Burrs, 200, 200
Butler's mouth gag, 112
Butorphanol, 117

Calcium hydroxide, 251
Calculus, 22, 74, 74, 76, 77
Callus formation, 72
Campylorrhinus lateralis, 55, 55–6, 207, 208–9
Canine teeth, 3, 22
  aging, 35
  examination, 108, 109, 118
  exodontia, 221, 223, 223
  floating, 186, 186, 195–6, 195, 204
  imaging, 143, 143, 147, 148
  nomenclature, 3
  orthodontics, 209, 210
  prophylaxis, 195–6, 195
Capping, endodontics, 251
Cap stage, tooth development, 5, 6, 8
Caps, 17, 22, 59, 59, 129
  examination, 108, 120
  orthodontics, 214, 214
  prophylaxis, 193–4, 193, 204
  tooth removal, 179, 227–30, 227–9
Carbide grit float, 188
Caries, 10, 17, 19, 52, 79–81, 80–1, 250
  charting, 123
Cariogenic acid, 79–80
Caudal hooks, 72–3
Cecal digestion, 4
Cellulitis, 83, 220
Cement, 4, 10, 11–12, 16–19, 17–18, 29
Cemental hypoplasia, 18–19, 51–2, 52, 59, 73, 80, 137
Cementoblasts, 8, 10, 15, 16, 17, 52
Cementogenesis, 49–51, 50, 52, 80
Cementoma, 86–7, 88–9, 89, 166
Cephalometric studies, 210, 213, 216
Cerebral infarction, 75
Cervical loop, 6
Charting, 122–3, 124–5, 185

Cheek
  anatomy, 60
  examination, 61
  retractor, 112, 119–20, 119, 176
  trauma, 62–5, 63–5
Cheek teeth, 3, 22–4
  imaging, 143–6, 143, 145, 148–52, 149–53
  instruments, 179
  removal, 221, 246
    lateral approach, 236–9, 237–9
    oral extraction, 230–35, 231 -35
    retrograde approach, 239–44, 240, 242–4, 248
  systematic effects of disease, 127, 129, 131, 132–4, 135
  wear, 70–1
Chewing
  rates, 33, 34
  see also Mastication
Chiffney, 61, 65, 69, 69
Chisels, 178
Chlorhexidine, 174
Choke, 134
Chondrosarcoma, 91
Cimetidine, 97
Cingula, 24, 187
Cisplatin, 95, 97
Clydesdale breed, 94
Cobalt60-teletherapy, 94
Col, 75
Colic, 110, 115, 134
Commissures, 60
Computerized
  dental charting, 122
  tomography, 121, 139, 167, 168
Conchal
  cysts, 85
  necrosis, 135
Condylar process, 259, 259, 261, 269
Condylectomy, 269
Congenital defects
  orthodontics, 207, 211–13, 212, 215, 216–7, 218
  prophylaxis, 203
Coronal see Crown
Coronoid process, 259, 259, 260, 261, 269
Cranial nerves, 30, 60
Craniofacial deformities, 206, 210, 215–6
Crib-biting, 21
Crown, 3, 8, 9
  loss, 53, 71, 71
Cryosurgery, 91, 97
Cups, aging, 36, 37, 41, 42, 43–5
Curette, 224, 226, 226, 231
Curve of Spee, 23
Curved arcade, examination, 109

Cushing's disease, 132
Cusps, 24, 187
Cysts, 122, 136
  dentigerous cysts, 86, 91, 100, 100, 156–7, 157
  eruption, 25, 58, 118, 136, 152
  imaging, 165–7, 166–7
  paranasal, 99
  periodontal, 185
  sinus, 85, 89, 91, 100, 166
Cytodifferentiative phase, embryology, 5

Dawn horse (Eohippus), 3–4, 29, 30
Debridement wound, 62–3, 65, 66
  fracture, 262, 269
Decay, 79–84
  endodontic disease, 51, 81–3, 81–3, 220
  see also Caries
Deciduous teeth, 3, 19–20, 22
  endodontic therapy, 251
  eruption, 35, 35, 40, 40
  examination, 108
  imaging, 147
  impaction, 58
  orthodontics, 206, 207, 209, 214, 214, 218
  prophylaxis, 199–200
  removal, 179, 220, 221, 227–30, 227–9
  see also Caps
Dehiscence, wound, 64, 65, 66, 67
Dental arcade, 60, 109, 120–21, 132, 209
  floating, 185, 186–7
Dental base plate wax, 231, 235, 236
Dental capping, 127
Dental follicle, 5, 6–8, 10, 10
Dental lamina, 5, 6
Dental sac, 5, 6–8, 10, 10
'Dental star', 13–14, 20
  aging, 36–7, 36–7, 40–2, 40–5
Dentigerous cysts, 86, 91, 100, 100, 156–7, 157
Dentin, 10, 13–15, 11–15, 16, 17, 19
  embryology, 5, 8, 9, 6–9
  endodontic disease, 81, 82, 84
  endodontics, 251
  sclerosis, 82
Dentofacial deformities, 210–11
Dentogenesis, 5
Dermatitis, 128
Detomidine, 117
Development, abnormalities, 49–59
  brachygnathia, 53–4, 54
  campylorrhinus, 55, 55–6
  embryology, 5–10, 6–10
  enamel hypoplasia, 53

eruption, 57–8, *57–8*
hypoplasia, cementum, 51–2, *52*
imaging, 154–7, *154–7*
impaction, 58–9, *58–9*
oligodontia, 52–3, *53*
physiology, 49–51, *49–51*
polyodontia, 53
prognathia, *54*, 55
rudimentary teeth, 55–7
Diarrhea, 134, *135*
Diarthrodial joint abnormalities, 211
Diastema, *17*, 23, 118, *137*, 259
orthodontics, *210*, 213
tooth removal, 221
Digastricus muscle, 30
Digital radiology, 121
Disarming, tooth removal, 220
Distal, nomenclature, 3
Dolicephalic, 23
Donkeys, 39
Draft horses, 210
Draft-horse halter, 173
Dremel-type instruments, 192, *193*,
196, 198, 200
Drug toxicity, 132
Dysmastication, 129, 130–34, *130–33*,
*135*, 136, 185
Dysphagia, 134, 136
trauma, 66, 67, 260
tumors, 92, 95
Dysprehension, 1297, *130*

Eating habits, 114, 117, 129
*see also* Mastication
Electrical testing, 83
Electromyographic data, 33, *34*
Elevators, 179, 224, 224, *226*, 226, 231,
*232*
Elodont teeth, 4, *5*
Embryology, 5–10, *6–10*, 81
Enamel, 4, 10–13, *11–12*, *17*, 19
embryology, *6–9*, 9
epithelium, *6–7*, 8
hypoplasia, 53
organ, 5, *6*, 8, *8*
points, 72, *73*
examination, 108, 109, 113,
116, 204, 230
floating, 178, 185, 186, 187–9,
197
orthodontics, 213, 217
systemic effect of, 127, 129,
132, 133–4
spot, 20
Enameloblastoma *see* Ameloblastoma
Endodontic disease, 51, 81–3, *81–3*, 220
Endodontic therapy, 250–57
acute pulp exposure,
management, 250–61

results, 256–7, *257*
surgical, 251–54, *254–6*
Endoscopic examination, 61, 66, 121,
142, 154, 230
Endotracheal intubation, 230, 231,
236, *237*, 239
Entrapment *see* Impaction
Environmental forces, dental
conformation, 212
Eohippus, 3–4, 29, *30*
Epiglottal entrapment, 62, 67
Epistaxis, 66, 136
Epithelial sarcoma, 96
Epulis, *86*, *93*, 100
Equichip chisel, 198
Equipment, examination, 110–13,
*111–13*
*see also* Instrumentation
*Equus*
*caballus*, 3, 30, 57
*cracoviensis*, 24
*mosbachensis*, 25
*Muniensis*, 25
Eruption
aging, 35–6, *35–6*, 40, *40*
abnormalities, 57–8, *57–8*
cyst, 25, 58, 118, 136, 152
examination, 108, 120
malocclusion, 207
physiology, 49–51, *49–51*
rate, 22
systemic effects of, 127, 128
Esophageal choke, 110, 115
Ethmoid hematoma, 91
Eugenol, 254
Evolution, 3–5
Examination, dental and oral,
107–25
adult performance horse, 108–9
ancillary diagnostic tests, 121–22
charting, 122–3, 185
equipment, 110–13, *111–13*
extraoral physical examination,
115–7, *116*
geriatric horse, 109–10
history, 113–14
mature horse, 109
oral examination, 117–11, *119–20*
patient observation, 114–5, *114–5*
prophylaxis, 203–4
records and treatment planning,
123, *124–5*
signalment, 113
trauma, 61
weanling examination, 108
young performance horse, 108
*see also* Imaging, Instrumentation,
Radiographic techniques
Exercise intolerance, 67

Exodontia, 220–48
cheek teeth, 230–44, *231–35*,
*237–40*, *242–4*
complications, 246–7, *248*
deciduous premolars, 179,
227–30, *227–9*
canines, 223, *223*
endodontia, compared, 251–52
incisors, 221–3, *222*
paranasal sinuses, 244–6, *245*
wolf teeth, 62, 179, 220, 221,
223–6, *224–7*, 229
Extraction forceps, 224, 226, *226*, 228,
*229*, 230, *231–3*, 234, 239
Eyes, 116

Facial
artery, 259
asymmetry, 108, 115
distortion and deformity, 135–6,
*137*
nerve, 63, 259
pain, 128, *128*
swelling, 228, *229*
vein, 259
Fiberoptic scope, 176
Fibroma, 88
Fibrosarcoma, 91
Fibrous dysplasia, *86*, 92, 100, *100*
Filing *see* Floating
Fissure, 24
Fistula, 136, *137*, 252
exodontia, 247, *248*
impaction, 58, 59
pulpitis, 83, *83*
trauma, 62, 63, *64*, 68
Fixation, 262, 266, 267, 268
Floating *see* Prophylaxis
Floats, 173, 176–8, *176–7*, 179–80, *180*
power, 193, *193*, 200, 203
S-float, *177*, 178, 191, 192, 196
Table float, 178, 189, *189*
Fluoroscopy, 121, 246
Fluorouracil cream, 95
Foley balloon catheter, 245–6
Food pouching, 130–1, *131*
Foreign bodies, 61, 62–3, 66
Forms, dental, 122–3, *124–5*, 185
Fossa, 24
Fracture, *137*
interdental space, 260, *260*, 263–6,
*263*, *265–6*
tooth removal, 220, 221
*see also* Mandible-fracture, Trauma
Full mouth speculum, 111–12, *112*,
174–5, *175*
exodontia, 231
floating, 186, 187–8, *189*, 189–90,
192, 204

Functional jaw orthopedics, 207
Functional orthodontic treatment, 206, 207, *208*, 217

Gag specula, 110–11, *111*
Gags, 61, 110–11, *111*, 112, 174, *175*
Galvayne's groove, 20, 38, *38*, *43–5*, 45
Gamma scintigraphy, 121, 128, 130
*Gastrophilus spp*, 132, *133*
Gel foam, 224, 226
Genetics *see* Congenital defects
Genioglossus muscle, 30
Geniohydeus muscle, 30
Geriatric horses, examination, 109–10
    *see also* Aging
Gingiva, 26–7, 35, 60, 74, 75–6
    hyperplasia, *99*
    sulcus, 26
Gingivitis, 72, 74, 76, 227
    examination, 108, 110, 117, 123, 204
Gingivosis, 74
Glossectomy, 65
Gouges, 224, 226, *226*
Granulation tissue, 85
Granulomatous abscesses, 66
Granulosa cell tumors, 102
Grinders, power instruments, 180–1, *181*
Guards, power instruments, 180, *181*
Guenther mouth speculum, 112
Guitta perdia, *235*
Gums *see* Gingiva
Gutta-percha, 252, 253–4

*Habronema musca*, 132, *133*
Halitosis, 76, 260
'Halo', 160
Halter, 110, *111*, 119, 173, *173*, 190
Hamartoma, 85, *86–7*, 89, 91, 92
Hard palate
    anatomy, 60
    trauma, 62, *65*, 66–7, *67*
Hausman mouth speculum, 112, *112*
Hausmann's gag, 61
Headshaking, 128, *128*
Hemangiosarcoma, 95, 99, 101
Hemimandibles, 25
Hemimandibulectomy, 93, 95
Hemorrhage, 67, 246
Hertwig's epithelial root sheath, 10
Histiocytes, 82
History, 107, 108, 113–14, 215
Hooks, 20, 54, 72–3, *72*
    aging, 38, *38*, *43–5*, 44–5
    examination, 109, 120
    floating, 178, 185, 191, 197–8, *197*, 204
    orthodontics, 207, 211, 213–5, *213*, 216, 217

Hydrostatic forces, eruption, 57
Hyoid apparatus, 60
Hypercementosis, 77, *83*
Hyperesthesia, *128*
Hyperkeratosis, *128*
Hyperparathyroidism, 131
Hyperptyalism, 66
Hyperthermia, 97
Hypsodont, characteristics, 3
    evolution, 3–5
    *see also* Brachydont
Hyracotherium (Eohippus), 3–4, 29, 30

Imaging, 139–69
    computed tomography, 121, 139, 167, *168*
    nuclear scintigraphy, 121, 139, 167–8, *168*
    *see also* Radiographic techniques
Immunomodulation, 95
Impaction, 58–9, *58–9*, 214, *214*
    alimentary tract, 134
    exodontia, 220, 227–8, *227*
    molar, 129
Impressions, orthodontics, 215, *215*
Incisal cup, 20
Incisive bone, 26
Incisivus muscle, 30
Incisors, 3, 19–22, *20–1*
    aging, 35–6, *35–6*, 37–8, *37–8*, 40–5, *40–5*
    behavioural consequences of disease, 127, 128*6*, 129
    endodontic therapy, 250
    examination, 109, 117
    exodontia, 221–3, *222*
    imaging, 143, *143*, 147, *148*
    mandible fracture, 260, 261–3, *261–2*
    orthodontics, 207, 209, 210, 211, 217
    prophylaxis, 199–203, *200–1*, *203*, 204
Indentation hardness-tests, 39
Infection, 66, 132, *133*, 136, *137*, 268
    imaging, 157, 159–65, *160–6*
    *see also* Sinusitis
Inflammation, pulp chamber, 81, 82
Infraorbital nerve, 128, *128*
Infundibular, 5, *17*, 18–19, 20, 37
    cement necrosis, 10
    cemental hypoplasia, 80
    necrosis, 10, *52*, 135, *137*
Initiating phase, embryology, 5
Instrumentation, 173–84
    basic equipment, 173–4, *173–4*
    cap extracting instruments, 179
    chisels, 178

floats, 173, 176–8, *176–7*, 179–80, *180*
    molar cutters, 178, *178–9*, 196–7, *197*, 199
    mouth gags and specula, 61, 110–11, *111*, 112, 174–5, *175*
    picks and molar fragment elevators, 176, 179
    wolf teeth extracting instruments, 179
    *see also* Power instruments
Interceptive orthodontics, 206, 220, 221
Interdental space, 23
    fracture, 260, *260*, 263–6, *263*, *265–6*
Interocclusal space, prophylaxis, 202
Interproximal, nomenclature, 3
Interbular dentin, *13*, 14
Intradental oral cavity (IDOC), 33, 34
Iridium, 95
Irritation dentin, 82
Isognathic, 23
Isthmus faucium, 60

Jaw growth, 211–12
Jeffery gag, 111, 174
Junctional cemental hypoplasia, 19
Jupiter Spool, 111, 174
Juvenile ossifying fibroma, *86*, *87*, 92–4, *93*, 96, 166, *166*

Keratin, 10, 80, 94
    pearls, 94
Keratinocytes, 94
Kirschner-Ehmer frame, 264, 266, *266*, 268
Knoop diamond indenter, 39

Labial
    apex, 43, *43–5*
    nomenclature, 3
Labii maxillaris muscle, 30
*Lactobacillus acidophilus*, 79
Lameness, 107
Lamina dura, 24
Lampas, 118, 129, *129*
Landmesser wedge, 174, *175*
Laparoscope, 112, 119
Laryngopalatal dislocation, 62
Lead, 110
Light source, 174, 176
Lingual, nomenclature, 3
    apex, 42–5
    frenulum, trauma, 62, 65
    power stroke, 25
    tonsils, 60
    *see also* Tongue
Lip tattoos, 116, *116*

Lipizzaners, 39
Lips
    anatomy, 60
    examination, 61
    trauma, 61, 62–5, *62–5*
Lophodont, 24
Lophs, 24, 30, 33
Lymphosarcoma, *86*, 102, *102*

McAllen mouth speculum, 112, 175, *175*
McClelen mouth speculum, 112
McPherson mouth speculum, 112, *112*, 175, *175*
Macrophages, 82
Maleruption, 121, 135, *137*, 155, *155*
Malformation *see* Development
Malocclusion
    developmental abnormalities, 53
    examination, 108–9, 203–4
    imaging, 155–6, *156*
    mandibular fracture, 260
    prophylaxis, 193, 196–7, *196*
    prognathia, *54*, 55, 70, 216
    Shear mouth, 73–4, 130, 213
    Step mouth, 72, *73*, 193
    tooth removal, 220, 221
    wear, 72–4, *73*
    Wave mouth, 52, 73, 109, 178
    Wry nose, 55, *55–6*, 207, *208–9*
    *see also* Beaks, Hooks, Orthodontics, Parrot mouth, Ramps
Mandible, 25
    aneurysmal bone cyst, *86*, 99–100
    cheek teeth, imaging, 145–6, *145*, 152–3
    fracture, 68–9, *69*
    osteosynthesis, 259–69, *259–63*, *265–7*
    glands, 27, 60, 68
    periapical disease, 163, 165, *165*
Mandibularis muscle, 30
Mandibulectomy, 266
Marks, aging, 37, 42–3, *41–5*
Masseter muscle, 25, 30, 34, 116, 267, *267*
Mast cell tumors, 97
Mastication, 29, 30–4, *31–4*
    examination, 115, 117
    muscles, 25–6
    orthodontics, 206
Masticatory surface *see* Occlusal surface
Maxillaris muscle, 30
Maxillary bone, 26
    cheek teeth, imaging, 143–5, *143*, *145*, 148–52, *148–53*
    fractures, 69

periapical disease, 157, 159–60, *160–63*
    sinus disease, 128, *128*
Maxillofacial surgery, 206
Meiers dental wedge, 111, 174
Meister speculum, 112
Melanoma, *86*, *92*, 97, 116
Mental nerve, 25
Mercuric blister, 132
Merychippus, 29
Mesenchyme, 5, *6*
Mesial
    drift, 209
    nomenclature, 3
Messer wedge, 111
Metaplastic calcification, 135, *135*
Mobile teeth, removal of, 220
Molar teeth
    aging, 35
    behavioural consequences of disease, 127, 128, 129
    cutters, 178, *178–9*, 196–7, *197*, 199
    eruption, 127, 128
    forceps, 226, 228
    fragment elevators, 179
    nomenclature, 3
    tables, 117
Molarization, 29, 30
Monkey mouth, *54*, 55, 70, 216
Morphogenetic phase, embryology, 5
Mouth speculum *see* Full mouth speculum
Mucus membrane, examination, 117
Musgrave elevator, 226
Mylohyoid muscles, 60
Myocardial infarction, 75
Myxofibroma, 87, 93
Myxoma, 85, 87, 93, *93*, 95–7, *96*

Nasal
    chambers, imaging, 144, 146
    disease, 127
    sepsis, 127
Nasogastric intubation, 67, 230, 236, 246
Neoplasia *see* Tumors
Nerves, teeth, 24, 25, 30, 60, 259
    headshaking, 128, *128*
    trauma, 63
Nomenclature, 3, 20, 122
Non-steroidal anti-inflammatory drugs, 66, 68, 132, 261
Nuclear scintigraphy, 121, 139, 167–9, *168*

Observation, 114–5, *114–5*
Obtura II system, 252, 254
Obturation, 253–4

Occlusal surface, 3, *8*, *17*, 18, *18*, 19, *20–1*, 30, *31*, 32
    aging, 35, 36–7, *36–7*, 43, *43–5*
    efficiency, 133
    examination, 108
    imaging, 151
    length, 72, *72*
    orthodontics, 206
    wear, 70–8
    *see also* Malocclusion
Odontoameloblastoma, 86
Odontoblast, 13, 14, 15, *14–15*, 16, 49, *49*
    embryology, *6*, *7*, *8*, *9*, *9*
    endodontic disease, 81, 82
Odontogenic tumors, 86–91, *86–91*
Odontoma, *86–7*, 89–91, *91*, 163–4
Oligodontia, 52–3, *53*
Omohyoideus muscle, 30
Oral microflora, 77
Oral cavity
    anatomy, 60
    examination, 61
Oral hemangiosarcoma, 99
Oral mucosa, 26–7, 63, 65, 69
Oral papilloma, *86*, *92*, 97–9
Oral ulceration, 61, 72, 129, 131–2, *132–3*
    examination, 118, 204
Orbicularis oris muscle, 30, 63
Organophosphate anthelmintics, 132
Orofacial fistula, *64*, 65
Oronasal
    fistula, 67
    neoplasia, 128, 136
Oropharyngeal foreign bodies, 61
Oropharynx, trauma, 65–6
Orthodontics, 206–18
    altered wear causing a shift in tooth movement, 213–15, *213–4*
    documentation, 215–6, *215*
    exodontia, 220, 221
    factors affecting head shape and dental conformation, 211–13, *212*
    parrot mouth, 54, 214–6
    principles, 206–11, *207–10*
    sequelae to malocclusion, 213
Orthognathic surgery, 206, 207, 216
Osseus carcinoma, 91
Osseous infection, 268
'Osseous tubercles', 25, 26
Ossifying fibroma, Juvenile, *86*, 87, 92–4, *93*, 96, 166, *166*
Osteitis, 59, 83, 84, 92, 136
    imaging, 145, 159, 160
Oseoblastoma, 91
Osteogenic tumors, 86, 91

Osteolysis, 135
Osteoma, *86*, 92
Osteomyelitis, *83*, 92, 220
Osteosarcoma, *86*, 87, 91
Osteotome, 231, 236, 241, 243–4
Overbite, 53, 70, 216, 217
Overjet, 53, 70, 211, 216, 217

Pain
    facial, 128, *128*
    pulpitis, 83
Palatal
    artery, 67
    nomenclature, 3
    ridges, 33, *33*
Papilla, 5, *6*, 81
Paranasal sinus, 127, 159, 243, 247
    cysts, 99
    drainage, 244–6, *245*
    imaging, 143, 144, 146
Parodontal disease, 74
Parotid ducts, 27, 60, 67–8, 259
Parrot mouth, 53–4, *54*, 70, 250
    examination, 174
    orthodontics, *208*, 210, 216–8
Pemphigus vulgaris, 132, *133*
Penicillin, 261
Periapical
    abscess, 83
    definition, 4
    granuloma, 83
    infection, 221
    mandibular disease, 163, 165, *165*
    maxillary disease, 157, 159–60,
        *160–3*
    sepsis, 68, 135
Periodontal cyst, 83
Periodontal disease, 74–8, *75*, 131, *137*
    charting, 123
    endodontic therapy, 256
    examination, 108, 109, 110, 120
    imaging, 83, 145, 151, 160, 165,
        *166*, *168*
    impaction, 58
    instruments, 179
    orthodontics, 212, *212*
    periodontal anatomy and
        function, 75–6, *76*
        clinical signs, 76, *76–7*
        etiology, 77
        treatment, 77–8
    prophylaxis, 199
    pulpitis, 250
    reluctance to eat, 129
    tooth removal, 220, 222, 223, 227,
        231
    wear, 72
Periodontal ligament, 57, 74, 75–6, *76*
    developmental abnormalities, 51

Periodontal pockets, 76, *77*, 78, 213
    tooth removal, 221, 246
Periodontitis, 74, 76, *77*, 80, *83*, 93
    charting, 123
    mandibular fracture, 261, 268
Periodontosis, 74
Periostitis, 74, 83, 223
Periradicular disease *see* Periodontal
        disease
Pertubular dentin, 13–14, *13*
Pharyngotomy, 66
Physiology, 29–34
    functional morphology, 29–30
    mastication, 30–4, *31–4*
Pica, 129
Picks, 176, 179
Pituitary adenoma-related Cushing's
        disease, *86*, 102
Plant irritations, 132, *133*
Plaque, 74, *74*, 76, 77, 118
Plexus of Raschkow, 24
Poisoning, 132, *133*
Polydioxanone, 63, *63–5*, 66, 67, *67*,
        261
Polyglactin 910, 63, 66, 68
Polymethmethacrylate (PMMA), 235,
        236, 247, *248*, 264
Polyodontia, 53
Polypropylene, 261
Power instruments, 83, 173, 179–82,
        *180–1*
    floats, 193, *193*, 201, 203
Predentin, *6–7*, *9*, *14*, 15, 81
Prehension, 117
Premolars
    aging, 35
    examination, 118
    imaging, 147, *147*
    nomenclature, 3
    *see also* Caps
Primary epithelial band, 5
Probes, 176
Prognathia, *54*, 55, 70, 216
Prophylaxis, 142, 185–204, 206
    bit seats, 190–3, *191–3*
    canine teeth, 195–6, *195*
    floating procedures, 185–9, *186–9*
    full mouth speculums, 189–90
    incisors, 199–203, *200–1*, *203*
    hooks, ramps and beaks, 197–8,
        *196*
    old horses, 198–9, *199*
    retained deciduous premolars,
        193–4, *193*
    safety, 203
    tall or long teeth, 196–7, *196*
    timetable for routine
        examination, 203–4
    wolf teeth, 194–5, *194–5*

Proximal, nomenclature, 3
Pseudocysts, 51, *51*
Pterygoid muscles, 25, 30, 34
Ptyalism, 128, 260
Pulp, 14, 15–16, *14–15*, 49, 81–2
    ablation, 250
    embryology, 5, *7*
    endodontic disease, 51, 81–3,
        *81–3*, 220
    *see also* Endodontic therapy
Pulpar nerve, 24
Pulpitis, 16, 79, 82–3, *83*, *137*
    endodontic therapy, 250
    exodontia, 223, 228
    mandibular fracture, 261, 268
Pulpo-dentinal complex, 14
Pulpotomy, 251
Punches, 240, *240*, 241, 242, *242*
Pyogenic membrane, 244

Quality evaluation, imaging, 146–7,
        *147*
Quarterhorses, 209–10
Quidding, 74, 115, 130, 131, *130–1*,
        132

Rabies, 117
Radiation, tumors, 88, 92, 94, 96, 97
Radiographic techniques, 121, 140–7,
        *143*, *145*
    cinical indications, 153–4, *154*
        mandible fracture, 261, 263
        orthodontics, 215
        pulpitis, 83
        temporomandibular joint
            degeneration, 130
        tooth removal, 221, 223, 226,
            230, 234, 236, 241, 246, 247
        trauma, 61, 68
    radiographic anatomy, 147–53,
        *147–53*
    radiological interpretation,
        154–67, *154–67*
Ramps, 73
    examination, 109, 120
    floating, 185, 196, 197–8
    parrot mouth, 217
Ramus, 25, 259, *259*, 260, 261, 266,
        *267*, 268
Rasping *see* Prophylaxis
Records, 107, 123
Renal failure, 132, *133*
Reparative dentin, 82, 251
Repulsion, cheek teeth, 239–44, *240*,
        *242–4*, 246
Reserve crown, 71, *71*, 72
Respiratory
    distress, *229*
    obstruction, 136

Restraint, 61, 142
Reynolds tooth extractors, 228, *229*
Rhinitis, 160, 163, *164*
Ridge, definition, 24
Root, definition, 4
    canal therapy, 250
    development, 51, 71
    slivers, 227, 228, 290
Root end resection *see* Endodontic
        therapy
Rostral
    hooks, 72–3, *72*
    teeth, examination, 119
Rostrocaudal movement, 5
Rudimentary teeth, 55–7, *57*

S-Type float, *179*, 178, 191, 192, 196
Saddlebreds, 216
Safety, prophylaxis, 203
Saggital fracture, *137*
Saliva, 62
Salivary
    adenocarcinoma, *86, 93*, 99
    fistula, 62, 63, 68
    glands, 27, 60, 116, 259
    trauma, 62, 67–8
Salivation, 128, 260
Sarcoid, *86, 93*, 95, 97, *97*
Sarcoma
    chondrosarcoma, 91
    epithelial, 96
    hemangiosarcoma, 97, 99, 101
    imaging, *166–7*
    lymphosarcoma, *86*, 101, *101*
    osteosarcoma, *86*, 87, 91
Schoupe mouth gag, 111, 174
Screening, 108
Secondary dentin, 82, 84
Sedation, 173–4, *173–4*
    examination, 117
    floating, 189–90, 204
    imaging, 142
    tooth extraction, 231
Sensory nerve, 24
Septicemia, tooth removal, 220
Seven-Year notch (Galvayne's
        groove), 20, 38, *38*, 43–5, 45
Sharpey's fibers, *15, 16, 17*, 24, 75
Shear mouth, 73–4, 130, 213
Shetland ponies, 39–45, *45*, 210
Sialoliths, 68
Signalment, 113
Sinography, 165
Sinus
    centesis, 121
    cysts, 85, 89, 91, 100, 166
    disease, 121, 122, 128, *128*, 135,
        220, 256
    empyema, 23, 83, *83*, 84, 253, 256

endoscopy, 121–2, 142, 154
    formation, 247
Sinusitis, 136, *136–7*
    examination, 122
    exodontia, 230, 236, 243, 244
    imaging, 157, 159, *168*
    impaction, 58
Smooth mouth, 18, 133
Snaffle bit, 191
Soft palate, trauma, 62, 66–7
Soft tissue
    trauma, 63–8, *63–5, 67*, 260
    tumors, 86, 92–8, *93–4, 96–9*
Sow mouth, *5*, 55, 70, 216
Speculum, 61, 110–12, *111–12*, 119,
        *119*, 173, 174–5, *175*
Spindle cell tumour group, 85
Spreader, molar, 230, 232–4, *232–3*,
        239
Squamous cell carcinoma, *86*, 87, *92*,
        94–5, *94–4, 96*, 99
Steinmann bone pins, 69
Stellate reticulum, *6, 7*, 8
Step mouth, 72, *73*, 193
Sternohyoideus muscle, 30
Stomatitis, 116, 132, *133*, 220
Stone castings, orthodontics, 215, *215*
Streptococcus, 79
Stubbs screw speculum, 112
Style, 24
Sub-epiglottal infection, 66
Sublingual glands, 27, 60, 68
Suckling, 211, 212
Supernumerary teeth, 135, *137*, 220
Swallowing, 117
Systemic effects, dental disease,
        127–37
    behavioural consequences, 127–9,
        *128*
    degenerative joint disease,
        temporomandibular joint,
        129–30, *130*
    dysmastication, 129, 130–4, *130–3,
        135*, 136, 185
    dysprehension, 129, *130*
    lampas, 118, 129, *129*
    secondary consequences, 135–6,
        *135–7*
    *see also* Dysphagia

Table float, 178, 189, *189*
Tartar, 110, 118, 223
Teething bumps, 51, *51*
Teletherapy, 95
Temperament, 115,
Temporal odontoma, *86*, 91, 100, *100*,
        156–7, *157*
Temporal terratoma, *86*, 91, 100, *100*,
        156–7, *157*

Temporalis muscle, 30, 116
Temporomandibular joint, 25–6, 30,
        34, 259
    disease, 129–30, *130–1*, 133
    evolution, 5
    fracture, 260–1, 266, 269
    observation, 116, 117
    tooth removal, 246
Tension band wiring, 216, 217, 261,
        262, 263, *265*
Teratogenic drugs, 53
Tertiary dentin, 82
Tetanus, 113, 261
Thermal effects, dental equipment,
        83, 181, 200
Thermal pressure, 83
Tomes' process, 8
Tongue
    anatomy, 60
    examination, 118, 203
    trauma, 61–2, 65–6, *65*
Tooth germ, 5
Tooth removal *see* Exodontia
Tranquilizers, imaging, 142
Trauma, 60–9, *62*
    imaging, 145, 146, 153–4, 157,
        *157–9*
    oral anatomy, 60
    oral environment and healing,
        62–3
    oral examination, 61
    orthodontics, 207, 212
    pulpitis, 82, 250
    tooth removal, 220
    treatment of soft tissue injuries,
        63–8, *63–5, 67*
    treatment of tooth and bone, 68–9,
        *69*
    ulceration, 132, *133*
    *see also* Mandible-fracture
Trephine openings, 121, 234, *235*,
        239–44, *240, 242–4, 245, 248*
Triadan system, dental
        nomenclature, 20, 122
Trituration, 33, 34
Trotter horse, aging, 39–45, *40–2, 44*
Tumors, 85–101, *86*
    enamel hypoplasia, 53
    examination, 110, 121, 122
    exodontia, 220
    imaging, 145, 165–7, *166–7*
    metaplastic calcification, 135, *135*
    neoplastic-like disorders of jaws
        and teeth, 99, *100*
    odontogenic tumors, 86–91, *87–91*
    odontoma, *86–7*, 89–91, *91*, 165–6
    oral ulceration, 132, *133*
    osteogenic tumors, 86, 91–2
    periodontal disease, 74

Tumors, *continued*
    secondary tumors of mouth and
        jaws, 101, *101*
    soft-tissue tumors, 86, 92–8, *93–4,*
        *96–9*
    systemic effects, 128, 136

U-bars, 263, 264, *266*
Ulceration, 61, 72, 118, 129, 131–2,
    *132–3,* 204
Ultrasonography, 121, 139
Underbites, 55, 70
Underjet, 70
United States Trotting Horse
    Association, 116
Urinary catheter, 244–5, *244*

Vaccination history, 113
Vascular forces, eruption, 57

Vascularization, *7–9,* 10, 24
Vernell's mouth gag, 112
Vesicular stomatitis, 116
Vestibular lamina, 5
Vincents infection *see* Gingivitis
Viral stomatitis, 132, *133*

Water retention, 134
Wave mouth, 52, 73, 109, 178
Weanling examination, 108
Wear, 70–8
    definitions, 70–4, *71–4*
    *see also* Periodontal disease
Wedge type, mouth gag, 110–11, *111,*
    174
Weight loss, 129, *130,* 131, 132–4, *135*
Williams operation, 236
Windsucking, 21
Wiring, 216, 217, 261, 262, 263–4, *265*

Wolf teeth, 23, 55–7, *57*
    behavioural consequences, 127, 128
    evolution, 4
    examination, 108, 117
    floating, 194–5, *194–5,* 204
    imaging, 150–1, *149–50*
    impaction, 58
    orthodontics, 209
    removal, 62, 179, 220, 221, 223–6,
        *224–7, 229*
Wound healing, tooth removal, 246,
    247
Wry nose, 55, *55–6,* 207, *208–9*

Xylazine, 117

Zinc oxide, 254
Zygomatic arch, *21,* 26
Zygomaticus muscle, 30